ACSM's
RESEARCH METHODS

ACSM's
RESEARCH METHODS

Editors

Lawrence E. Armstrong, PhD, FACSM

Professor
Department of Kinesiology
University of Connecticut
Storrs, Connecticut

William J. Kraemer, PhD, FACSM

Professor
Department of Human Sciences
The Ohio State University
Columbus, Ohio

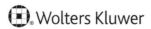

Philadelphia · Baltimore · New York · London
Buenos Aires · Hong Kong · Sydney · Tokyo

Acquisitions Editor: Michael Nobel
Product Development Editor: Staci Wolfson
Marketing Manager: Shauna Kelley
Production Project Manager: David Orzechowski
Design Coordinator: Holly McLaughlin
Manufacturing Coordinator: Margie Orzech
Prepress Vendor: Absolute Service, Inc.

9 8 7 6 5 4 3 2 1

Printed in China

Library of Congress Cataloging-in-Publication Data

ACSM's research methods / editors, Lawrence E. Armstrong, William J. Kraemer.
   p. ; cm.
  American College of Sports Medicine research methods
  Research methods
  Includes bibliographical references.
  ISBN 978-1-4511-9174-5
  I. Armstrong, Lawrence E., 1949- , editor. II. Kraemer, William J., 1953-, editor.
III. American College of Sports Medicine. IV. Title: American
College of Sports Medicine research methods. V. Title: Research methods.
  [DNLM: 1. Research Design. 2. Sports Medicine. 3. Exercise. 4.
Physical Fitness. QT 261]
  RC1210
  617.1'027--dc23
                    2015024261

DEDICATION

To my family members April, Jim, Jamie, and Stephen;
my mentors David L. Costill and Roger W. Hubbard;
my father, Edward L. Armstrong; and to Liz, who has
encouraged excellence with kindness and patience.
To the many undergraduate, master's, and
doctoral students who have made scientific research
an exciting, creative, and enjoyable experience.
— Lawrence E. Armstrong

To my wife, Joan, and my children, Daniel, Anna, and
Maria, for their love and support in life's journey.
To the many students and colleagues who have allowed
the research process to come to life and made the
long journey over my career to be filled with
excitement and the joy of discovery!
— William J. Kraemer

ACSM's Research Methods—Reviewers

George Abboud, PhD, MA
Associate Professor
Sport and Movement Science Department
Salem State University
Salem, Massachusetts

Kristal Anderson, PhD, CSEP-CEP, CSEP-CPT
Instructor
Exercise & Wellness
Camosun College
Victoria, British Columbia, Canada

William R. Barfield, PhD, FACSM
Professor
College of Charleston
Charleston, South Carolina

Susan A. Bloomfield, PhD, FACSM
Professor
Kinesiology
Texas A&M University
College Station, Texas

Edward F. Coyle, PhD, FACSM
Professor
Kinesiology and Health Education
University of Texas at Austin
Austin, Texas

Anne Crecelius, PhD, MS, BSE
Assistant Professor
Health and Sport Science
University of Dayton
Dayton, Ohio

Paul Cutrufello, ATC, CSCS, PhD
Assistant Professor
Department of Exercise Science and Sport
University of Scranton
Scranton, Pennsylvania

Tania Flink, PhD
Assistant Professor
Sport and Exercise Science
Gannon University
Erie, Pennsylvania

Michael G. Flynn, PhD, FACSM
Professor
Health and Human Performance
College of Charleston
Charleston, South Carolina

Charles Fountaine, PhD, MS, BA
Associate Professor
Health, Physical Education and Recreation
University of Minnesota Duluth
Duluth, Minnesota

Andrea Fradkin, PhD
Associate Professor
Exercise Science
Bloomsburg University of Pennsylvania
Bloomsburg, Pennsylvania

Diane L. Gill, PhD, FACSM
Professor
Kinesiology
University of North Carolina at Greensboro
Greensboro, North Carolina

Jason Gillis, PhD
Assistant Professor
Sport and Movement Science
Salem State University
Salem, Massachusetts

Allan H. Goldfarb, PhD, FACSM
Professor
Kinesiology
University of North Carolina at Greensboro
Greensboro, North Carolina

Kevin S. Heffernan, PhD
Assistant Professor
Health and Exercise Science
Syracuse University
Syracuse, New York

Vicci Hill-Lombardi, EdD, ATC
Associate Professor
Athletic Training, School of Health and Medical Sciences
Seton Hall University
South Orange, New Jersey

Alan Jung, PhD
Associate Professor
Kinesiology
Samford University
Birmingham, Alabama

Jill A. Kanaley, PhD, FACSM
Professor
Nutrition & Exercise Physiology
University of Missouri
Columbia, Missouri

H. Scott Kieffer, EdD, FACSM
Exercise Science Assistant Department Chair
Health and Human Performance
Messiah College
Mechanicsburg, Pennsylvania

Lisa Kihl, PhD
Associate Professor
School of Kinesiology
University of Minnesota
Minneapolis, Minnesota

James J. Laskin, PhD
Associate Professor
Physical Therapy
The University of Montana
Missoula, Montana

Manon Lemonde, RN, PhD
Associate Professor
Health Sciences
University of Ontario Institute of Technology
Oshawa, Ontario, Canada

J. Timothy Lightfoot, PhD, FACSM, RCEP, CES
Professor
Health and Kinesiology
Texas A&M University
College Station, Texas

Yit Aun Lim, PhD
Faculty
Sport Health Science
Life University
Marietta, Georgia

Jennifer Livingston, PhD, ATC
Associate Professor
Exercise and Sport Science
Azusa Pacific University
Azusa, California

Rebecca Lopez, PhD, ACSM-HFS, ATC, CSCS
Assistant Professor
Department of Orthopaedics and Sports Medicine
University of South Florida
Tampa, Florida

Jeff McNamee, PhD
Associate Professor
Health, Human Performance, and Athletics
Linfield College
McMinnville, Oregon

Robert Murray, PhD, FACSM
Managing Principal
Sports Science Insights
Crystal Lake, Illinois

Robert A. Oppliger, PhD, FACSM

David D. Pascoe, PhD, FACSM
Professor
Kinesiology
Auburn University
Auburn, Alabama

Sally Paulson, PhD, ATC, CSCS*D
Associate Professor
Exercise Science
Shippensburg University
Shippensburg, Pennsylvania

Reid Perry, MS
Health Fitness Specialist Executive Program Chair
Health, Wellness and Fitness
Globe University
Woodbury, Minnesota

John Quindry, PhD, FACSM
Associate Professor
Kinesiology
Auburn University
Auburn, Alabama

William Russell, PhD
Associate Professor
Health, Physical Education, and Recreation
Missouri Western State University
Saint Joseph, Missouri

Michael Sachs, PhD
Professor
Kinesiology
Temple University
Philadelphia, Pennsylvania

Duncan Simpson, PhD, MS
Assistant Professor
Sport & Exercise Psychology
Barry University
Miami, Florida

John R. Stofan, MS
Senior Manager
Gatorade Sports Science Institute at PepsiCo
Barrington, Illinois

Gary Van Guilder, PhD
Assistant Professor
Health & Nutritional Sciences
South Dakota State University
Brookings, South Dakota

Christian M. Westby, PhD

Malcolm Todd Whitehead, PhD, CSCS, EP-C
Associate Professor
Department of Kinesiology and Health Science
Stephen F. Austin State University
Nacogdoches, Texas

Phillip Wilson, BSc, MSc, PhD
Associate Professor
Kinesiology
Brock University
St. Catharine's, Ontario, Canada

Kathleen Y. Wolin, ScD, FACSM
Associate Professor
Preventive Medicine
Northwestern University
Evanston, Illinois

Jeffrey J. Zachwieja, PhD, FACSM
Dairy Research Institute

Gerald Zavorsky, PhD
Associate Professor
Department of Health and Sport Sciences
University of Louisville
Louisville, Kentucky

Contributors

Lawrence E. Armstrong, PhD, FACSM
Professor
Department of Kinesiology
University of Connecticut
Storrs, Connecticut

William J. Kraemer, PhD, FACSM
Professor
Department of Human Sciences
The Ohio State University
Columbus, Ohio

Brent A. Alvar, PhD, FACSM
Professor and Vice-President of University Research
Rocky Mountain University of Health Professions
Provo, Utah

Matthew D. Barberio, PhD
Center for Genetic Medicine Research
Children's National Medical Center
Washington, D.C.

Jenna M. Bartley, PhD
Center on Aging and Department of Immunology
University of Connecticut School of Medicine
Farmington, Connecticut

Margaret K. Bradbury, MS, CGC, MSHS
Senior Genetic Counselor
GeneDx
Gaithersburg, Maryland

Douglas Casa, PhD, ATC, FACSM, FNATA
Professor, Department of Kinesiology
Chief Operating Officer, Korey Stringer Institute
University of Connecticut
Storrs, Connecticut

Brett A. Comstock, PhD
Division of Kinesiology and Sport Science
University of South Dakota
Vermillion, South Dakota

Craig R. Denegar, PhD, PT, ATC, FNATA
Professor
Department of Kinesiology
University of Connecticut
Storrs, Connecticut

Michael R. Deschenes, PhD
Professor and Chair
Department of Kinesiology and Health Sciences
College of William & Mary
Williamsburg, Virginia

Daniel J. Dodd, PhD, CSCS*D
Exercise Physiology Laboratory
School of Kinesiology and Recreation
Illinois State University
Normal, Illinois

Courtenay Dunn-Lewis, PhD
Assistant Professor
Department of Sports Medicine
Merrimack College
North Andover, MA

J. Larry Durstine, PhD
Distinguished Professor of Exercise Science
Department of Exercise Science
University of South Carolina
Columbia, South Carolina

Joan M. Eckerson, PhD, FACSM
Professor
Department of Exercise Science and Pre-Health Professions
Creighton University
Omaha, Nebraska

Shawn D. Flanagan, MA, MHA
Department of Human Sciences
The Ohio State University
Columbus, Ohio

Andrew C. Fry, PhD, CSCS*D, FNSCA
Department of Health, Sport, and Exercise Sciences
University of Kansas
Lawrence, Kansas

Andrew J. Galpin, PhD, CSCS
Center for Sport Performance
Department of Kinesiology
California State University, Fullerton
Fullerton, California

Matthew S. Ganio, PhD
Associate Professor, Exercise Science
Director, Human Performance Laboratory
Department of Health, Human Performance and Recreation
University of Arkansas
Fayetteville, Arkansas

Benjamin T. Gordon, PhD
Department of Exercise Science
University of South Carolina
Columbia, South Carolina

Daniel J. Henkel, BA, APR
ACSM National Office
Indianapolis, Indiana

David R. Hooper, MA
Department of Human Sciences
The Ohio State University
Columbus, Ohio

Monica J. Hubal, PhD
Department of Exercise Science and Nutrition
Department of Integrative Systems Biology
George Washington University
Washington, D.C.

Julie M. Hughes, PhD
US Army Research Institute of Environmental Medicine
Natick, Massachusetts

Courtney Jensen, PhD
Health, Exercise, and Sport Sciences
University of the Pacific
Stockton, California

Evan C. Johnson, PhD, CSCS
Division of Kinesiology and Health
University of Wyoming
Laramie, Wyoming

Elaine C. Lee, PhD
Assistant Professor
Department of Kinesiology
University of Connecticut
Storrs, Connecticut

David P. Looney, MS, CSCS
Department of Kinesiology
University of Connecticut
Storrs, Connecticut

Carl M. Maresh, PhD, FACSM
Department of Kinesiology
University of Connecticut
Storrs, Connecticut

Amy L. McKenzie, PhD, ATC, PES
Department of Kinesiology
University of Connecticut
Storrs, Connecticut

Jason P. Mihalik, PhD, CAT(C), ATC
Assistant Professor, Department of Exercise and Sport Science
Co-Director, Matthew Gfeller Sport-Related Traumatic Brain Injury Research Center
University of North Carolina at Chapel Hill
Chapel Hill, North Carolina

Melinda L. Millard-Stafford, PhD, FACSM
Professor
School of Applied Physiology
Georgia Institute of Technology
Atlanta, Georgia

Colleen X. Muñoz, PhD
Department of Kinesiology
University of Connecticut
Storrs, Connecticut

Robert Newton, PhD, FESSA, FNSCA
Professor
Edith Cowan University Health and Wellness Institute
Joondalup, Western Australia

Bradley C. Nindl, PhD, FACSM
Professor and Director
Neuromuscular Research Laboratory/Warrior Human Performance Research Center
Department of Sports Medicine and Nutrition
School of Health and Rehabilitation Sciences
University of Pittsburgh
Pittsburgh, Pennsylvania

Kent B. Pandolf, PhD, MPH, FACSM
U.S. Army Research Institute of Environmental Medicine
Natick, Massachusetts

Linda S. Pescatello, PhD, FACSM, FAHA
Distinguished Professor of Kinesiology
Department of Kinesiology
University of Connecticut
Storrs, Connecticut

Mark D. Peterson, PhD, MS
Assistant Professor
Department of Physical Medicine and Rehabilitation
University of Michigan—Medicine
Ann Arbor, Michigan

Lori L. Ploutz-Snyder, PhD
Division of Space Life Sciences
Universities Space Research Association
NASA Johnson Space Center
Houston, Texas

Jessica M. Scott, PhD
Division of Space Life Sciences
Universities Space Research Association
NASA Johnson Space Center
Houston, Texas

Jill M. Slade, PhD
Associate Professor
Department of Radiology
Michigan State University
East Lansing, Michigan

Teresa K. Snow, PhD
School of Applied Physiology
Georgia Institute of Technology
Atlanta, Georgia

Rebecca L. Stearns, PhD, ATC
Assistant Professor
Department of Kinesiology
Vice President of Operations and Education
Korey Stringer Institute
University of Connecticut
Storrs, Connecticut

Tunde K. Szivak, MA
Department of Human Sciences
The Ohio State University
Columbus, Ohio

Beth A. Taylor, PhD
Director of Exercise Physiology Research
Department of Preventive Cardiology
Hartford Hospital
Associate Professor
Department of Kinesiology
University of Connecticut
Hartford, Connecticut

Baylah Tessier-Sherman, MPH
Occupational and Environmental Medicine Program
Yale University School of Medicine
New Haven, Connecticut

Raymond W. Thompson, PhD
Department of Exercise Science
University of South Carolina
Columbia, South Carolina

Maria L. Urso, PhD, FACSM
Smith & Nephew
Biotherapeutics
Fort Worth, Texas

Gordon L. Warren, PhD
Distinguished University Professor
Department of Physical Therapy
Georgia State University
Atlanta, Georgia

Kathrine R. Weeks, PhD
University of Connecticut
Storrs, Connecticut

Joseph P. Weir, PhD, FACSM
Department of Health, Sport, and Exercise Sciences
University of Kansas
Lawrence, Kansas

Mark T. White, MS
Vencore, Inc.
Arlington, Virginia

Andrew J. Young, PhD, FACSM
U.S. Army Research Institute of Environmental Medicine
Natick, Massachusetts

Jorge M. Zuniga, PhD
Assistant Professor
Department of Exercise Science and Pre-Health Professions
Creighton University
Omaha, Nebraska

Preface

The first edition of *ACSM Research Methods* offers a wealth of essential information that spans the entire research process, from initial concept to final scientific publications. The breadth of chapter topics is illustrated by the following diagram of the research process. This diagram serves to provide context for each chapter, illustrating its place in the research process.

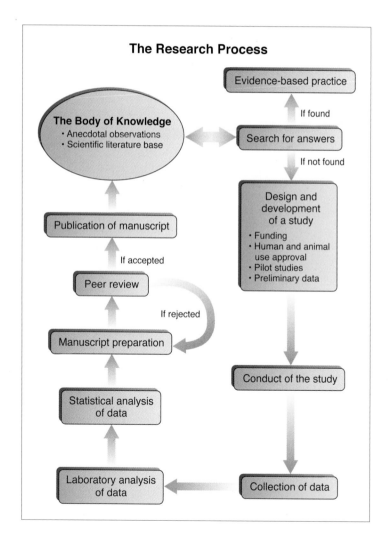

The Research Process

Evidence-based practice

If found

The Body of Knowledge
· Anecdotal observations
· Scientific literature base

Search for answers

If not found

Design and development of a study
· Funding
· Human and animal use approval
· Pilot studies
· Preliminary data

Publication of manuscript

If accepted

Peer review

If rejected

Manuscript preparation

Conduct of the study

Statistical analysis of data

Laboratory analysis of data

Collection of data

The authors of this book include scientists who are affiliated with universities, corporations, and government and private research institutions; clinical investigators who conduct research in hospitals; statisticians; scientists who specialize in human and animal studies; graduate students; and media specialists. They bring decades of experience and insight to the chapters that follow.

Written for graduate students, this book presents the essential aspects of valid, well-designed scientific experiments and describes the advancement of scientific knowledge. The purpose of this book will be fulfilled if the reader contributes to the scientific literature in the fields of exercise science, sports medicine, clinical exercise physiology, biomechanics, motor control, sport nutrition, sport psychology, or genomics. We hope this extensive volume guides, stimulates, and enhances your future research efforts.

—**Lawrence E. Armstrong and William J. Kraemer**
Editors

Acknowledgments

I gratefully acknowledge the efforts of Dr. William J. Kraemer, my colleague and friend of many years. Bill assembled an excellent list of contributors and guided this book, using the wisdom gained by countless experiences as a scientist, professor, and editor.

I also appreciate the managerial and editorial expertise of Staci Wolfson, Angela Chastain, and Katie Feltman.

— **Lawrence E. Armstrong**

I, too, gratefully acknowledge the efforts of Dr. Lawrence E. Armstrong who has been a colleague and a supportive friend for over three decades. Larry shared the belief in this approach to teaching the research process and with his attention to detail, exquisite focus, and organization acted as an ideal collaborator in this very demanding process of putting such a seminal book together. I also want to acknowledge the support and friendship of Dr. Carl Maresh who has always supported my work in science these many years, including taking on such a demanding editorial task.

I, too, so appreciate the managerial and editorial expertise of Staci Wolfson, Angela Chastain, and Katie Feltman, especially for their patience and professionalism in helping to mediate this process.

— **William J. Kraemer**

Contents

ACSM's Research Methods Authors

Chapter 1: Introduction to Research Methods
Lawrence E. Armstrong, PhD, FACSM
William J. Kraemer, PhD, FACSM

Chapter 2: The Importance of Research for Evidence-Based Practice
Amy L. McKenzie, PhD, ATC, PES
Evan C. Johnson, PhD, CSCS
Lawrence E. Armstrong, PhD, FACSM

Chapter 3: Choosing Your Research Project: Framing the Problem, Research Hypotheses, and Predictions
Maria L. Urso, PhD, FACSM
Julie M. Hughes, PhD

Chapter 4: Searching the Scientific Literature
Joan M. Eckerson, PhD, FACSM
Jorge M. Zuniga, PhD

Chapter 5: Fundamentals of Study Design
Brent A. Alvar, PhD, FACSM
Mark D. Peterson, PhD, MS
Daniel J. Dodd, PhD, CSCS*D

Chapter 6: Understanding Research: A Clinician's Perspective of Basic, Applied, and Clinical Investigations
Craig R. Denegar, PhD, PT, ATC, FNATA
Courtney Jensen, PhD

Chapter 7: Experimental Design I—Independent Variables
Melinda L. Millard-Stafford, PhD, FACSM
Teresa K. Snow, PhD
Gordon L. Warren, PhD

Chapter 8: Experimental Design II—Dependent Variables, Blinding, Randomization, and Matching
Andrew J. Galpin, PhD, CSCS
Andrew C. Fry, PhD, CSCS*D, FNSCA

Chapter 9: The Unique Challenges of Field Research
Douglas Casa, PhD, ATC, FACSM, FNATA
Rebecca L. Stearns, PhD, ATC
Jason P. Mihalik, PhD, CAT(C), ATC
Matthew S. Ganio, PhD

Chapter 10: Veracity of Data: Understanding Validity and Reliability
Lori L. Ploutz-Snyder, PhD
Jessica M. Scott, PhD

Chapter 11: Unique Features in Animal Research
Michael R. Deschenes, PhD

Chapter 12: Ethical Principles in Human and Animal Research
Matthew D. Barberio, PhD
Margaret K. Bradbury, MS, CGC, MSHS
Monica J. Hubal, PhD

Chapter 13: Developing a Funding Base for Your Research
William J. Kraemer, PhD, FACSM
Shawn D. Flanagan, MA, MHA
Mark T. White, MS
Brett A. Comstock, PhD
Courtenay Dunn-Lewis, PhD

Chapter 14: Conducting a Study: Pilot Testing, Sampling, and Data Collection
Jill M. Slade, PhD

Chapter 15: Instrumentation: Calibration and Standardization
Robert Newton, PhD, FESSA, FNSCA

Chapter 16: First Analyses After Data Collection
Elaine C. Lee, PhD
Kathrine R. Weeks, PhD

Chapter 17: Database Development and Management
Beth A. Taylor, PhD
Baylah Tessier-Sherman, MPH
Linda S. Pescatello, PhD, FACSM, FAHA

Chapter 18: Statistical Approaches to Data Analysis
Joseph P. Weir, PhD, FACSM

Chapter 19: Drawing Inferences, Logical Fallacies
J. Larry Durstine, PhD
Raymond W. Thompson, PhD
Benjamin T. Gordon, PhD

**Chapter 20: Writing a Research Manuscript
and Determining Authorship**
Carl M. Maresh, PhD, FACSM
Jenna M. Bartley, PhD
Colleen X. Muñoz, PhD

**Chapter 21: Submitting a Manuscript for Publication:
Finding the Publication Outlet**
William J. Kraemer, PhD, FACSM
David P. Looney, MS, CSCS
David R. Hooper, MA
Tunde K. Szivak, MA
Shawn D. Flanagan, MA, MHA

Chapter 22: Demands of the Peer Review Process
Bradley C. Nindl, PhD, FACSM
Andrew J. Young, PhD, FACSM
Kent B. Pandolf, PhD, MPH, FACSM

**Chapter 23: Building the Science Buzz: Working with Media
to Create a Lay Translation of Your Discovery**
Daniel J. Henkel, BA, APR

CHAPTER 1

Introduction to Research Methods

Lawrence E. Armstrong, PhD, FACSM, and William J. Kraemer, PhD, FACSM

INTRODUCTION

The purpose of this textbook is to take a student in his or her first experience with research through the research process from the development of the question to the publication of a scientific manuscript. To do this, we start at the beginning with the research question and the development of the various hypotheses from our current understanding arising from current scientific literature and anecdotal evidence. The research process is driven by the desire to solve problems and answer questions in order to gain greater understanding about a particular topic. As we shall see in this book, the use of the **scientific method** typically allows for the generation of a factual understanding by testing our hypotheses and thereby answering questions in which we are interested. Any new student first starting out in research will learn that this can be a slow and tedious process, but the joy and satisfaction of gaining new insights and answering questions about the world around us is both an exciting and exhilarating experience.

Although there are numerous approaches to problem solving, the scientific method offers a superior, objective approach. The scientific method, which underpins the research process (Fig. 1-1), is recognized as the cornerstone of modern research methodology. Therefore, a primary goal of *ACSM's Research Methods* is to help the student understand each step in the research process.

In the chapters of this book, as we have noted earlier, you will learn that scientific research cannot exist without one or more questions to direct the course of study. Upon completion of this text, you also will come to appreciate that scientific discoveries influence accepted ideas, change behaviors, and modify everyday practices such as exercise prescription and injury treatments. In addition, new insights into the molecular, cellular, and physiologic mechanisms that explain such practices are elucidated. The outcomes of research are what represent the most valuable and exciting products of scientific inquiry (1).

In order to properly test a hypothesis, an appropriate experimental design must be developed, which reflects the context of the question and the study's purpose. For example, if one is attempting to determine the effects of exercise training, then the experimental design must have exercise training as an element in its design. As we shall see in this textbook,

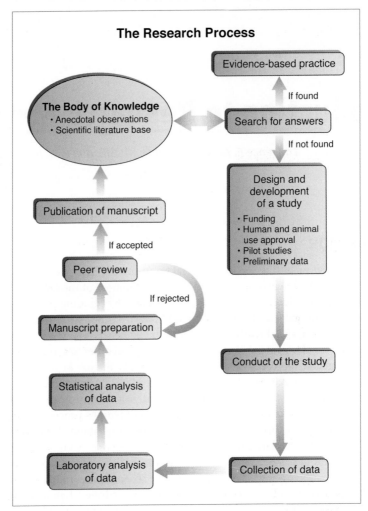

FIGURE 1-1:   Follow this diagram of the scientific method throughout each chapter as you learn about the processes of research from start to finish.

there are many details and requirements in the research process which are needed in order to answer a question and test a hypothesis correctly. This textbook will get into these basic research elements including how to read and understand the scientific literature in the search for existing answers to your question, what goes in to the development of a proper experimental design for your hypotheses, the importance of reliable and valid laboratory techniques, the need for proper data acquisition and analytical systems, the use of appropriate statistical techniques matching your design, proper interpretation and generalization of findings, the development of a manuscript for the body of knowledge (*i.e.*, scientific literature), and dissemination of your findings to the lay public. Each of these research elements plays a vital role in your understanding of the research process. Therefore, this book provides a context for the scientific method by describing the essential qualities of valid, well-designed scientific experiments as well as the techniques which advance scientific knowledge.

THE SCIENTIFIC METHOD

After you pose a question (Step 1), you should seek an answer in existing scientific literature (Step 2). If you learn that no answer exists or if research findings are ambiguous, one can then formulate a possible answer to the question. This tentative answer is then used to develop a **hypothesis** (Step 3) that can be experimentally tested. This hypothesis is simply an educated guess based on your present knowledge of the phenomenon and the interpretation of the scientific literature. Ironically, a hypothesis can be disproven, but it cannot be proven. If a hypothesis or group of hypotheses is supported by repeated experimental testing by multiple investigations and laboratories, it can become a **theory**. Next, you test your hypothesis by conducting experiments (Step 4). When all data is collected, you then analyze the data using appropriate statistical methods (Step 5) and then draw conclusions (Step 6). Finally, because research unpublished is research undone, you disseminate your findings (Step 7) to other scientists and the general public. Because of the fact that dissemination in a scientific journal requires peer review and approval, this aspect of the process helps to validate the research.

Figure 1-1 illustrates the research process in the form of a flow diagram. For purposes of providing a "roadmap" for the research process, this figure appears on the first page of every chapter in *ACSM's Research Methods* to let you know where you are and give you some context in relationship to the other aspects of scientific research. The cyclic structure of this diagram emphasizes that research is ongoing, dynamic, and evolving as new questions arise in a field of study.

However, scientific research today requires much more than a systematic approach to answering questions. A successful scientist uses many different talents and personal interaction skill sets to conduct research to a successful conclusion. This is because in today's world of research, it takes a team, from laboratory assistants, research technicians, and medical support to graduate students and postdoctoral scholars. Many scientists today, in addition to conducting a research program within a university or research institution, also serve as laboratory directors, small group leaders, grant managers, accountants, academic advisors, lecturers, writers, content specialists, authors, media spokespeople, and/or editors. Thus, in this book we just start with the fundamentals of the research process which has even more dimensions and complexity as one progresses in their careers in research. This in part helps to explain some of the complexity of the content presented in the following chapters.

As you progress through learning the material presented in the chapters in this book, you also will discover that the scientific method is not infallible. The findings, as we will learn, are framed by a set of independent variables and the dependent variables that are measured. No scientific investigation has been or will be perfect. Each experiment is conducted within a specific laboratory, field setting, country, or environment. The findings, therefore, apply to those specific settings, but they may or may not be extended to other environments. Thus, the generalization of research findings is specific to the study design and its experimental characteristics. Also, each experiment uses specific methods, which may or may not generate the same outcomes when different techniques, instruments, or participants are involved.

TYPES OF RESEARCH

Interestingly, the steps in the research process (see Fig. 1-1) can be accomplished in various locations using a myriad of experimental interventions, involving different test participants, controlling numerous factors across days, and selecting appropriate statistical analyses. These many design options can make it difficult to classify research studies.

For the exercise scientist and sports medicine clinician, two types of research are most relevant. The first, **experimental research**, is undertaken to explain mechanisms or cause and effect (*i.e.*, doing x results in y). This is accomplished by controlling (holding constant) as many factors across trials (independent variables such as air temperature, time of day, diet, entering hydration status, exercise, etc.) as possible, except one (the intervention). The intervention is the factor being investigated (*e.g.*, present during one test but not during another). Measurements (dependent variables such as strength, endurance, oxygen consumption, etc.) inform the investigator if the intervention altered relevant characteristics as hypothesized. Examples include the effect of a dietary supplement on exercise performance (2) or a comparison of two resistance training programs on muscle hypertrophy (3).

The second type might be called **descriptive research**. Although everything is descriptive to a certain extent in any research study, true descriptive research just describes characteristics and phenomena but does not explain how something works or its underlying/causal mechanism. Examples include body composition characteristics of professional football players, changes in body water during ultra-endurance cycling, and training characteristics of elite marathon runners. Although descriptive research provides only a profile of characteristics, it may provide a basic scientist with clues regarding which dependent variables should be measured to determine cause and effect or to explain mechanisms (*e.g.*, which mechanisms mediate the development of high levels of muscle mass in bodybuilders).

In addition, the following dual classifications are often used to distinguish various types of research:

- Laboratory (indoor site which enhances potential control of experiments) versus field (road race, gymnasium, athletic field, mass participation event, etc.; involves less experimental control)
- Basic (data collection without concern for how the information will be used) versus applied (designed to answer real-world practical questions that improve quality of life)
- Quantitative (numerical data are recorded to explain the effect of an intervention, to describe relationships, or to infer cause and effect) versus qualitative (involving case studies, narrative records, or interviews which are coded to provide a detailed description of a phenomenon); quantitative research converts generalities into specific findings (deductive reasoning), whereas qualitative research converts specific observations into generalities (inductive reasoning)

These categories are described in greater detail and are accompanied by examples in several of the chapters which follow the current chapter.

NON-SPECIFIC APPROACHES TO SOLVING PROBLEMS

In contrast to the research process (see Fig. 1-1), three non-scientific processes provide solutions (both valid and invalid) to problems and answers to questions. These are the empirical method, the rationalistic method, and trial and error. The **empirical method** is part of the research process (see Fig. 1-1) that involves personal observations but are linked to scientific method that one cannot just use *a priori* reasoning to come up with the answer, thus it differs considerably from accepted research practices if not properly quantified and analyzed (*e.g.*, making a decision on a question based only on your own inherent observations). Thus, improper empiricism can be summarized as "it worked for me, and it will work for you." Depending on one's background and individual experiences, this method may or may not provide correct answers to questions.

The **rationalistic method** employs reasoning and logic to produce facts. The truth and validity of premises and their relationships to each other are the keys to this process. Rationalism grew out of the philosophical arguments which involved metaphysical and epistemologic problems that needed a foundation of basic principles to start with. If one started with a fundamental principle, then one could deductively derive the rest of the needed knowledge of a particular problem. Some philosophers thought that all knowledge could be gained through reason alone, but this proved to be impossible for certain aspects of the human condition; albeit the best application was in mathematics. Thus, rationalism might be viewed as explaining things based on logic alone.

Trial and error refers to trying multiple actions randomly until one action results in the desired outcome. Although this random process does not involve the scientific method or true experiments, it may provide useful information if guided by scientific facts. None of these three processes is considered a valid scientific research method.

Many different influences can affect the research process or are used by practitioners not familiar with a scientific approach to problem solving. In contrast to the scientific method, personal perspectives and thought patterns influence solutions to problems and answers to questions. For example, some people rely on tradition, superstition, authority, or bias. In the case of **tradition**, a previous course of action (either rational or irrational) worked successfully across months, years, decades, or centuries, and there appears to be no present reason to change. **Superstition**, in contrast, is a belief that one action influences another event positively (*i.e.*, the alignment of planets influences life events) without natural causes; the influence is believed to be supernatural. In the latter case, an **authority** figure or organization is allowed to control, command, or exert power. Furthermore, **bias** may be present when decisions are made or when questions are considered. Bias is a tendency to accept one answer to a question without weighing all possible options or answers equally. A biased viewpoint usually relies on past experiences rather than objectivity and neutrality. Notably, bias often occurs as an unknowing consequence of the research process.

REPORTING SCIENTIFIC FINDINGS TO THE WORLD

At scientific conferences such as the annual meetings of the American College of Sports Medicine, investigators convey research findings to their peers in the form of oral slide presentations or board-mounted posters. Because annual meetings are attended by a limited number of professionals, the most effective means of disseminating scientific information is to publish in a scientific journal. As noted before, a peer-reviewed scientific journal gives a degree of credibility to the work, yet it is not perfect, and poor studies find their way into the literature. Nevertheless, historically it was through the use of books and research papers that scientists communicated with each other before the days of telephones and sophisticated communication networks of today. Still, reporting your research findings in a suitable scientific publication is what allows others to learn from, evaluate, and advance your findings.

As a student starting out in the study of the research process, you might have observed throughout your education that oral communications, poster presentations, and manuscripts use a common format to convey scientific information. All three begin with an **introduction**, which presents the scientific question and develops the hypothesis to be studied by using support from the relevant studies already in the literature. In doing so, one sets up the rationale(s) for the study and ends with the primary purpose(s) of the investigation. The introduction establishes the context and importance of the research. Next, the **methods** section describes the approach to research problem(s), test participants, the experimental design, techniques and procedures, key independent and dependent variables, and statistical or qualitative analyses. Other scientists should be able to follow written methods such that they could reproduce all aspects of the study in order to confirm or refute its findings. Human subject testing is another important component of this section in that the text should explain that (a) the protocol was reviewed and approved by a human subjects review board or institutional review or ethics board; (b) that participants gave full informed voluntary consent to participate after hearing the risks, benefits, and procedures; and (c) that participants could withdraw from testing at any time without negative repercussions. The **results** section presents descriptive and experimental findings. In experimental studies, numerical values are presented for each dependent variable in the form of text, tables, and figures. The **discussion** is where one brings it all together and explains the results from its relationship to the existing literature. In many cases, it also supports and explains the physiologic or biomechanical aspects of the results, especially in basic research studies. It is vital to let the reader understand the importance of the study to the topic and field under investigation. In the discussion, one must also integrate into the discussions of how the study answered the question and tested the hypotheses. In part, future questions and directions are briefly discussed to inspire others to do more work on the topic. Finally, **references** allow other scientists to locate relevant publications. Each journal has a format, but the list typically provides author name(s), article title, journal name, volume, page numbers, and year of publication for each citation.

As shown in Figure 1-1, publication is the final critical step in the cycle of research. Publication of an investigation in a peer-reviewed journal is respected throughout the scientific world as the standard for others' considerations of the findings. **Peer review** (*i.e.*, evaluation of a manuscript on the basis of its scientific merit) is the process by which a manuscript is evaluated in order to limit the studies that have "fatal" flaws in their experimental designs or methodologies, or less so, their interpretations of their results. As you will see in a later chapter, the process of peer review is a systematic approach of submission and management by an editor with a set of reviewers who work in the same field of study, yet should have no conflict of interest in the paper being reviewed (4). A review process may proceed in one of three ways: the authors know the identities of the reviewers and vice versa (very rare in the review process); the authors do not know the reviewers but the authors' names are revealed to the reviewers (**single-blind review**); or neither the authors nor the reviewers know the identities of the other parties (**double-blind review**).

Evaluating Journal Articles

The relevance and value of a published article to your research depends on many factors, but similarity of purpose and the methods employed are key factors. If an article focuses on the same research question as your research and that article used a similar approach, it is likely that you will include it in the reference, introduction, and discussion sections of your manuscript. But before you use information from another investigation, you should consider several features of each publication.

- What is the context of the study?
- Are the statements, interpretations, and conclusions logical and valid?
- Were statistical analyses appropriate?
- Can I generalize the findings to my research?
- Does the paper contain internal contradictions?
- Are previous publications accurately summarized?
- Does the discussion section address all discrepancies or similarities to the findings of other research studies?

These considerations will guide your thinking, inform your interpretations of data, and facilitate development of valid conclusions. Thus, selected reviewers evaluate the purpose, rationale, methods, analyses, results, figures, tables, and conclusions, and they submit required revisions and send a decision to the editor.

A decision may be any one of the following: accepted with no revisions (a rare circumstance), accepted with minor revisions, accepted with major revisions, or rejected. Ultimately, it is the editor who determines the fate of the submitted manuscript with reviewers acting as a type of advising body in the process. Thus, the editor can go along with the reviewers' recommendations or decide differently or in opposition to the reviewers' decisions. Typically, only in rare circumstances does an editor act alone in opposition to his or her expert reviewers. The accepted manuscript is then sent to the publisher for production. If the manuscript is not accepted for publication, the authors usually submit the manuscript to a different peer-reviewed journal.

SUMMARY

Research results in answers to questions and the testing of hypotheses. The research process and practices are based on the scientific method. Understanding the research process (see Fig. 1-1) allows you to evaluate published research, determine if it applies to your situation, or to reject the findings as irrelevant to your needs. It is important as a young student investigator to understand the basics behind the research process. Furthermore, it is important to demonstrate in student research that you can develop a focused study that adheres to the fundamental principles of the scientific method outlined in this textbook. As one grows in the field of science as an investigator, one begins to take on more and more sophisticated studies requiring a team of experts involved in its conduct. The results of a study can have important impacts on practice in a variety of fields used by athletes, soldiers, laborers, coaches, dietitians, physicians, athletic trainers, and physical therapists to enhance performance, reduce the risk of injury, apply the best treatment, and use the most effective techniques.

GLOSSARY

Authority: a person or organization that is allowed to control, command, or exert power

Bias: a perspective that thwarts unprejudiced assessment

Descriptive research: a study that is not experimental; involves either a one-time interaction with participants (cross-sectional study) or observation of individuals over time (longitudinal study)

Discussion: concluding section of a scientific paper which explains the meaning and importance of the results, describes the limitations of the study, and suggests future lines of research

Double-blind review: neither the authors nor the reviewers know the identities of the other parties

Empirical method: data are collected to answer specific research questions, with the goal of developing or testing a theory or hypothesis

Experimental research: controls variables, measures precisely, and seeks to understand cause-and-effect relationships

Hypothesis: a clear statement as to the expected outcome of a phenomenon based on insights from the current literature that can be experimentally tested using scientific method

Introduction: initial section of a manuscript which provides the research question(s), hypotheses, rationale, and purpose(s) of the study

Methods: section of a manuscript which describes the experimental design, test participants, techniques and procedures, key independent and dependent variables, and statistical analyses

Peer review: assesses the quality of articles submitted for publication in a scholarly journal; this is performed by professionals of similar competence to the authors of the work

Rationalistic method: employs reasoning and logic to produce facts

References: a list of publications that includes author name(s), article title, journal name, volume, page numbers, and year of appearance; this allows scientists to locate observations that are relevant to their research

Results: presents descriptive and experimental findings (numerical values) in the form of text, tables, and figures

Scientific method: a systematic approach to solving a problem or answering a question

Single-blind review: the authors do not know the reviewers, but the authors' names are revealed to the reviewers

Superstition: a belief that is based on fear of the unknown or faith in magic or luck

Theory: an explanation that is well supported by evidence and is verified repeatedly

Tradition: a previous course of action (either rational or irrational) worked successfully across months, years, decades, or centuries, and there appears to be no present reason to change

Trial and error: trying multiple actions randomly until one action results in the desired outcome

REFERENCES

1. Kraemer WJ, Fleck SJ, Deschenes MR. *Exercise Physiology: Integrating Theory and Application.* 2nd ed. Baltimore (MD): Lippincott Williams & Wilkins; 2015.
2. Jackman SR, Witard OC, Jeukendrup AE, Tipton KD. Branched-chain amino acid ingestion can ameliorate soreness from eccentric exercise. *Med Sci Sports Exerc.* 2010;42(5):962–970.
3. Kraemer WJ, Nindl BC, Ratamess NA, et al. Changes in muscle hypertrophy in women with periodized resistance training. *Med Sci Sports Exerc.* 2004;36(4):697–708.
4. Tipton CM. Publishing in peer-reviewed journals. Fundamentals for new investigators. *Physiologist.* 1991;34(5):275, 278–279.

The Importance of Research for Evidence-Based Practice

Amy L. McKenzie, PhD, ATC, PES, Evan C. Johnson, PhD, CSCS, and Lawrence E. Armstrong, PhD, FACSM

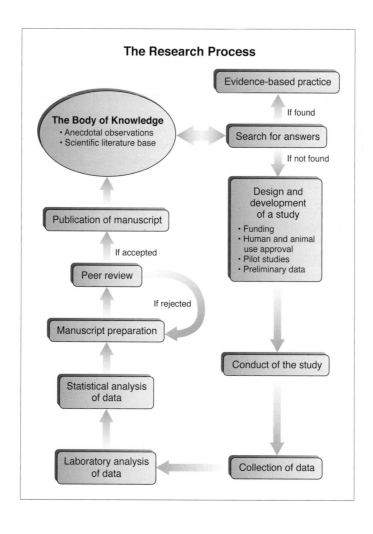

WHAT IS EVIDENCE-BASED PRACTICE?

Evidence-based medicine is the integration of best research evidence with clinical expertise and patient values.

Sackett DL, Straus SE, Richardson WS, Rosenberg W, Haynes RB.
Evidence-Based Medicine: How to Practice and Teach EBM. 2nd ed.
Edinburgh, United Kingdom: Churchill Livingstone; 2000.

Although the above definition refers to medicine, several other clinical fields rely on scientific evidence. Thus, the word *practice* is appropriate in this chapter and may refer to a therapy, intervention, or service. This concept applies to any field that involves choosing a course of action to solve a problem or accomplish a goal, including but not limited to a:

- physician, athletic trainer, or physical therapist deciding how to best repair and rehabilitate a collegiate soccer player recovering from anterior cruciate ligament reconstruction surgery
- clinical exercise physiologist implementing a cardiac rehabilitation program for a patient with coronary artery disease
- personal trainer designing an exercise program for a middle-aged man who competes in adventure races.

The concept of evidence-based practice extends beyond the membership of the American College of Sports Medicine (ACSM) and is used in fields such as education, psychiatry, substance abuse rehabilitation, and social work. But in all professions, observation and analysis of published research replaces anecdotal evidence, single observations, rules, traditions, and lore.

Obviously, evidence is the foundation of **evidence-based practice (EBP)**. The word "evidence" refers to the best, most current scientific research that informs the question, problem, or goal at hand. The definition of "best research" varies across professions. Sometimes, a well-constructed meta-analysis provides a clear direction for clinical decisions. When a meta-analysis is not available or does not answer a specific question, individual research studies contribute to a decision regarding practice. For example, if a meta-analysis does not exist for a rehabilitation program following suprascapular nerve decompression surgery, individual research studies and case reports must be reviewed to edify the decision.

Beyond evidence and practice, two other components of EBP exist—the clinician and the client. The **clinician** may be any professional making a recommendation regarding the care, treatment, service, or plan for a client or group; the **client** is the person or people to whom the care, treatment, or plan is applied.

THE HISTORY OF EVIDENCE-BASED PRACTICE

Evidence-based medicine (EBM) by name was not introduced to the public until the early 1990s (21). Today, EBP is similar to the scientific method, involving a controlled study and a comparison among different treatment options. Reviewing a few historic examples of EBP helps us understand that the principles underlying EBP are similar to the procedures underlying great medical advances of the past.

The Ancient History of Evidence-Based Practice

Claridge and Fabian (14) provide an outline of different medical eras and how EBP has been involved in each of them. One of the first examples of a successful but rudimentary use of evidence-based reasoning appears within the Bible (Daniel 1:11–17, English Standard Version):

> *Then Daniel said to the steward whom the chief of the eunuchs had assigned over Daniel, Hananiah, Mishael, and Azariah, "Test your servants for 10 days; let us be given vegetables to eat and water to drink. Then let our appearance and the appearance of the youths who eat the king's food be observed by you, and deal with your servants according to what you see." So he listened to them in this matter, and tested them for 10 days. At the end of 10 days it was seen that they were better in appearance and fatter in flesh than all the youths who ate the king's food. So the steward took away their food and the wine they were to drink, and gave them vegetables.*

At the time of this example, a diet similar to that of the king (*e.g.*, consisting of meat, rich foods, and only wine to drink) was considered to be desirable and a luxury for servants. The clinical problem involved Daniel's sense that the king's food was "defiling him." Besides his moral objections based on religious belief, Daniel's objection can be viewed as an act that would influence human health. Although Daniel did not have access to 21st century nutritional research, his intelligent guess (*i.e.*, hypothesis) was that a better diet would improve the health of his fellow servants. Next, he proposed to test the hypothesis with an experiment in which one group ate the king's lavish diet and a second group ate only vegetables and drank no wine. The outcome in this example was that the latter group was " . . . better in appearance and fatter in flesh . . . " Following the experiment, the steward critically assessed the evidence. He realized that feeding the servants was relevant to the population and that the new practice had value for all servants in terms of improved health and productivity. Thus, the new treatment was implemented into everyday practice; the king prescribed the healthier diet. This is likely not the first, but it provides an early, elementary example of successful evidence-based reasoning.

The modern principles of EBP indicate that without follow-up experiments, it is impossible to determine if the outcomes were due to a diet of vegetables, reduced alcohol consumption, the combination of both, or another uncontrolled factor. This is precisely why the final step of EBP (Fig. 2-1) emphasizes the importance of evaluating the performance of a practice and revising the practice if new evidence is published.

Although similar experiments occurred during the ancient era, they were not commonplace. Tradition and ritual reigned supreme in all parts of life. The physiologic basis of medicine was primarily drawn from the ancient Greek physician, surgeon, and philosopher

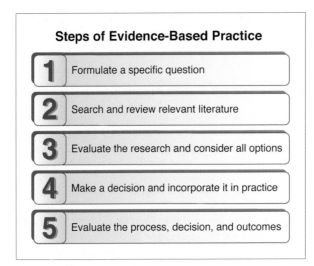

FIGURE 2-1: Steps of evidence-based practice.

Galen of Pergamon (circa 170 A.D.). Although he was far ahead of his time, he was strongly influenced by Hippocrates' theories of humoralism, which described health as a balance of four bodily substances known as "humors." Especially within the medical community, which was highly unregulated, healing methodologies were passed down from generation to generation, physician to physician, as best practices of the day (23). Even 1,500 years after Galen, a majority of ailments were assumed to be due to a disturbance of bodily humors or an invasion of evil spirits, and treatments were designed to rebalance or purge the body (27). It was not until the Scientific Renaissance (15th–17th centuries) that this paradigm fell out of favor.

Renaissance Era Evidence-Based Medicine

From approximately 1600–1900, evidence emerged to aid medical decision-making. As with any change, initial proclamations were often rejected despite sound evidence. However, the power of numbers and their relation to treatment options, as observed during systematic observations, eventually began to gain acceptance. Two well-known successes of EBM define the Renaissance era—the elimination of bloodletting as a treatment for a variety of illnesses and the discovery that scurvy resulted from a vitamin C deficiency.

In 1628, William Harvey published a then-controversial book entitled, *On the Motion of the Heart and Blood in Animals.* Galen's physiology had previously described a unidirectional flow of blood (1). Harvey challenged this concept by using the volume of the heart chambers multiplied by heart rate to elegantly calculate the enormous daily blood volume production needed to sustain life and health. These calculations allowed Harvey to logically discredit Galen's concepts and to describe blood flow moving away from the heart in the arteries and back to the heart via veins. Over 200 years later, French physician Pierre Charles Alexandre Louis combined this physiologic knowledge with mounting evidence against bloodletting to develop a new technique that evaluated medical treatments ("la method numérique") (12). Louis produced detailed tables that compared mortality outcomes for different treatments. His calculations provided substantial evidence that bloodletting was not an effective treatment.

In addition to removal of poor treatments and programs, EBP is also useful in the introduction of novel practices. As the Age of Exploration continued and shipboard voyages became more frequent and longer in duration, scurvy became commonplace among sailors. Now known to be caused by a deficiency of vitamin C, scurvy is characterized by oral lesions, recession of the gums, and eventually joint and cardiac complications that can lead to death. Although anecdotal evidence for the benefits of citrus fruits aboard ships existed, it was not until 1747 that Sir Gilbert Blane and Sir James Lind of the British Navy described a systematic method to evaluate various scurvy treatments (26). They divided 12 scurvy patients into six different treatment groups containing two men each. This allowed Blane and Lind to compare the best practices of that day (*e.g.*, gargling with sea water, drinking cider, or consuming 25 servings of "elixir of vitriol" which contained sulfuric acid) to a treatment which required eating two oranges and one lemon per day. As we know today, the fruits were "the most effectual remedy for this distemper at sea" (26). Despite this evidence, many years passed before this therapeutic nutritional intervention became standard practice, due to previous etiologic misconceptions and poor record keeping. Thus, the systematic and accurate recording of patient outcomes became a central theme of EBP (see Fig. 2-2).

The Era of Evidence-Based Practice Transition

From approximately 1900–1970, the emergence of the **randomized controlled clinical trial** (**RCT**) impacted EBP greatly because a standardized approach to the evaluation of procedures was not in place, and follow-up interventions were rare. If a treatment or service was not effective, many clinicians believed that the patient was beyond treatment and would not benefit from this intervention. The EBP transition era involved a shift in this mindset toward one of increased experimentation which advanced treatments without duplicating mistakes of the past.

Ernest Amory Codman (16) introduced an era of standardized practice, accountability, and transparency to the medical field. Early in his surgical career, Codman began documenting on index cards the pre-care, post-care, and outcomes of his surgeries. Additionally, he followed up with patients a year after treatment and determined if errors or negative outcomes had occurred. Codman's goal was to allow public access to these records so that individuals would be able to choose their surgeons based on data and not solely by reputation. Codman championed the creation of the American College of Surgeons and established the first outcome-based hospital. He may also be considered to be a forefather of malpractice, as he considered hospitals to be responsible for the care

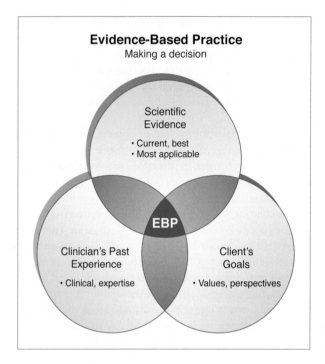

FIGURE 2-2: Evidence-based practice.

they provided. Once again, a controversial individual changed the landscape of what was then common practice.

Soon after Codman's paradigm-shifting work, the Medical Research Council of the United Kingdom began completing RCT in which patients were randomly allocated to either a treatment or control group. The two benefits of this model were (a) treatment bias was reduced and (b) outcomes were compared to either no treatment or the best practice of that day. As RCT became more common, research procedures ensured that physicians were unaware of the treatment group (double-blinding), further decreasing experimental bias. Also, physicians and researchers were accurately and objectively documenting treatment outcomes. Most importantly, medical journals published the results of RCT, and professionals shared lessons throughout the world. Publication and the spread of research findings became the backbone of today's EBP (see Fig. 2-2).

The Modern Era of Evidence-Based Practice

Although most authorities believe that the modern era began in approximately 1970, the name of EBP became commonplace in 1992 and 1993 due to the efforts of Archie Cochrane, David Sackett, and Gordon Guyatt. This era marked the incorporation of technology and initiated the widespread dissemination of research findings. The importance of technology in EBP continues to grow as therapies, services, and programs become more complicated and diverse.

In the 1980s, David Sackett popularized the concept of clinical epidemiology. He brought to light the importance of meshing the art and science of medicine and the need for clinicians to stay abreast of evolving trends in patient care. In 1992, proceedings of an EBM working group led by Guyatt were published in the *Journal of American Medical Association* (21). The group announced, "Evidence-based medicine de-emphasizes intuition, unsystematic clinical experience, and pathophysiologic rationale as sufficient grounds for clinical decision-making and stresses the examination of evidence from clinical research." Following a flurry of critical editorials published in *The Lancet* (20), EBM experienced a difficult birth.

In 1993, the Cochrane Collaboration was formed in Oxford, England, by Iain Chalmers as a response to a call by Archie Cochrane (15). Cochrane's call for increased use of research findings in clinical decision-making created a paradigm shift toward EBP. This effort was realized by the formation of the Cochrane Collaboration, facilitating the increased distribution of quality systematic reviews. These reviews were used to consolidate RCT outcomes into evidence-based recommendations for treatment. Today, the voluntary independent work of the Cochrane Collaboration is accomplished by more than 31,000 individuals in over 120 countries. This widespread membership reduces bias and expands the breadth of evaluated evidence. The resulting database provides a central resource for clinicians to begin their quest for relevant, objective information regarding treatment options. With the present exponential increase of published RCT, the importance of this organization grows each year.

A 1996 paper, "Evidence-Based Medicine: What It Is and What It Isn't," published by Sackett and colleagues (33) in the *British Medical Journal*, responded to many of the criticisms that had arisen over the previous years. The seemingly logical suggestion to base medical treatment decisions on "an integration of individual clinical expertise and the best available external clinical evidence from systematic research" was met with great disapproval. EBM was viewed by critics as arrogant and as an attempt to limit clinical freedom. This debate continues today.

Since the introduction of modern EBP to the medical and research lexicon, RCTs have become the gold standard. Considering the ever-growing number of clinical trials, it is fortunate that the spread and navigation of information have been aided by electronic databases. Search engines such as PubMed.gov, which is maintained by the U.S. National Library of Medicine of the National Institutes of Health, place vast amounts of information at the fingertips of physicians and researchers. However, the rapidly rising number of publications also makes it difficult to determine the quality of experimental designs and author inferences. It is potentially overwhelming for a new researcher or clinician to work through all publications independently, so institutions such as the Cochrane Collaboration are integral to the success of evidence evaluation. However, Guyatt and Sackett would be the first to counter that the data must be interpreted and evaluated carefully to ensure that decisions are appropriate to patient/client goals, values, and expectations.

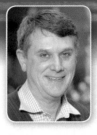

CONCEPT BOX 2-1   Pioneer of Evidence-Based Medicine

Dr. Gordon Guyatt *is a distinguished professor in the Department of Clinical Epidemiology and Biostatistics at McMaster University located in Hamilton, Ontario, Canada. He was the chair of the Evidence-Based Medicine Working Group that produced the seminal publication in 1992 through the Journal of the American Medical Association entitled "Evidence-Based Medicine: A New Approach to Teaching the Practice of Medicine" (21). He shared the following insights regarding the past, present, and future of EBM.*

Q: *What was the initial inspiration for the EBM working group?*

GG: It began with my mentor Dr. David Sackett and his work in the critical appraisal of medical literature. We began to take that concept and apply it to the patient bedside to make it relevant for patient care. We quickly found that we had something of importance because it was different than the current model. Dr. Sackett had previously authored publications specific to critical appraisal; however, we both recognized the limitations. We set out to create the EBM working group, consisting of many different types of clinicians and medical professionals, with the goal of developing a new model with a broad background and application.

Q: *What was the initial reaction to the first publication?*

GG: The responses ranged from euphoria to outright hostility. I can remember that it was less than a year following the publication that I received a newsletter which described our community as being in the "age of evidence-based medicine." This made it quite evident that the time had come. We were developing a new model that challenged very well-established doctors while trying to alert them that there was something fundamentally limited in how we had been practicing to date. We realized that one should not expect rejoicing. However, most of the criticisms about EBM being "cookbook medicine," or placing an overemphasis on randomized control trials, are misinterpretations of what we were and are still trying to accomplish.

Q: *What changes have occurred within evidence-based medicine since the beginning of your career?*

GG: Two major changes have occurred. First, there has been a shift in the original hierarchy of evidence. Originally, there was much emphasis on the literature. Now

we know that taking the context of the situation, as well as the values and preferences of the patient, into consideration is just as important. We know that the evidence alone never directs what to do. Secondly, optimal practice or health policy requires a systematic summary of the best available evidence. The GRADE system provides a sophisticated understanding of what "best available evidence" entails. We now consider not only study design and other aspects of risk of bias but also precision, consistency, directness, and publication bias when rating the literature. This leaves room for not only the evidence of randomized control trials but also the valuable contributions from well-performed observational studies.

Q: *What is the future of EBM?*

GG: We recognize how crucial the values and preference of the patient are. However, we don't yet know how to best apply these factors. We have started to include them through shared decision-making with both the clinician and the patient. In the future, this will become not only a larger focus for teaching medicine but also will help guide research. Additionally, we have come a long way in terms of the efficiency of the pre-processed information that is disseminated to clinicians. It will not be long until the best available evidence is supplied automatically to doctors, for each patient in their electronic medical records. This will allow the doctor to decide exactly how deep into the literature he or she wants to go. They can look at the overall statement, go deeper into some of the reviews, or if desired, pull out individual studies.

Q: *You have been practicing and teaching EBM for more than 20 years. What issues continue to be exciting to you?*

GG: Despite its age, we are still making methodological advances in EBM. The GRADE system has really moved things forward, and we are currently preparing a 20-part series in the *Journal of Epidemiology*, 15 of which are already published. These types of analysis are sufficiently challenging to keep life interesting. Also, we now are starting research projects that will analyze different evidence presentation techniques. This will allow us to understand physician and patient preferences for how we present evidence summaries. EBM has taught us that there is never an absolutely perfect treatment. Treatments are always dependent on people's values and preferences. Describing average personal values is very complicated, but I believe this will help to optimize medical decision-making.

THE PROCESS OF EVIDENCE-BASED PRACTICE

In clinical practice, questions arise that must be answered to optimize therapy, an intervention, or a service. These questions often develop from a single event or a string of similar events. An experienced, effective clinician seeks to find an answer that will provide each client with the best outcome. At this point, the professional employs the following procedures, as illustrated in Figure 2-1.

Step 1. Formulate a Specific Question

This process strongly resembles developing the research question of a scientific investigation and should be specific to the problem and client. The question should include the problem; the population; possible therapies, interventions, or services; a comparison intervention, if one exists; the outcome measures of interest; and the time frame. If the question is too broad, the interventions and outcome measures may be irrelevant to a client. Professionals should bear in mind that the client's goals and expectations will guide which outcome measures are of interest and how much change in the outcome measure is practical. Defining a question that is too narrow may result in finding too little evidence and may render the question unanswerable, as described in the following example.

An athletic trainer works with a sophomore collegiate baseball player whose primary diagnosis is suprascapular nerve pathology with a secondary diagnosis of slight degenerative fraying of the labrum. This baseball player considers the options of surgery for suprascapular nerve decompression and debridement of the labrum versus conservative rehabilitation. He is concerned about recovery time and the impact of surgery on the remaining years of his sport eligibility. In this case, the athletic trainer might ask, "In baseball players, how does surgical intervention for suprascapular nerve pathology and labrum debridement compare to conservative treatment in terms of length of recovery, time to return to play, and performance upon return?" However, realizing that this question is too specific, the athletic trainer divides into one for suprascapular nerve decompression surgery and one for labrum debridement surgery in order to gather relevant information.

Step 2. Search and Review Relevant Literature

When reviewing the literature, a professional should consult databases that are relevant and specific to an answerable question. Commonly used databases include Evidence-Based Medicine Reviews, Clinical Evidence, MEDLINE, PubMed, the Cochrane Library, PEDro, SportDiscus, Scopus, and CINAHL. These databases allow the professional to conduct a thorough, focused literature review.

For example, consider a clinical exercise physiologist who is caring for a patient with peripheral artery disease and wants to include resistance training in the exercise plan. This physiologist might develop the question, "What benefit does resistance training, compared to other exercise interventions, provide to a peripheral artery disease patient in six months and after 1 year?" The physiologist might begin a search by referring to the "peripheral artery disease" entry in Clinical Evidence, a database containing peer-reviewed systematic reviews of common medical disorders. He or she then might follow the literature search with a more focused question using another clinical database.

Step 3. Evaluate the Research and Consider All Interventions

The professional should (a) select the best, most current, and most relevant publications; (b) note the individual features of each article (*i.e.*, test participants, interpretation of data); (c) consider reported outcomes; and (d) determine if this publication applies to the client's goals. A meta-analysis or RCT may not be available to address every clinical question, so searching for the best available literature on the topic is critical. Levels of evidence and quality of research are discussed in Chapter 6.

Step 4. Make a Decision and Incorporate It in Practice

After the relevant research has been evaluated, this research is combined with clinical expertise and the goals and expectations of the client to make an informed, evidence-based decision for clinical practice (see Fig. 2-2). Decisions regarding clinical practice should always consider multiple factors. *Even the best research studies (alone or combined) can't fully obviate a clinician's experience with the problem or what is important to the client, so each clinical decision should be a combination of those inputs.* Sometimes, the treatment or plan with the most evidence or the one with the best overall outcomes will not be the best option for a particular client.

Step 5. Evaluate the Process, Decision, and Outcomes

The final step of EBP involves evaluating the outcomes that result from a clinical decision. Did the implementation of this decision elicit the expected and desired outcomes? Was the client satisfied with the outcomes of the decision? Were barriers or problems encountered during the implementation of the decision? Is new information available that may change the clinical decision for a similar client in the future?

EVALUATING PUBLISHED EVIDENCE

In published journal articles, the methods range from scientific experiments to expert group consensus opinion. This continuum necessitates evaluation of all publications in terms of levels of evidence, strong to weak. In most professions, the RCT is considered to be the epitome of evidence types. However, even RCT should be evaluated on strict criteria, such as effectiveness of concealing the treatment group from test participants and individuals assessing the outcome.

Thorough evaluation of published evidence requires meticulous scrutiny of the background information, evidence of confounding variables, the experimental design, controls, methods, instrumentation, test participant sample, comparison group, outcome variables, statistical analyses, sample size, interpretation of data, and inferences made. This process may indicate that published conclusions are not valid or appropriate to the goals and values of a client. Furthermore, discovery of possible mental or physical harm to clients must be a major consideration in each therapeutic decision.

Regardless of experimental design and methods, the findings of each study should be evaluated on the basis of pre-established criteria. This reduces the likelihood that poor quality or incomplete evidence will be considered. More than 100 professional organizations and research consortia have developed grading systems that are intended to optimize EBP decision-making (35). Table 2-1 presents seven widely used evidence evaluation systems: University of Oxford Centre for Evidence-Based Medicine: Levels of Evidence; Strength of Recommendation Taxonomy (SORT); Physiotherapy Evidence Scale (PEDro); Grading of Recommendations, Assessment, Development, and Evaluation (GRADE); U.S. Preventive Services Task Force grading system; the Cochrane Library grading system; and the National Registry of Evidence-based Programs and Practices (NREPP).

Easy access to evidence (*e.g.*, via internet or mobile device) optimizes decision-making at the point of care. Tools to assist evaluation and application of published medical literature to clinical practice are available at the website of the *Journal of the American Medical Association* (24).

ARCHIVED DATABASES

Professionals may access online information that assists decision-making, such as the NREPP (see Table 2-1), which prescribes an RCT evaluation system (28). This online database includes only treatments that have one or more reports of positive outcomes, have been published in a peer-reviewed journal or formal evaluation report, and have training materials available. Similarly, the PEDro database provides an archive of RCT and non-randomized controlled clinical trials and uses an original rubric, the PEDro scale, to help users identify which clinical trials are likely to be internally consistent, interpretable, and generalizable. The PEDro scale is not intended to measure the validity of a study's conclusions. This is true for a number of reasons, including (a) significant effects ($P < .05$) and a high PEDro scale score do not necessarily indicate that a treatment or program is clinically worthwhile; (b) treatment effects may not be large enough to warrant clinical use; (c) negative effects may outweigh positive effects; and (d) a treatment may not be cost-effective (32). Other archived databases are noted in Table 2-1.

SYSTEMATIC REVIEW AND META-ANALYSIS

EBM relies heavily on systematic reviews of RCT. A systematic review provides a comprehensive synthesis of numerous studies that are relevant to a single question in a manner that is

Table 2-1   Systems That Evaluate Published Evidence

System	Level and Type of Evidence	Organizations and Journals That Have Adopted This System	Supporting Information
University of Oxford Centre for Evidence-Based Medicine: Levels of Evidence	Levels (10) of evidence range from systematic reviews of RCT (strongest) to expert opinion without explicit critical appraisal (weakest). These levels of evidence are considered from the perspective of therapy, etiology, potential for harm, prognosis, diagnosis, and cost.	Centre for Evidence-Based (CFE-b) Dermatology, CFE-b Child Health, CFE-b Dentistry, CFE-b Mental Health, CFE-b Nursing (all are within the United Kingdom)	Source: http://www.cebm.net/oxford-centre-evidence-based-medicine-levels-evidence-march-2009/ The Centre for Evidence-Based Medicine (CEBM) promotes evidence-based healthcare. The CEBM provides free support and resources to doctors, clinicians, teachers, and others interested in learning more about EBM. The University of Oxford is one of several similar sites in the United Kingdom.
Strength of Recommendation Taxonomy (SORT)	Three levels of evidence: (a) good-quality, patient-oriented evidence; (b) inconsistent or limited-quality patient-oriented evidence; (c) other evidence including consensus, disease-oriented evidence, usual practice, expert opinion (or case series for studies of diagnosis, treatment, prevention, screening).	American College of Sports Medicine, *American Family Physician*	Source: http://www.aafp.org/afp/2004/0201/p461.html Developed by the American Academy of Family Physicians (AAFP), the SORT scale addresses the quality, quantity, and consistency of evidence; it allows authors to rate individual studies or bodies of evidence. The AAFP journal (*American Family Physician*) also offers point-of-care guides and summaries of patient-oriented evidence.
Physiotherapy Evidence Scale (PEDro)	The PEDro scale considers test participant inclusion–exclusion criteria, random and concealed assignment to treatments, group similarity at baseline, blinding of participants and researchers, between-group statistical comparison, treatment effect size, and key outcome variables.	American Physical Therapy Association, *British Journal of Sports Medicine*, Chartered Society of Physiotherapy (United Kingdom), Australian Physiotherapy Association	Source: http://www.pedro.org.au/ PEDro is managed by the Centre for Evidence-Based Physiotherapy at The George Institute for Global Health, Sydney, Australia. The randomized physiotherapy trials on PEDro (>25,000) are independently assessed for quality. These ratings guide users to trials that are more likely to be valid and trials which contain sufficient information to guide clinical practice.
Grading of Recommendations, Assessment, Development, and Evaluation (GRADE)	Four levels of evidence exist: high (further research is very unlikely to change confidence in the estimate of effect); moderate (further research may change the estimate of effect); low (further research is very likely to have an important impact on confidence in the estimate of effect); and very low (any estimate of effect is very uncertain).	Cochrane Library, World Health Organization, American College of Physicians, European Society of Thoracic Surgeons, U.K. National Institute for Clinical Excellence, Canadian Cardiovascular Society, American Red Cross, *British Medical Journal*	Source: http://www.gradeworkinggroup.org/ The GRADE Working Group, an informal collaboration of more than 180 professionals, developed a transparent approach to grading quality of evidence and strength of recommendations. International organizations have contributed to the development of the GRADE scale. A software application facilitates use of the GRADE scale and allows the development of summary tables.

Table 2-1 Systems That Evaluate Published Evidence

System	Level and Type of Evidence	Organizations and Journals That Have Adopted This System	Supporting Information
U.S. Preventive Services Task Force (USPSTF)	Services are graded by the USPSTF at five levels: A (there is high certainty that the net benefit is substantial); B (there is high certainty that the net benefit is moderate); C (there is at least moderate certainty that the net benefit is small); D (there is moderate or high certainty that the service has no net benefit or that the harms outweigh the benefits); and I (current evidence is insufficient to assess the balance of benefits and harms of the service).	World Health Organization, American College of Physicians, Centers for Disease Control and Prevention, Centers for Medicare and Medicaid Services, Department of Defense Military Health System, Department of Veterans Affairs Center for Health Promotion and Disease Prevention, National Institutes of Health, and U.S. Food and Drug Administration	Source: http://www.uspreventiveservicestaskforce.org/ The USPTF is an independent, non-government, volunteer panel of experts that formulates evidence-based recommendations about clinical preventive services (*e.g.*, screenings, counseling services, and preventive medications). Recommendations apply only to people who have no signs or symptoms of a specific disease or condition and address only services offered in the primary care setting or services referred by a primary care clinician.
The Cochrane Library grading system	Levels of evidence are determined by considering strength of the evidence, relevance of evidence, size of effect, and statistical confidence intervals.	World Health Organization Assembly, National Institute of Diabetes and Digestive Kidney Disease, Agency for Healthcare Research and Quality	Source: http://www.cochrane.org/cochrane-reviews/cochrane-database-systematic-reviews-numbers The Cochrane Collaboration is an international network of more than 31,000 individuals from over 120 countries. This online collection of databases brings together research on the effectiveness of healthcare treatments and interventions as well as methodology and diagnostic tests. Over 5,000 reviews are currently available in the Cochrane Library. Also, a central registry of RCT and abstracts of external reviews are available.
National Registry of Evidence-based Programs and Practices (NREPP)	Each NREPP reviewer evaluates quality of research for an intervention using the following criteria: reliability of measures, validity of measures, intervention fidelity, missing data and attrition, potential confounding variables, and appropriateness of analysis. Reviewers use a scale of 0.0 (lowest rating) to 4.0 (highest rating).	NREPP is an arm of the Substance Abuse and Mental Health Services Administration, U.S. Department of Health and Human Services, Rockville, MD.	Source: http://nrepp.samhsa.gov/ViewAll.aspx NREPP is a searchable online registry of more than 300 interventions supporting mental health promotion and substance abuse prevention and treatment. NREPP connects citizens to intervention developers, allowing them to learn how to implement these approaches in their communities.

RCT, randomized controlled clinical trial; EBM, evidence-based medicine.

similar to the "discussion" section of a scientific article. In any systematic review, the authors should describe all journals and databases that were searched; pre-determined criteria for inclusion, exclusion, and relevance; and the system that was used to evaluate published evidence.

However, researchers usually find it difficult to integrate and interpret dozens or hundreds of publications which focus on a single question. In such cases, or when the literature base is small or weak, a statistical meta-analysis can be employed to develop a stronger conclusion. Meta-analysis is a method that codes relevant data from multiple investigations and transforms these data into a common factor, which is analyzed statistically to determine effect size. In any meta-analysis, the analyst should describe inclusion and exclusion criteria, statistical power, significant findings, as well as the validity and reliability of measurements. The final conclusion regarding the effectiveness of a therapy or service is based on greater diversity of test participants and greater statistical power (*i.e.*, due to increased sample size) than any single publication. However, the selection of studies for inclusion in a meta-analysis is critical to a valid outcome. If poorly designed or small sample studies are included, the validity of the conclusions is threatened. Heterogeneity in participant or patient selection, intervention, and outcome measures can also lead to erroneous conclusions.

Also, EBP may be controversial. The most common controversies involve the time required and the relevance of a recommendation for a specific client or patient (18). Table 2-2 presents many present-day arguments for and against EBP. As you review this table, determine whether the positive or negative points of view incorporate all EBP steps, especially the final steps as shown in Figure 2-1.

EVIDENCE-BASED PRACTICE IN AMERICAN COLLEGE OF SPORTS MEDICINE POSITION STANDS

Beginning in 2004, ACSM began writing and publishing position stands using an evidence-based model (Table 2-3). The authors of this chapter interviewed Lynette Craft, PhD, who is the ACSM Vice President for Evidence-Based Practice and Scientific Affairs, to determine what influenced the ACSM to create an EBP model for positions stands, the benefits of an EBP approach, and the future of EBP with ACSM. The following discussion resulted from that interview.

Despite its widespread use in medical fields such as surgery and nursing, EBP was not common in sports medicine prior to 2002. Investigators and authors were limited by their own memory and exposure to the scientific and clinical literatures. During those years, the best practice involved expert group consensus that included systematic reviews of published evidence. However, as digital search engines grew in size and ease of access, ACSM position stands were modified to include specific questions and a systematic review of all available literature. The goal was to produce documents of the highest possible quality. As seen in the third column of Table 2-3, ACSM position stands now employ sound EBP (2–11,13,17,19,22,25,29–31,34).

Recently, ACSM has implemented a standard protocol manual for all position stand working committees. This entails a uniform grading rubric, an evidence grading system, and a clear description of methods that allow researchers to replicate experiments. In addition to convenience for clinicians and practitioners, the EBP approach allows gaps in the literature to be identified, including questions which have not been answered.

Table 2-2 The Pros and Cons of Evidence-Based Practice

Theme	For	Against
Time	• Improves efficacy and efficiency of clinicians by eliminating ineffective treatments	• It is time-consuming to perform a literature search and to implement new treatment protocols.
Statistical	• Decisions are based on rubric-guided interpretation of multiple data sets.	• Mean values may represent a bimodal rather than a normal distribution, limiting the applicability of the findings (external validity). • Extremes of the distribution of data may be ignored or excluded.
Creativity	• Allows clinicians to draw on the objective experience of many researchers and accepted scientific standards • Encourages clinicians to observe treatment outcome after implementation to evaluate its credibility	• Limits clinical judgment and creativity • May encourage algorithm ("cookbook") interventions • EBP is perceived as not allowing for differing treatments.
Research	• Helpful in identifying gaps in the literature or treatment • Promotes scientific studies and collection of data in areas which are lacking information • Encourages outcome-focused research questions • Supports appropriate research design	• May suppress research interventions for which funding is difficult to obtain • Overemphasis on RCT • Study populations may be too narrow
Policy	• Provides a scientific basis for the construction of departmental decisions and healthcare policy • Facilitates accountability and increased credibility, which in turn may lead to additional resources	• Some health insurance organizations may not reimburse treatments that have no EBP evidence. • Focuses on therapeutic interventions vs. prevention, prognosis, or diagnostic strategies
Education	• Promotes better practice • Promotes better quality of student management • Facilitates clinical reasoning and informed decision-making	None
Patient	• Encourages monitoring and review of practice • Promises to better inform patients and clinicians about clinical practices and treatment options	• Increased expectations from consumers or colleagues that all interventions must be justified

EBP, evidence-based practice; RCT, randomized controlled clinical trial.

Craft envisions that as literature becomes more available over a broader range of research topics, future ACSM position stands will become intentionally narrower. For example, since the 2004 position stand entitled "Exercise and Hypertension," thousands of publications have altered the landscape of available evidence. In the future, this topic may be separated into multiple position stands regarding several different populations, or it may be written to focus on specific modalities of exercise. Also, ACSM hopes to begin including executive summaries because current documents are lengthy and extremely dense by design, resulting from an effort to evaluate each question comprehensively. However, for the instructor looking to expose students to a number of position stands or the clinician who requires a rapid answer, an executive summary will meet these needs efficiently. Executive

Table 2-3 American College of Sports Medicine Position Stands and Evidence-Based Practice, as of November 2013

Year	Position Stand Title (Reference)	Evidence-Based	Evaluation System	Categories
1987	*The Use of Anabolic-Androgenic Steroids in Sports* (7)	No	Based on comprehensive literature survey and careful analysis of claims	
1994	*Exercise for Patients with Coronary Artery Disease* (8)	No		
1996	*The Use of Blood Doping as an Ergogenic Aid* (34)	No		
1996	*Weight Loss in Wrestlers* (30)	No	Previous research had not investigated the relationship between wrestling performance and weight loss.	
1998	*AHA/ACSM Joint Position Statement: Recommendations for Cardiovascular Screening, Staffing, and Emergency Policies at Health Fitness Facilities* (10)	No	Recommendations were based on a review of literature and consensus of the writing group.	
2002	*Automated External Defibrillators in Health Fitness Facilities* (3)	No		
2004	*Physical Activity and Bone Health* (25)	No		
2004	*Exercise and Hypertension* (31)	Yes	SORT	A, B, C, D
2006	*Prevention of Cold Injuries during Exercise* (13)	Yes	SORT	A, B, C
2007	*Exercise and Fluid Replacement* (9)	Yes	SORT	A, B, C
2007	*Exertional Heat Illness during Training and Competition* (5)	Yes	SORT	A, B, C
2007	*Exercise and Acute Cardiovascular Events: Placing the Risks into Perspective* (4)	No		
2007	*The Female Athlete Triad* (29)	Yes	SORT	A, B, C
2009	*Exercise and Physical Activity for Older Adults* (6)	Yes	SORT	A, B, C, D A, B, C, E
2009	*Nutrition and Athletic Performance* (11)	Yes	U.S. Preventive Service Task Force	I, II, III, IV, V
2009	*Progression Models in Resistance Training for Healthy Adults* (2)	Yes	SORT	A, B, C, D
2009	*Appropriate Physical Activity Intervention Strategies for Weight Loss and Prevention of Weight Regain for Adults* (19)	Yes	SORT	A, B, C, D
2010	*Exercise and Type 2 Diabetes* (17)	Yes	SORT	A, B, C, D A, B, C, E

Table 2-3   American College of Sports Medicine Position Stands and Evidence-Based Practice, as of November 2013

Year	Position Stand Title (Reference)	Evidence-Based	Evaluation System	Categories
2011	*Quantity and Quality of Exercise for Developing and Maintaining Cardiorespiratory, Musculoskeletal, and Neuromotor Fitness in Apparently Healthy Adults: Guidance for Prescribing Exercise (22)*	Yes	SORT	A, B, C, D
2013	*Prevention, Diagnosis, and Treatment of the Overtraining Syndrome: Joint Consensus Statement of the European College of Sport Science and the American College of Sports Medicine*	Yes		

ACSM, American College of Sports Medicine; AHA, American Heart Association; SORT, Strength of Recommendation Taxonomy.

summaries may also expose a broader audience, including mass media outlets, to the best available interpretation of published evidence.

The leaders of ACSM also plan to develop an EBP library, similar to the Cochrane Library (see Table 2-1) but with a sports medicine focus. With the aid of technology, users of this ACSM library will be able to select individual references to see exactly how the evidence from each was graded. Needless to say, educators will be able to use this database to teach students the process of evaluating published evidence and the relationship of published evidence to clinical practice (see Figs. 2-1 and 2-3).

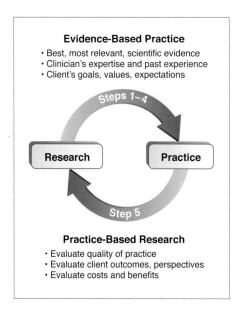

FIGURE 2-3:   The research–practice cycle.

OPTIMIZING EVIDENCE-BASED PRACTICE: EVALUATION AND EDUCATION

As illustrated in Figure 2-1, EBP involves more than evaluating the scientific-clinical literature (step 3), making a decision, and incorporating that decision in practice (step 4). EBP also involves evaluating the original question. A thorough assessment of a service or of therapeutic outcomes (step 5) begins a new series of events which are guided by a modified question (step 1).

Depending on the training, interests, and motivation of the professional, an evaluation of the treatment decision and outcomes also may stimulate an original study or RCT. Known as "practice-based research," this systematic process evaluates the quality of practice, outcomes, achievement of client goals, and the cost-to-benefit ratio of a treatment or service. The interactions of EBP and practice-based research are illustrated in Figure 2-3. When published in a peer-reviewed journal, practice-based research becomes the evidence that informs EBP. In fact, EBP cannot evolve without the new clinical information and perspectives that are generated by practice-based research. Occasionally, the clinician and researcher are one in the same; these individuals participate in all aspects of the research–practice cycle (see Fig. 2-3).

Finally, as all outstanding clinicians realize, excellent EBP requires intellectual curiosity and continuing self-education with the goal of discovering new treatments or practices that benefit clients. These requirements can be met by self-study, continual use of the complete EBP process, conference attendance, journal clubs, and grand rounds. Researchers also require continuing self-education. This typically occurs when they communicate with clinicians (see Fig. 2-3) to (a) identify new therapies, instruments, and services; and (b) understand clinical problems, failures, successes, and original ideas. These are the ingredients of new and effective EBP.

ACKNOWLEDGMENTS

The authors appreciate the technical support of Lindsay Ellis, who assisted with manuscript preparation, editing, and reference formats.

GLOSSARY

Clinician: in evidence-based practice, the professional who makes a recommendation regarding the care, treatment, service, or plan for a client or group

Client: the person or people to whom the care, treatment, or plan is applied

Evidence-based practice (EBP): practice in education, psychiatry, substance abuse rehabilitation, and social work that incorporates research evidence with patient values and clinical expertise

Randomized controlled clinical trial (RCT): experiments in which participants are assigned randomly to the treatments being studied; such protocols are considered to be the gold standard of all research

REFERENCES

1. Aird WC. Discovery of the cardiovascular system: from Galen to William Harvey. *J Thromb Haemost.* 2011;9(suppl 1):118–129.
2. American College of Sports Medicine. American College of Sports Medicine position stand. Progression models in resistance training for healthy adults. *Med Sci Sports Exerc.* 2009;41(3):687–708.

3. American College of Sports Medicine, American Heart Association. American College of Sports Medicine and American Heart Association joint position statement: automated external defibrillators in health/fitness facilities. *Med Sci Sports Exerc.* 2002;34(3):561–564.

4. American College of Sports Medicine, American Heart Association. Joint position statement: exercise and acute cardiovascular events: placing the risks into perspective. *Med Sci Sports Exerc.* 2007;39(5):886–897.

5. American College of Sports Medicine; Armstrong LE, Casa DJ, Millard-Stafford M, et al. American College of Sports Medicine position stand. Exertional heat illness during training and competition. *Med Sci Sports Exerc.* 2007;39(3):556–572.

6. American College of Sports Medicine; Chodzo-Zajko WJ, Proctor DN, Fiatarone Singh MA, et al. American College of Sports Medicine position stand. Exercise and physical activity for older adults. *Med Sci Sports Exerc.* 2009;41(7):1510–1530.

7. American College of Sports Medicine; Sawka MN, Burke LM, Eichner ER, et al. American College of Sports Medicine position stand. Exercise and fluid replacement. *Med Sci Sports Exerc.* 2007;39(2):377–390.

8. American College of Sports Medicine position stand. Exercise for patients with coronary artery disease. *Med Sci Sports Exerc.* 1994;26(3):i–v.

9. American College of Sports Medicine Position Stand and American Heart Association. Recommendations for cardiovascular screening, staffing, and emergency policies at health/fitness facilities. *Med Sci Sports Exerc.* 1998;30(6):1009–1018.

10. American College of Sports Medicine position stand on the use of anabolic-androgenic steroids in sports. Med Sci Sports Exerc. 1987;19(5):534–539.

11. American Dietetic Association, Dietitians of Canada, American College of Sports Medicine. American College of Sports Medicine position stand. Nutrition and athletic performance. *Med Sci Sports Exerc.* 2009;41(3):709–731.

12. Bollet AJ. Pierre Louis: the numerical method and the foundation of quantitative medicine. *Am J Med Sci.* 1973;266(2):92–101.

13. Castellani JW, Young AJ, Ducharme MB, Giesbrecht GG, Glickman E, Sallis RE. American College of Sports Medicine position stand: prevention of cold injuries during exercise. *Med Sci Sports Exerc.* 2006;38(11):2012–2029.

14. Claridge JA, Fabian TC. History and development of evidence-based medicine. *World J Surg.* 2005;29(3):547–553.

15. Cochrane AL. *Effectiveness and Efficiency: Random Reflections on Health Services.* London: Nuffield Provincial Hospitals Trust; 1972. 92 p.

16. Codman EA. The classic: a study in hospital efficiency: as demonstrated by the case report of first five years of private hospital. *Clin Orthop Relat Res.* 2013;471:1778–1783.

17. Colberg SR, Albright AL, Blissmer BJ, et al. Exercise and type 2 diabetes: American College of Sports Medicine and the American Diabetes Association: joint position statement. Exercise and type 2 diabetes. *Med Sci Sports Exerc.* 2010;42(12):2282–2303.

18. Croft P, Malmivaara A, van Tulder M. The pros and cons of evidence-based medicine. *Spine.* 2011;36(17):E1121–E1125.

19. Donnelly JE, Blair SN, Jakicic JM, Manore MM, Rankin JW, Smith BK. American College of Sports Medicine Position stand. Appropriate physical activity intervention strategies for weight loss and prevention of weight regain for adults. *Med Sci Sports Exerc.* 2009;41(2):459–471.

20. Evidence-based medicine, in its place. *Lancet.* 1995;346(8978):785.

21. Evidence-Based Medicine Working Group. Evidence-based medicine. A new approach to teaching the practice of medicine. *JAMA.* 1992;268(17):2420–2425.

22. Garber CE, Blissmer B, Deschenes MR, et al. American College of Sports Medicine position stand. Quantity and quality of exercise for developing and maintaining cardiorespiratory, musculoskeletal, and neuromotor fitness in apparently healthy adults: guidance for prescribing exercise. *Med Sci Sports Exerc.* 2011;43(7):1334–1359.

23. Hajar R. The air of history: early medicine to galen (part I). *Heart Views.* 2012;13(3):120–128.

24. Journal of the American Medical Association Evidence Web site [Internet]. New York (NY): Journal of the American Medical Association Evidence; [cited 2013 Nov 1]. Available from: http://jamaevidence.com

25. Kohrt WM, Bloomfield SA, Little KD, Nelson ME, Yingling VR. American College of Sports Medicine position stand: physical activity and bone health. *Med Sci Sports Exerc.* 2004;36(11):1985–1996.

26. Lind J. Nutrition classics. A treatise of the scurvy by James Lind, MDCCLIII. *Nutr Rev.* 1983;41(5):155–157.

27. Missios S. Hippocrates, Galen, and the uses of trepanation in the ancient classical world. *Neurosurg Focus.* 2007;23(1):E11.

28. National Registry of Evidence-Based Practices and Programs Web site [Internet]. Rockville (MD): SAMSHA's National Registry of Evidence-based Programs and Practices; [cited 2013 Nov 1]. Available from: http://www.nrepp.samhsa.gov/courses/Implementations/resources/imp_course.pdf

29. Nattiv A, Loucks AB, Manore MM, Sanborn CF, Sundgot-Borgen J, Warren MP. American College of Sports Medicine position stand. The female athlete triad. *Med Sci Sports Exerc.* 2007;39(6):1867–1882.

30. Oppliger RA, Case HS, Horswill CA, Landry GL, Shelter AC. American College of Sports Medicine position stand. Weight loss in wrestlers. *Med Sci Sports Exerc.* 1996;28(6):ix–xii.

31. Pescatello LS, Franklin BA, Fagar R, Farquhar WB, Kelley GA, Ray CA. American College of Sports Medicine position stand. Exercise and hypertension. *Med Sci Sports Exerc.* 2004(3);36:533–553.

32. Physiotherapy Evidence Database Web site [Internet]. Sydney, Australia: Physiotherapy Evidence Database; [cited 2013 Nov 1]. Available from: http://www.pedro.org.au/

33. Sackett DL, Rosenberg WM, Gray JA, Haynes RB, Richardson WS. Evidence based medicine: what it is and what it isn't. *BMJ.* 1996;312(7023):71–72.

34. Sawka MN, Joyner MJ, Milles DS, Robertson RJ, Spriet LL, Young AJ. American College of Sports Medicine position stand. The use of blood doping as an ergogenic aid. *Med Sci Sports Exerc.* 1996;28(6):i–viii.

35. U.S. Department of Health and Human Services, Agency for Healthcare Research and Quality. *Evidence Report/Technology Assessment Number 47: Systems to Rate the Strength of Scientific Evidence: Summary.* Rockville, MD: U.S. Department of Health and Human Services, Agency for Healthcare Research and Quality; 2002. 11 p. Available from: U.S. AHRQ publication No. 02-E015. Accessed May 24, 2015, at: http://archive.ahrq.gov/clinic/epcsums/strengthsum.htm

Choosing Your Research Project: Framing the Problem, Research Hypotheses, and Predictions

Maria L. Urso, PhD, FACSM, and Julie M. Hughes, PhD

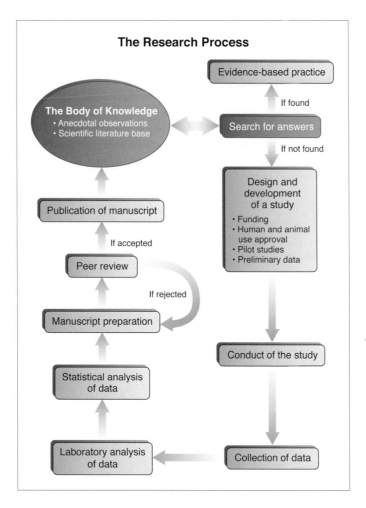

The Research Process

INTRODUCTION: JOIN THE SCIENTIFIC CONVERSATION

Advancing knowledge through scientific inquiry can be thought of as contributing to a conversation. It's an ongoing conversation among curious individuals seeking questions as to why and how things work. This community of interacting scientists is composed of many different sub-disciplines, each with a particular enduring conversation. If you were to eavesdrop on a cardiovascular physiology conversation, you might overhear several scientists discussing the role of inflammation in plaque rupture. If you were to listen in on a conversation among biomechanists, you may overhear a discussion regarding gait changes in runners switching to barefoot-style shoes. In yet another conversation, physicists can be overheard discussing the revolutionary implications of the discovery of the Higgs boson particle. The fuel for these conversations is the research findings that are shared at scientific conferences, in peer-reviewed scientific journals, over wine in European cafés, among residents in teaching hospitals, and in journal clubs in academic settings.

When it is time for you to design, complete, and share the findings of your own research project, whether you are a graduate or advanced undergraduate student, you are inserting yourself into the conversation. A seamless transition requires that you first learn what has been discussed in the previous conversation. Fortunately, the historical transcripts are archived in the published scientific literature. By taking the time to familiarize yourself with the existing literature, you will gain important insight into the questions that remain to be asked in your field, thus providing a critical foundation for developing an impactful research project.

If you are embarking on your first empirical solo mission, the journey that begins with identifying a research question and ends with the publication of your results can seem overwhelming. Even pioneering physiologists agree that investigators do not march straight to their goal with ease and directness. Obstacles and difficulties are sure to be encountered (1). In this chapter, it is our goal to demystify the first steps of the research process by sharing everyday skills and techniques involved in developing a quality research project. Specifically, we outline a process that guides you through defining your topic area of interest, becoming familiar with the existing literature, and identifying gaps in the literature. We then provide recommendations for defining your specific research project by bridging together your ideal project with some practical temperaments. We conclude this chapter with recommendations for writing solid purpose statements, objectives, and hypotheses so that you can clearly express what you will be doing (and why you will be doing it) to your graduate advisor, your committee members, a grant reviewer, a journal editor, or (most importantly) your own mother. With this approach, your attempt to understand a certain scientific phenomenon will be likened to a series of adventures rather than a string of unpleasant misadventures.

This chapter walks you through the rationale behind building a strong research foundation and how you can develop that foundation to get the most out of your first research project. The highlighted boxes throughout the chapter allow for an excursion from the straight and narrow and provide personal and anecdotal insight into each of the research steps. Additionally, they suggest exercises that will help you develop your research idea. By the end of this chapter, it is our hope that you will have some tools in your research toolbox to identify a research problem, develop a research question, and formulate appropriate hypotheses. Bear in mind that one day, after you have completed this process several times, you can refine and pass these techniques on to future research scientists as a mentor.

BUILDING THE FOUNDATION FOR YOUR RESEARCH PROJECT

The foundation of a good research project is a good **research question**, which originates from a strong understanding of the past and current literature in your field. When you have identified a field of study that interests you, it is then your duty as a researcher to become familiar with the findings of other researchers in your field. One of the benefits that comes with dedicating time to aggressively learning the relevant literature is that you will begin to detect **gaps in the literature**, and you will inevitably find yourself asking a question about a phenomenon in the field that has yet to be answered. You must first gain experience in reading and understanding the current literature and what we know scientifically about a topic. As time goes on and your career progresses, you then start to have the potential to ask even more insightful questions that eventually may lead you to be a thought leader and innovator in a particular field of research. If you have the practical means to empirically address the question, then you have successfully identified your research project. (See Fig. 3-1 for a visual roadmap of the steps taken to identify your research project.) In the following sections, we guide you through this process.

Identifying Your Topic Area: Choosing the Conversation You Want to Join

The first step in the research process is to choose your topic area of interest. You can think of this as choosing the conversation you will be joining. Of course, most of us like to join a conversation in which we are interested. Sometimes you have a specific research topic assigned to you for a class project or a research assistantship which may not be initially interesting to you. However, once you get started, you may find that the conversation unexpectedly piques your curiosity.

In most cases, you will have some room to choose your topic area. If you are at the place in your education when you are deciding what your topic area will be (particularly if you are deciding what laboratory to join based on the research focus), there are four questions that will help you determine what topic area will best fit you. The first question to ask yourself is the most important one—what are my interests? Designing your study, analyzing your results, and sharing your findings are all much more enjoyable when you are truly interested in a topic. Often, events in your life will lead you to an area of interest. Perhaps your father has been diagnosed with diabetes, and you are interested in the role of nutrition and exercise in managing the condition. Maybe you are a competitive athlete with an interest in coaching and are curious about sports psychology. Maybe a physical disability with which you have lived piqued your interest in motor control. Some researchers will find their area of interest during prior education. It is possible that in a biochemistry class, a future researcher becomes interested in the mechanisms of muscle or bone anabolism. Perhaps in a physics class, a student becomes interested in studying how the human body

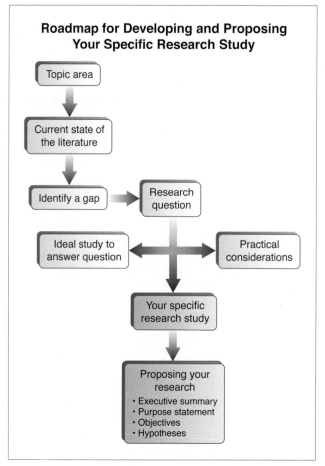

FIGURE 3-1:   This roadmap is meant to be used by a young investigator as a guide to lead to a specific research project. When planning your first study, we recommend familiarizing yourself with the literature in your field of interest so as to identify a gap in the literature. Once you formulate a specific research question based on this gap, your ideal study design must be tempered by practical considerations. This process should help you identify a project that is novel and will contribute to the existing literature.

moves most efficiently during different activities. Take your time to find a topic area that truly interests you.

Another important question that you want to ask is, "What am I good at?" Some people have the aptitude for basic science research, whereas some people are better tailored to work with human subjects. Some scientists begin in basic research and will make a partial shift to applied science in their career, or vice versa. However, by knowing your strengths and choosing a topic area and type of research geared toward your strengths, you are setting yourself up for a successful career.

A third question that you want to ask is, "What research topics have practical implications in society?" Will your research contribute to solving a problem in the world? Will it

Concept Box 3-1 Justifying Your Research: Who Does It Benefit?

As a researcher, you should *always* be able to reply clearly and concisely to the question, "Why does your research matter?" This is true whether you are studying the acute signaling dynamics of a specific molecule or characterizing an organ-level response to a chronic stimulus. Simply put, your research should matter. It should be relevant to society in general, or it should benefit a specific population. By following the steps outlined in this chapter, including identifying a gap in the understanding of a problem, you can ensure your work will be relevant and justifiable. John E. Greenleaf, a prolific and internationally renowned physiologist, had several research tenets that should be adopted by young investigators (3).

These included that research should have some application to human well-being and that taxpayer-funded research should benefit, in order: the country, the institution, and the research team. You should be able to justify your research in terms of these stakeholders, and if your research is funded by a special interest group, you should have a good understanding of how your research will help your sponsoring organization reach its goals. Being granted resources by an institution, your mentor, and/or your country to conduct research is a privilege, and it is your solemn duty as a researcher to understand the context of it and be able to justify the importance of your work in relation to a societal problem.

help in understanding the mechanisms of a certain disease? Will your research advance the performance of athletes? If so, does this matter? To whom does it matter? Will your research improve the quality of life of people? If your research is relevant, you will have an easier time finding funding for your research from government sources or from special interest groups. You will also have more success when publishing your findings. In general, the more people who will benefit from your research, the more support you will find for your research (See Box 3-1 for further discussion on why your research should impact society.)

A final question that you may ask yourself is, "How many other people are conducting research in the same topic area?" Through advancing common knowledge, scientists work as a team. However, it is also true that scientists constantly compete over resources to support their work. For this reason, finding your niche is essential when considering a career in research. This does not mean that it is necessary to find an obscure topic to study; rather, identifying a sub-topic within a broader topic area can ensure that your work will be unique.

Your research topic area does not have to meet all of these criteria—to be of interest to you, geared toward your personal strengths, relevant to society, and unique. However, if you do find a research area that fulfills these criteria, then you have set yourself up for a successful research experience.

Another important consideration when determining your research focus is selecting an appropriate advisor. When you join a research laboratory, your research will be intrinsically linked with the focus area of your advisor. When you have identified an area of research in which you are interested, you have the aptitude for it, and the work is relevant to society and novel, it is time to find a mentor who can help you grow as a scientist and provide you with the tools necessary to study your chosen topic. When searching for a mentor, there are a few key attributes to keep in mind. Your advisor should have a research focus in your area of interest and should have a good reputation for publishing in this area. Your advisor should have the funding and resources to support you. You should interview other students working for your potential advisor and confirm that he or she is a good mentor. If you plan to pursue a line of research in a topic of interest to you, finding the right mentor to guide you will be a critical step in becoming a successful and independent researcher. Once you have identified your area of interest, you are ready to take the next step in identifying your first research project—reading the relevant literature.

Current State of the Literature: Listening to and Learning from the Past Conversation

Once you have identified the conversation you want to join, it is now time to become familiar with the past conversation. Fortunately, the history of the conversation in your field is recorded in the scientific literature. Therefore, you must first identify in which journals the scientists in your field of interest publish most frequently and begin your literature search with these. If your topic area is broad, however, the amount of published research can be overwhelming. For this reason, it is best to narrow your research focus to a manageable level. For example, say you are a student in a laboratory studying the role of exercise in aging. Because there is an immense amount of literature on this broad topic, you want to narrow your focus, and consequently, your literature search, to a more specific topic such as the role of exercise in preventing falls in the elderly. You may even want to further narrow your focus to the role of strength training in preventing falls in the elderly. Once you have a manageable topic, you must then read the relevant research papers in your topic area to learn what has been done before, who has done it, and what remains to be done.

When you are reading the relevant literature, there are a few tips that will help you be efficient. One tip is to stay focused on your particular sub-topic to prevent getting overwhelmed by the amount of literature. As you will find in a research course and in this textbook, just because a paper is published does not mean it explains everything on a topic or was done correctly as it may have experimental errors. Finding reviews on a topic by a top investigator or position stands by organizations such as the American College of Sports Medicine can be one way to jump into the literature and get a feel for a particular topic in the field. Then you must understand that in science, there can be many different views on a particular topic, even opposing ones. The individual papers and their evaluation and interpretation are the direct way to sort it out for yourself, but again, it takes time. Many times other people's interpretations can also be false. When you start with individual papers at first, you may find it helpful to read just the abstracts of the papers in your topic area to get a broad overview of what has been done. Then, as you identify papers that are most relevant, take time to read the full text and study the figures and data tables. As you become more familiar with the literature, you will notice that some papers are cited more than others. Often, these are landmark papers with which you should become familiar. Take time to study these papers, as they have provided the foundation for more recent research. Another tip is to pay attention to the authors of the papers that you are reading. Pay particular attention to the order of the authors. The first author is typically the person who wrote the bulk of the paper. The last author is often the senior author. The senior author is commonly the principal investigator of the study and the leader of the laboratory that conducted the research. If you stay in the field, you will likely interact professionally with the authors whose work you have read.

When reading the literature, review articles can be helpful in providing a summary of the relevant literature. Another benefit of a literature review is that it can provide an unbiased review of your research topic area. In these articles, the authors are likely experts in the field, and their summaries and interpretations can guide you through learning the state of the literature on a topic. In the field of science, reviews are typically only thought of as being important if the author(s) has had extensive experience doing research in that area of study. One can see this by looking at the review's literature base, and if the author(s) does not show up, it is not considered a high-level review. Although you may write a review of literature as part of a thesis or dissertation, its merit to the outside world of science will only be valued if your major professor is an expert in the field and publishes the paper with you. Writing a literature review is a lot of work but will ensure that you have a strong grasp of the literature in your field. This exposure will ensure that your research is comprehensive enough to form appropriate hypotheses.

As you become more familiar with the literature, you will begin to understand the history of the field. You will learn who has done what research in the field and how their research was used as a foundation for further research. You will start to pick up on important theories in the field and see how they have changed as new evidence has become available. You may even find yourself developing your own theories and asking questions that have not been asked yet. These are good indications that you are now ready to start contributing to the conversation in your field by developing your own research question. However, a common misconception is that this process is relatively easy and can be accomplished with a few hours of focused searching. Becoming familiar with the literature to the degree that you begin to identify new research questions takes dedication far beyond performing a simple electronic search. Not only will you need to work hard to initially build a foundation of understanding of the relevant work in your field but also you will find that throughout your career, you will continuously study the relevant literature in your field to stay current in your knowledge.

Identifying a Gap in the Literature: What's Missing in the Conversation?

Now that you have reviewed the existing literature on the topic, you are ready to start contributing to the conversation with your own ideas and questions. To do this, you will have to identify something that is missing from the current conversation—a gap you can fill. Typically, the laboratory you work in will have a line of research going on. You may then see how some of the work can be extended with your own individual novel twist to it and have the technology to undertake it and then, as you will read in this book, search for funding to pursue it. While you were conducting your literature review, you may have begun to ask questions or wonder why certain research studies have not yet been performed. If you have become well read in your area, you may have even developed a specific idea about a certain problem or an explanation for a natural phenomenon that is consistent with previous experimental evidence. In other words, you may have developed a theory. At this point, you can begin to refine your theory so that you are eventually in a position to ask a specific research question and embark on your own research project. If you have developed a new theory or even a new way to look at an old theory, this will provide the fuel to generate a novel research question. However, you do not necessarily need to develop a new theory to generate a research question that addresses a gap in the literature; rather, other ideas for research projects may have developed during your literature review.

Collectively, prior research can be categorized as previous experience; it identifies experimental designs that were successful, those that failed (or did not properly address the research question), highlights what a logical (or necessary) next step would be, and indicates what gaps need to be filled and how one can approach those gaps. From this literature, you may have gathered that it is necessary to repeat a series of experiments with additional measures at more frequent time points or to repeat an experiment in a higher-order organism in order to understand if similar results would be obtained. For example, a study may have demonstrated interesting findings in mice and now needs to be replicated in humans. Advances in technology may also shape how you interpret previous research and develop a research question that was not practicable several years prior. Asking yourself what new questions you can ask based on new technology with higher resolution is a fantastic way to generate a research question that is novel. However, the new technology should not be the main driver of your current and future research. Such research is termed **methods-driven research**, and we caution against this type of research if you plan to have a career as a research scientist. (See Box 3-2 for a discussion on **hypothesis-driven research**.) By basing your research questions on previous work (rather than on availability of new technology), you will develop a series of research studies that tell a focused and interesting story. However, technological capabilities and funding limit what questions can be addressed, and here is where the laboratory you work with during your educational career will frame what you can do. The line of research you pursue is most often an extension of your mentor's laboratory technologies and general interests. The productivity of a particular laboratory and the dynamics of the laboratory group will in part influence your career and its trajectory.

All of these approaches are capable of filling a gap in the literature—improving on previous studies, doing so with novel technology or other variations in study design, and starting from scratch with a new experimental design to test a new theory. Once you have identified a gap in the literature that you would like to fill, you are ready to formulate your research question.

Formulating Your Research Question: What Will You Add to the Conversation?

You have identified a gap in the literature; you have found a place where you can contribute new knowledge. Remember you may find a gap in the literature and ask why this has not been done before. Then when trying to pursue it, you find out that it may not be technologically possible and that there was a good reason why the gap remains. Conversely, you may now be able to overcome the past limitations and fill the gap with the new data that had been waiting for you to produce. Now it is time to ask a specific question that you will seek to answer with your research project. It is best if your research question is narrowed as far as possible, such that it can begin to be answered with a single research study. For example, say that your initial topic area of interest was the role of physical activity in the academic success of children. You may have found some background literature on this topic but realized there was a gap in evidence regarding the relationship between the amount of time spent in physical education classes and how students perform on standardized academic tests.

CONCEPT BOX 3-2 **Telling a Story with Your Research**

In this chapter, we outline the process of identifying a novel first research project. However, if you choose a career in research, you will have the opportunity to make the decisions outlined in this chapter over and over again. (See Fig. 3-2 for major research decisions.) Your first research study will not necessarily determine the trajectory of your entire research career. It is possible that you may choose a different research focus as you advance to graduate school, a postdoctoral fellowship, to an academic position, or into private industry. Each career move may come with a shift in focus depending on the objectives of the laboratory research group or institute you join. It is not uncommon to change postgraduate institutions three or more times before settling into a more permanent research position (4). As noted before, when you join a laboratory group, you will most

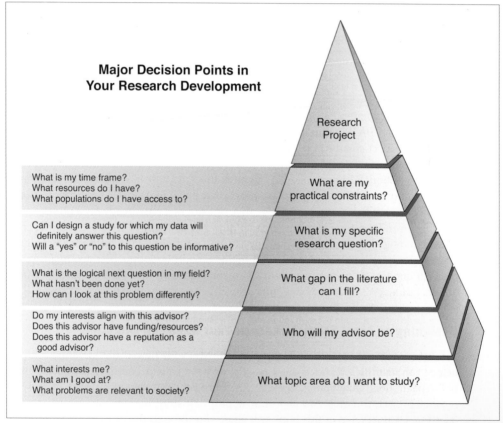

Major Decision Points in Your Research Development

Research Project

What is my time frame?
What resources do I have?
What populations do I have access to?

What are my practical constraints?

Can I design a study for which my data will
    definitely answer this question?
Will a "yes" or "no" to this question be informative?

What is my specific research question?

What is the logical next question in my field?
What hasn't been done yet?
How can I look at this problem differently?

What gap in the literature can I fill?

Do my interests align with this advisor?
Does this advisor have funding/resources?
Does this advisor have a reputation as a
    good advisor?

Who will my advisor be?

What interests me?
What am I good at?
What problems are relevant to society?

What topic area do I want to study?

FIGURE 3-2: There are several important decisions you will have to make on your journey as a young scientist. One of the most important decisions you will make is what topic area you would like to study. Another important decision you will make is who to choose as a research advisor. You will then have to make decisions for each new research project you undertake, including choosing what gap in your field to fill with your project, how to narrow your project down to a specific research question, and then you will have to consider your practical constraints when designing your specific research study. Here, we outline some important questions to ask yourself along the way.

(Continued)

Concept Box 3-2   Telling a Story with Your Research

(Continued)

likely take on what your mentor or the principal investigator does in his or her line of research and be asked to use your own creativity to work from the cutting edge that the laboratory is working from. Many times that is why you pursue working with that laboratory group in the first place. Independent of your shifts in research focus, your work should be aimed at telling a story. When you've identified a societal problem your work can contribute to solving, then you may choose multiple approaches to solving the problem, including developing cellular-, organ-, system-, and organism-level models to study the problem. Your results from one study may provide the stimulus for a new hypothesis to be tested

in a subsequent study. By conducting hypothesis-driven work aimed at solving a specific problem, the body of work you produce will tell a compelling story that you can share in the literature and at conferences. For this reason, we promote hypothesis-driven research over methods-driven research. The latter type of research can be seductive when you acquire a novel piece of technology or a new research technique. Don't let your resources drive your research, but rather try to find the resources needed to answer your research questions. Doing so will help distinguish you as an expert in a specific area and will ensure that your research career contributes to solving an important societal problem.

Now that you have refined your interests and found a gap, you will want to state the purpose of your research in question form: Does the amount of time spent in physical education classes affect standardized academic test performance? You will know your research question is specific enough if the data you collect will provide a definitive answer to your research question. Furthermore, you can be assured you have a novel research question if a "yes" or a "no" to your question will be informative either way. This is a good indication that the work you are doing will not be repetitive of work that has already been done.

Once you have formulated a research question that will address a gap in the current understanding in your field, it is now time to start considering the methods you will use to address this question. We recommend thinking broadly about the best way to answer your research question first, and then we recommend adjusting your project based on practical considerations. We discuss these points next.

Designing an Ideal Study to Answer Your Research Question

You have identified your topic of interest, and you've reviewed the literature which has helped you identify a research question that addresses a gap. You have completed the initial steps in identifying your specific research project. However, in order to propose your research project, you must first choose an appropriate study design to answer your research question. Chapters 5–8 in this book will guide you through the process of designing your study. Here, we give you a few suggestions for beginning this process. You will have to fully characterize and refine your study design before you can write the initial components of your research proposal—your executive summary, objectives, and hypotheses.

When designing your study, we recommend performing an academic exercise. Open a notebook to a blank page or stand in front of a whiteboard and start brainstorming and recording your ideas. Think about your specific research question. Ask yourself, "If I had unlimited resources and time, what study design would I use to *best* answer my research question?" Think big and resist the temptation to consider barriers such as time, money, and ethical considerations (you will *have* to consider these things eventually, but not yet). What population would you study? Elite cyclists? Astronauts? Deep sea divers? Would you test animals? Would you follow a group of people prospectively? Would you simply observe natural phenomena, or would you intervene? Perhaps you would randomize participants to an exercise group or a control group. Would you give participants a performance-enhancing drug? Would you follow participants for a year, a decade, or from childhood until death? This exercise is integral to the research process for many reasons.

The first reason is that this practice will allow you to be creative and will help you become better at identifying novel experimental designs in the future. Once you have completed a brainstorming session, you can prioritize your ideas and research questions from the most complex to the most basic. You may find that you will be able to answer one or more questions with a simple experimental design, but other questions will require a series of experiments to take place before you are able to address them. This is not just an exercise for students—the proverbial cocktail napkin brainstorming session has been the foundation of success for many scientists, entrepreneurs, and writers. Using creative designs from the prior literature even from other fields may allow one to address questions in their own field in a new and novel way and provide important new knowledge to the field.

This brainstorming practice will also make you keenly aware of how your final research project is different from what you would do if you did not have limitations. This process identifies what aspects of your research question *cannot* be answered with the data that you will collect. This is a normal part of research. In fact, it is wise to include these limitations in your research proposal. Also, when writing your final report, whether a manuscript or a term paper, you should address the impact of the limitations on your data interpretation. For example, you would ideally study the effects of an intervention in humans but for practical reasons (*e.g.*, one cannot cut out a human's kidneys to study them) can only study the intervention in mice. You can state the obvious that a limitation of your study is that findings are not generalizable to humans but can acknowledge they do provide insight into certain phenomena that are similar across species. However, this should be obvious to most readers based on their understanding of research generalizations. This way, you are not discounting your research or your data, but you will not be criticized for overstating your findings. In the real world of science, there is no such thing as a "perfect" study, but one can have a tightly designed and justified study that has well defined controls and constraints. However, it cannot answer every question for every part of the total population, and thus limitations exist in its generalization. However, in a paper, these limitations need to be more carefully dealt with so as not be thought of as "red flags" or "fatal flaws" in the experimental design.

Finally, this exercise will allow you to sketch out an experimental design that is appropriate to answer your research question. Although many research questions seem great in theory, once you draft a plan of *when* you will collect data for each of your criterion measures, you may realize that your data collection timeline is not practicable. For example, you may have planned to take blood samples from your subjects every day at 6 a.m. after a 12-hour fast for one month straight. You then realize that it will be difficult to do this over the weekend when the dining hall does not start serving dinner until 6 p.m. Refining your design at this stage is ideal because you will then be able to construct the most accurate **hypothesis** and not have to change it according to changes in your experimental design.

Another reason for this exercise is that you may identify a study that you will be able to complete down the road when you find yourself replete with resources. If you do this exercise correctly, you should be able to develop some unique and creative ways to answer your research question. When you have identified an ideal study design (or close to it), it is time to start writing down those ideas that you have committed to and consider what you are able to do with the resources and time frame you have.

Practical Considerations

There are a number of practical considerations that will shape your research design. Perhaps the most important consideration in your research design is whether or not your research methods will be ethical. Pretend you would like to study the effects of smoking cigarettes on the ability to perform certain physical tasks required of firefighters. Scientifically, it would be ideal to design a study in which you have one group of firefighters smoke for several months and compare their ability to perform certain physical firefighting tasks to a control group of firefighters that do not smoke during the study. For obvious health reasons, this study would not be ethical. Most research you conduct will require approval from an institutional review board (IRB), otherwise known as a "Human Use in Research Committee" (HURC) or "Institutional Animal Care and Use Committee" (IACUC). An IRB must approve all research, even survey research. The responsibility of the IRB is to make sure that the research tools, data collection techniques, data analysis procedures, and dissemination of results do not put the human subject at a risk that outweighs the potential benefit of the research. Although harm to a research subject participating in invasive research (*e.g.*, muscle biopsy is obtained) is obvious, sensitive topics that are addressed in survey research may also put a subject at risk. In the case of animal research, it is important to identify how the investigator plans to minimize distress to the animal and reduce the number of animals needed for an experiment. The ethical aspects of research and research clearance are discussed in depth in Chapter 12.

Getting your research approved by an IRB can be a time-intensive process you will have to consider when developing your research methods. This brings us to another important practical consideration—being realistic about the time you have to complete your research. For example, if you are conducting research as an academic requirement and will only receive credit in one course, you will need to structure your research differently than someone who is developing a thesis and has several months or years to complete the research project. If this is your first research project, it is easy to underestimate the amount of time necessary to take your project from conception to completion. A major determinant of the amount of time it takes to complete your research project will be how you choose to design your study. If you have a year or more to complete your study, you may choose to design a prospective study in which you follow people over time and record certain behaviors and measurements. If you are on a short time frame, you may choose a cross-sectional design in which you compare two groups with a difference in a variable relevant to your research question. A more in-depth discussion of study design can be found in Chapters 7 and 8.

Besides choosing an appropriate design for your timeline, you will also have to consider the funding you have available for your study. You may not have any money for your study, in which case, your design may be drastically different than a study that is funded by a major National Institutes of Health grant. You will have to consider the costs that are associated with research. Potential items and services that you should factor into your budget are the costs of equipment that you will need, transportation for participants to and from your laboratory, and monetary compensation of participants for their time (this is not always necessary). There are many other financial considerations that you will have to make when considering the design of your research study. Chapter 13 covers the financial aspects of research in more depth.

A final practical consideration is whether you have the research equipment you need to appropriately answer your research question. If you are a member of an established laboratory, and your research focus is aligned with the goals of your laboratory, then you likely have the equipment you need. If you have finances available, you may be able to purchase the equipment you need. If you do not have what you need, you may need to be creative, you may need to change your research question, or you may need to choose an alternate measurement. For the latter scenario, suppose you would like to measure muscle fatigue but do not have equipment necessary to perform electromyography; instead, you may have to be creative and come up with an alternate measure of muscular fatigue, such as the ability to perform a muscle-fatiguing physical test. Coming up with new ideas within the capabilities and research lines of the laboratory you are working in can allow you to carve out your own ideas and content expertise.

All of these practical considerations will shape your ultimate study design. If this is your first research study, we recommend keeping your study design as simple as possible while still addressing your research question (see Box 3-3 for more on keeping your first study simple). No matter the size of your research study, you will obtain skills and experiences that will start to shape your research career. These skills and experiences are essential components of a solid research foundation.

When you have settled on an experimental design that answers your research question while adhering to your practical constraints, you have successfully identified a research project. Furthermore, if you are answering a novel research question born out of a gap in the existing literature, then your research project will be relevant and justifiable—both important criteria for writing a compelling research proposal. Below, we share some guidelines for drafting the first sections of your research proposal.

PUTTING IT DOWN ON PAPER: DRAFTING YOUR PROPOSAL

Whether you are proposing your research to your research advisor, a granting agency, or your doctoral supervisory committee, most proposals consist of a standard set of sections, including the executive summary of the research, a purpose statement, a list of your objectives, and your hypotheses. We provide some guidelines in the following text for drafting these preliminary sections of your research proposal. The remainder of your proposal will likely consist of your literature review, your study design, and your specific methods. These topics are covered extensively in Chapters 4–8 in this book. Figure 3-3 provides a template for the initial sections of your research proposal.

Concept Box 3-3 Dr. Maria Urso on Keeping Your First Project Simple

Starting graduate school was an exciting prospect. I had been exposed to research at many levels. There were the first movies I watched when I was younger, and I aspired to be like the young heroine who collected samples from animals in the wild to draw grand conclusions about that species. Of course, those conclusions always changed our way of thinking. To be a scientist meant conducting glamorous research, obtaining groundbreaking results, and becoming a household name after making a fantastic discovery. This was why I counted the minutes until graduate school began. I was going to be a scientist—I had work to do!

Fast-forward 15 years. Graduate school worked out and I became a scientist, but I have long since abandoned my hopes for a glamorous existence as a scientist. Sure, whenever someone asks what I do and I reply, "I am a scientist," I can see the wheels turning. They, too, have me in a white lab coat conducting grand science experiments at a bench top over an Erlenmeyer flask filled with a smoking, colored liquid. While this is hardly the case, the profession is one of great rewards as long as you have patience and can appreciate the importance of all the small steps that contribute to the big picture.

Although everyone has the potential to conduct groundbreaking research that changes the way we think about things, treat a disease, or address a problem, it is important to first build a research foundation. Like any magnificent skyscraper, the foundation is the most important part. This is a hard concept for many graduate students to acknowledge, and they try and start with the fine-pointed needle at the top of the skyscraper. Unfortunately, this line of thinking has stalled and even halted many blossoming research careers. *Do not be afraid to keep it simple and design your research questions as a series of small steps, rather than one big step. Your initial research plan does not need to be all-encompassing for it to be successful.*

Writing Your Executive Summary

An **executive summary** is a brief synopsis of your research plan that is written in simple language. An executive summary is usually less than one typed page. When writing your executive summary, your goal should be to describe your study purpose, hypothesis, methods, and anticipated outcomes without losing the interest of your reader in the minutia. These details will be in your proposal and should not be necessary to describe your research. Therefore, your challenge when writing your executive summary is to grab the reader's attention by describing to them what you plan to do, why it is important, how you plan to do it, and why your results will further the existing knowledge in your subject area. If you do this correctly, you will entice the reader to read the rest of your proposal. Most importantly, if you do this well, a reader who was unable to review your proposal beyond the executive summary will have a general understanding of your research project. If your proposal is a grant application, you may want to think of your executive summary as a sales pitch. Another advantage of the executive summary is that it will allow you to identify what the clearest aspects of your research are and which aspects or methods will need more clarification in the proposal. As you do this, you will develop a stronger vision of your research project and you will become better at telling your story. This is critical when seeking research funding, proposing your project to a committee, or when describing your study to potential participants.

Your Title Here: The Effects of (Independent Variable) on (Dependent Variable)

Principal Investigator: Your name here, your degree(s)

Associate Investigators: The names of others helping you with your research, their degree(s)

Executive Summary

Statement of the bigger picture/problem: Lorem ipsum is a major public health concern associated with XX dollars in healthcare costs and XX days in lost productivity.

Statement of what is known in the literature: Previous research has demonstrated that lorem ipsum is associated with dolor sit amet, consectetur, and adipscing elit.

Statement of what is unknown (the gap you will be filling): However, it is unclear what the role of donec veneatis is in the onset of lorem ipsum.

Purpose statement: Therefore, the purpose of this study is to determine if increases in donec veneatis is associated with increases in lorem ipsum.

Statement of the major methods you will be using: The diam a gravid tool will be used to stimulate donec veneatis, and the ultricies method will be used to measure lorem ipsum.

Statement of the benefits/what the reviewers/world will gain from this research: The findings from this study will help us better understand the role of donec veneatis in lorem ipsum. Ultimately, this work will help identify countermeasures for prevention of lorem ipsum.

Objectives

The primary objective of this study is to pellentesque fermentum lacus sed consequat gravida.

The secondary objective is to nam elementum ligula ut quam tempor mattis sed dignissim nec odio eget dictum.

Hypotheses

The primary hypothesis is that as that as donec veneatis increases, lorem ipsum will increase.

The secondary hypothesis is that lorem ipsum will increase when donec elementum metus erat but not when sit amet ultricies quam rhoncus.

FIGURE 3-3:   Template for the initial sections of your research proposal (Latin used as placeholders). The executive summary should be written simply, following the order of statements in this figure. Your objectives should be focused and simply written, and your hypotheses should state exactly what you predict your outcomes will be in relation to the manipulations in your experiment.

Writing Your Purpose Statement

Your purpose statement should be a declarative sentence or two that summarizes the goal of your research. The purpose statement will appear in your executive summary, in the body of your proposal, and in the abstract and introduction of the research paper you submit for publication. A well-written purpose statement will let the reader know what they will gain from supporting the research study or reading your research paper. The most effective purpose statements are specific, precise, clear, and goal-oriented. You should write exactly what you plan to do. Scientific writing is straightforward and does not leave a lot of room for embellishment, and when writing your purpose statement, you must heed this rule of thumb. In fact, the common introductory phrase for a purpose statement is, "The purpose of this research is to . . . " You should not hesitate to write all of your purpose statements this way.

Writing Your Objectives

The objectives of your research are the concrete steps that will ensure that you address the concepts and theories that helped to shape your research question. Collectively, your objectives are the plan that you will follow to accomplish your aims. Although the overall aim of your research is broad in nature, as depicted in the purpose statement, the objectives should be focused and practical. When you write your objectives, they should be a list of practical steps that you will take to meet your aims and overall purpose. You can start simply by numbering each specific objective. This will ensure that each objective stands alone with its own concrete method. This is when it is critical to have a research timeline in mind (or drafted out from your brainstorming session). The timeline will help you list your objectives sequentially with appropriate methods for each. Similar to the purpose, your objectives should be concise and directly relate to your aims. It is common to have several objectives for each aim.

The advantage of writing your objectives in your proposal is that you will immediately identify if you have the appropriate resources available to address your aims. Also, this portion of your proposal will let the reader, whether your advisor or the granting agency, know exactly how you intend to approach a given subject, how you plan to get access to data (*e.g.*, human subjects or animals), and how your resources will fit into your experimental design. Finally, objectives may identify any ethical or logistical problems that you may encounter.

Writing Your Hypotheses

Your research problem cannot be scientifically solved if it is not reduced to hypothesis form. A hypothesis is a concise statement of what you plan to investigate, and it must be testable. The latter part of this statement is the most critical. Although a hypothesis can never be too general or too specific, you must be able to reasonably test for the occurrence, or lack thereof, of the outcomes that you are predicting. First, your prediction is based on what you think will happen. This should be based on your preliminary research, your understanding of the science, and the scientific principles that are relevant to your proposed experiment or study. When you factor these components in, your prediction becomes a well-formulated and educated guess.

When it comes to proposal writing, one of the most important things you will do is write your hypothesis. This is the fundamental aspect of your research, and it needs to be precise and easy to interpret. If you are unable to concisely state what you are setting out to do, what you are testing, and what you think will happen, the people who review your proposal will lose confidence in your ability to conduct and complete a successful research study that answers your research question. That said, it is remarkable how often the hypothesis is the most poorly constructed aspect of a research proposal. Your hypothesis should be written in clear and simple language and define exactly what you think will happen—*before* you begin your experiment.

Writing a well-constructed hypothesis should not be difficult to do, but you must follow some specific rules and resist the temptation to enhance your hypothesis statement to make your writing more appealing. Additionally, it should be reiterated that your hypothesis comes after you have developed your research question. The hypothesis is a prediction statement based on your research question. Thus, your hypothesis should always be a statement and not a question.

A simple exercise to practice constructing hypotheses is to complete the following sentence that should be the skeleton of any good hypothesis: "If I do X, then Y will happen." This is a good strategy to use because it will ensure that you have the fundamentals for a good hypothesis statement before you start to complicate the task by adding technical information. The technical information that comprises the rest of your hypothesis statement is a result of the variables that you will include in your experimental design.

When you developed your research question, you identified the variables of your experimental design. Variables include any factor, condition, or trait that exists in your experimental design in various amounts or types. A well-designed experiment will usually have independent, dependent, and control variables. As the investigator, you will manipulate the **independent variable**. As you change the independent variable, you will observe what happens to the **dependent variable**. The value of the dependent variable will depend on the value of the independent variable, and there will typically be more than one dependent variable. It is always necessary to include a control variable so that you have a constant in your experiment. Observations of the control variable are just as important as the dependent variables.

For example, if you roll a ball down a hill with a certain slope (the independent variable), the speed of the ball (dependent variable) changes in response. Your observation is that the speed of the ball increases. If we repeated this experiment on hills with various slopes (changing the independent variable), the dependent variable will change as a result. There is usually more than one dependent variable, and distance that the ball rolled at the end of the hill could be a second dependent variable in this experiment. As mentioned, it is important to have a control variable. In this example, the control could be the terrain and the position where you released the ball. By keeping the terrain and the position where you released the ball constant, you know that the dependent variables (speed and distance the ball traveled) were a direct result of the slope of the hill and not the smoothness of the terrain or the point on the hill at which the ball was released.

Although the discussion of variables may seem out of place when developing a strategy to construct a good hypothesis, the variables are critical aspects of any good hypothesis statement. In most cases, you must be able to quantify each variable in your experiment by a unit of measure. The exception to this is in qualitative and mixed-methods research. Research of this nature is inductive, and the goal is to understand processes, meanings, cultures, and so on within a particular social context. Therefore, hypotheses for qualitative and mixed-methods research will not necessarily follow the structure we provide here. This type of research is reviewed in depth elsewhere (2).

In the aforementioned experiment, speed and distance are easy variables to measure. If you cannot reasonably quantify a variable with a scientific tool or unit of measure and you are conducting quantitative research, it is a poor variable and should not be included in your experiment or your hypothesis statement. A good hypothesis will define your variables in easy-to-measure terms such as who your research subjects will be, what you are manipulating during the testing, and what you predict the effect(s) of these manipulations will be.

Now that you have an appreciation of the components of a well-written hypothesis, below are some examples of good and bad hypotheses based on a single research scenario. As you read through the examples, try to identify the variables (independent and dependent). The goal of this exercise is to help you appreciate the importance of a testable hypothesis.

Example: You are a coach working at a fitness center for children. One of your responsibilities is to increase the amount of time that children spend being active. You design an experiment to determine if the athletic shoe that a child wears affects the amount of time spent being active. You give the children choices of four different athletic shoes (shoe A, shoe B, shoe C, and shoe D). All shoes are equally comfortable for the children. Shoe A is the same shoe that a popular basketball athlete wears. Shoe B is white and plain. Shoe C is covered in images of superheroes. Shoe D is the same shoe that a popular tennis athlete wears. You offer the children all four shoes and document which shoe they choose to wear and how much time they spend being active.

This study provides several different scenarios for you to formulate different experimental hypotheses:

- *When offered all four types of shoes, the children will choose shoe B.*

  This hypothesis satisfies the two criteria for experimental hypotheses. It is a prediction because it predicts the anticipated outcome of your experiment, and it is *testable*. It is testable because once you have collected and evaluated your data (which shoe the children choose when all four shoes are offered), you know whether or not more children chose shoe B more than the other types of shoes. This hypothesis is incomplete, however, because it does not address your research question related to how much time children will spend being active.

- *When offered all four shoes, the children who pick shoe A will spend the most time being active because they feel more like professional athletes.*

  This hypothesis is partially correct because it is a *predictive* statement and it has a measurable dependent variable (how much time spent active). However, it is not entirely *testable*, at least not based on your criterion measures (you did not ask the children how they felt or what their motivation was for being more active). Your data will show you *whether* the children were more active when they wore a certain shoe, but it will not tell you *why* they were more active. Therefore, it can be concluded that the second half of this hypothesis statement is an assumption rather than a hypothesis.

- *When offered all four shoes, which shoe will the children choose to wear?*

  This is not a hypothesis because it is not *predictive* statement. A question is not a hypothesis.

- *When offered all four types of shoes, children will preferentially choose shoe A, and they will spend the most time being active in this shoe.*

  We have now come full circle. This hypothesis meets all criteria. It is *predictive* and *testable*. It is also specific because it has an independent variable (shoe type) and a dependent variable (time spent being active). You can also repeat this experiment many times over and obtain additional data. A reader evaluating your research proposal will know exactly what you plan to do.

Although your hypothesis statement must be perfected for your research proposal, the hypothesis should be a recurring theme in your research. When you write the methods section of your proposal, you should include the hypotheses and how each part of your experimental methodology helps you address your hypothesis. For instance, in the study example earlier, you may do the following in your proposal:

- *When offered all four types of shoes, children will preferentially choose shoe A, and they will spend the most time being active in this shoe.*

  To test this hypothesis, all children will wear an activity monitor that will track the amount of time spent moving. Data will be analyzed according to shoe type and the overall time spent being active.

One strategy that is helpful when designing research proposals is to sketch your graphs before you collect any data. These graphs are simply a visual representation of your hypothesis. When you have completed your data collection, you will replace these hypothetical data with your actual data. This is an excellent way to identify your independent and dependent variables. Additionally, because you have your results section outlined before you begin your research, this is a reliable way to keep your research on course. Overall, these methods are simple ways to help shape your research proposal and ensure that your methods are appropriate for the research question being asked. When it comes time to write your manuscript, restating the hypothesis throughout the results helps guide the reader through your data analysis and interpretation.

Making Predictions

Now that you have identified your research question, hypothesis, experimental design, and independent and dependent variables, there is a final exercise that will complete your roadmap and prove invaluable when developing your research study, analyzing your data, and preparing your final report. As you noticed in your literature review, most of the research papers have figures that are graphical representations of the data. Independent and dependent variables are plotted on the x- and y-axes, respectively. With the information you have collected to outline your research project, you should be able to sketch a separate graph for each hypothesis that illustrates the independent and dependent variables. You can then use these graphs to plot your anticipated outcomes. As you collect data, you can modify these graphs with your actual data. Not only is this an easy way to monitor how well your dataset aligns with your hypothesis but it may also identify methodologic issues with your measurements. For example, do your data make sense? Do they follow the anticipated pattern? Are the data points that you collect physiologically acceptable? This topic will be reviewed in further detail in Chapters 14–16.

Chapter 14 will also discuss the importance of pilot data. Pilot data is a cursory dataset from a small number of subjects or experiments that demonstrates your ability to collect the data that you have planned in your research study. At this stage of your career, these data will not have the statistical power to support or refute hypotheses, but they will demonstrate to your advisor or a granting agency that you have the tools and skills to address your hypotheses. You may also be fortunate to work in a laboratory that has some preliminary data related to your research question. Although these data are precious in forming research hypotheses and obtaining support for your research study, it should be your responsibility to practice these methods on your own as you develop your research project. This is absolutely critical if you are repeating methods from a research paper in your own laboratory. Sometimes, the most difficult part of a research study is obtaining the necessary data collection tools and confirming that they are valid and reliable in your laboratory. An extensive review of validity and reliability is covered in Chapter 10.

SUMMARY

One of the great privileges of being a young scientist is being able to join an ongoing conversation among some of the finest scientific minds by contributing your own novel perspective. The research findings from your own research project will give you the opportunity to add value to this conversation. In this chapter, we reviewed the steps to seamlessly join this conversation—learning what the previous conversation has been through reading the relevant literature and finding where you can contribute to the conversation by identifying gaps in the literature. These initial steps are critical for identifying a research question that is novel and relevant. Once you have a research question, your next step is to determine how you can address your question by branching ideal research methods with practical considerations to identify a feasible research project. The next step is to propose your project by writing a clear research proposal consisting of your executive summary, purpose statement, objectives, and hypotheses. Although this process may seem overwhelming initially, if you invest the time to follow each step of the process, you will be surprised how prepared you are to describe what you are doing and why you are doing it. In the following chapters, you will learn about subsequent steps in your research process such as learning how to design your study, collect data, interpret your results, and craft a manuscript for publication. All of these next steps, however, hinge on identifying an important research project and being able to clearly propose your research. We hope we provided you with a roadmap and the necessary skills to do so in this chapter.

GLOSSARY

Dependent variable: the response or output variable in an experiment

Executive summary: the first and most important section of a research proposal consisting of a brief overview of the research you will be doing, a description of your main methods, and a statement of the benefits of the research

Gaps in the literature: a phrase referencing a missing piece of information in the existing literature that provides an opportunity for a novel research project

Hypothesis: a concise statement of the predicted results of your study; must be testable

Hypothesis-driven research: research that is designed to test a hypothesis

Independent variable: the predictor or manipulated variable in an experiment

Methods-driven research: research that is designed based on available research equipment or techniques

Research question: a statement that probes an aspect of a study or a broad topic

ACKNOWLEDGMENTS

This material is based on work supported by appointment to the Postgraduate Research Participation Program (JMH) funded by the U.S. Army Research Institute of Environmental Medicine and administered by Oak Ridge Institute for Science and Engineering.

Disclaimer: The opinions or assertions contained herein are the private views of the author(s) and are not to be construed as official or as reflecting the views of the Army or the Department of Defense.

REFERENCES

1. Cannon WB. *The Way of an Investigator: A Scientist's Experiences in Medical Research.* New York (NY): Hafren; 1968.
2. Creswell JW. Research Design: *Qualitative, Quantitative, and Mixed Methods Approaches.* London, United Kingdom: SAGE Publications; 2013.
3. Ritchie J, Lewis J. *Qualitative Research Practice: A Guide for Social Science Students and Researchers.* London, United Kingdom: SAGE Publications; 2003.
4. Watenpaugh DE. John Greenleaf's life of science. *Adv Physiol Educ.* 2012;36:234–245.

CHAPTER 4

Searching the Scientific Literature

Joan M. Eckerson, PhD, FACSM, and Jorge M. Zuniga, PhD

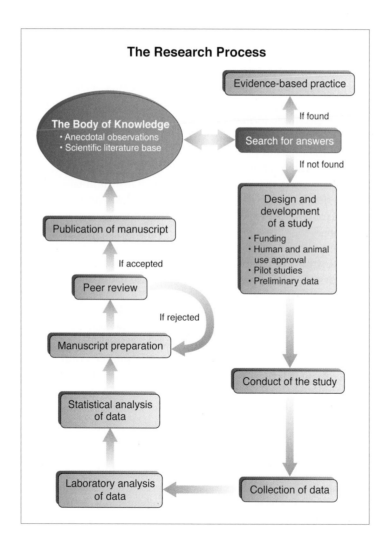

INTRODUCTION

Searching the scientific literature is an essential part of the research process and a critical step in the process of writing a review of literature as part of a class assignment, capstone course, or developing a research question as part of a thesis proposal. The **scientific literature** may be defined as a collection of all of the scholarly writings on a specific topic and can include original research articles, review articles, meta-analyses, books, conference proceedings, and scientific abstracts. This chapter provides a guideline for performing a comprehensive, reproducible, and systematic search of the scientific literature to identify high-quality resources and gives practical advice on how to conduct an efficient search.

SEARCHING SCIENTIFIC DATABASES

Conducting a thorough scientific review of the literature starts with selecting the most appropriate scientific databases and is largely dependent on the topic of interest or research question, which was the focus of Chapter 3. **Scientific databases** are electronic indexes that provide information about a particular source such as subject, author, and title that are linked to a particular set of periodicals giving a full citation for each article and an **abstract** in an electronic format. PubMed and Google Scholar are examples of public databases that are free to anyone who has access to a computer. University libraries provide free access to hundreds of private online bibliographic databases, such as SPORTDiscus and Academic Search Premier, which are both maintained by EBSCO Information Services (www.ebsco.com) and require an annual institutional subscription. In addition to offering scientific databases, many private database providers such as EBSCO have several other product lines and services including e-journals, e-books, dissertation orders, and publishing.

When searching for studies related to human healthcare and interventions for prevention, treatment, and rehabilitation, MEDLINE/PubMed, EMBASE, and the Cochrane Database of Systematic Reviews are commonly used databases. Databases with a narrower focus include SPORTDiscus (exercise science), PsycINFO (psychology and psychiatry), CINAHL (nursing and allied health professions), MANTIS (osteopathy and chiropractic), and AMED (complementary medicine). Although the names of some databases indicate what type of information can be found (*e.g.*, MEDLINE, PsycINFO), others are not as clear (EMBASE, MANTIS). Therefore, you may need to find descriptions of the various databases to determine which ones are most appropriate for your search. Table 4-1 includes a list and description of common electronic databases used in exercise science, the biomedical sciences, and the allied health professions.

University libraries typically maintain a complete list of scientific databases by subject area, which can be accessed via the web both on and off campus, so visit your university homepage to find out which databases for which your library currently has subscriptions. Librarians are very helpful in getting the right key words that can help dramatically with a search and thus are great resources to use to help conduct a scientific search of the literature. Many universities also offer research assistance from reference librarians to help guide students through the scientific review process.

Table 4-1 Common Electronic Bibliographic Databases Used in Exercise Science

Databases	Description
Annual Reviews	Critical reviews of the most significant primary research literature for disciplines within the biomedical and life sciences, physical sciences, and social sciences
Cochrane Library	The Cochrane Library is a collection of six databases including the Cochrane Database of Systematic Reviews, Cochrane Central Register of Controlled Trials, the Cochrane Methodology Reviews, and the Database of Abstract of Reviews and Effects. This is an excellent database for locating randomized controlled trials related to healthcare interventions (www.thecochranelibrary.com).
FedStats	Provides current statistics from over 100 different agencies with links to their websites. The site also provides statistical profiles from all 50 states.
Web of Knowledge/ Web of Science	This database provides researchers, administrators, faculty, and students with quick, powerful access to the world's leading citation databases. Authoritative, multidisciplinary content covers over 10,000 of the highest impact journals worldwide, including open-access journals and over 110,000 conference proceedings. You'll find current and retrospective coverage in the sciences, social sciences, arts, and humanities.
EMBASE	Biomedical and pharmacologic database that provides over 25 million indexed records with citations, abstracts, and indexing derived from articles in peer-reviewed journals, with a primary focus on drug and pharmaceutical research
Academic Search Premier (EBSCO)	A multidisciplinary database designed specifically for academic institutions that includes a large collection of peer-reviewed full-text journals. The database offers information in several areas of academic study including engineering, physics, chemistry, and medical sciences.
SPORTDiscus	This database offers a multidisciplinary aggregation of unique and extensive coverage of key aspects of sport medicine and research. This includes content from therapy to recreation, focusing on all aspects of fitness and health relating to sports medicine and related fields. SPORTDiscus database offers records with journal coverage going back to the 1800s, which includes dissertations, theses, and references to articles in 60 languages. There is a broad selection of material consisting of international references from journal and magazine articles, books, conference proceedings, and more.
ScienceDirect	The Health and Life Sciences Edition of this database contains over 25% of the world's science, technology, and medicine full-text and bibliographic information. More than 2,000 journals from Elsevier are available on ScienceDirect. Most journal articles become available immediately after peer review and before the printed versions are issued. Additionally, they gain online access to multimedia features not available in print journals, such as video, audio, and spreadsheet files.
Cambridge Scientific Abstracts	Provides detailed fact sheets for primary databases in a variety of subject areas, including the natural sciences. The fact sheets include sample records and information relevant to searching a specific database.
R2	R2 is a web-based application that aggregates health sciences book content from leading publishers in a single platform. This service is available exclusively through hospital, academic, and institutional libraries.
Health Source: Nursing/ Academic Edition	This database covers approximately 550 scholarly full-text journals as well as abstracts and indexing for nearly 850 journals. Multiple medical disciplines are covered with strong nursing and allied health. This database also includes Clinical Pharmacology Database as well.

(Continued)

Table 4-1 Common Electronic Bibliographic Databases Used in Exercise Science *(Continued)*	
Databases	**Description**
Health Source: Consumer Edition	This is a consumer-health database that provides information on health-related issues. Health topics include the medical sciences, food sciences and nutrition, childcare, sports medicine, and general health. Available full text for approximately 190 journals as well as abstracts for over 200 general health, nutrition, and professional healthcare publications including 1,190 health-related pamphlets.
CINAHL	This is a cumulative index database with focus in nursing and allied health literature; bibliographic and full text for approximately 800,000 records including nursing, allied health, biomedicine, and healthcare. Full text is included for several state nursing journals and some newsletters, standards of practice, practice acts, government publications, research instruments, and patient education material.
AltHealth Watch	This database provides full text for articles from more than 180 international journals, consumer newsletters, pamphlets, booklets, special reports, and original research.
AMED (Alternative Medicine)	This database is mainly used by physicians, therapists, medical researchers, and clinicians regarding alternative medicine including complementary medicine, physiotherapy, occupational therapy, rehabilitation, podiatry, and palliative care. AMED contains records from over 500 journals and is produced by the Health Care Information Service of the British Library.
Academic OneFile	Academic OneFile has an extensive coverage of the physical sciences, technology, medicine, social sciences, the arts, theology, literature, and other subjects; it is both authoritative and comprehensive. With millions of articles available in both PDF and HTML full-text with no restrictions, researchers are able to find accurate information quickly.
MANTIS	The MANTIS Database (Manual, Alternative, and Natural Therapy Index System) is an index of biomedical journal articles with a primary focus on chiropractic, osteopathic, and alternative medicine.
WorldCat	WorldCat is a large network of library content and services. WorldCat libraries are dedicated to providing access to their resources on the web, where the majority of people start the search for information. It allows the user to search libraries' collections in local communities and many more around the world. Users can search for popular books and videos of about almost any topic. Students and scientists may also find article citations with links to full text and other research materials, such as documents and photos, as well as digital versions of rare items that aren't available to the general public.

Types of Scientific Literature

An early step in searching the scientific literature is to determine if your search should include primary literature, secondary literature, or both. **Primary scientific literature** includes original scientific research such as journal articles that contain methods, results, and discussion sections; conference papers; technical reports; theses; and dissertations. **Secondary scientific literature** includes publications and journal articles that synthesize what is already known about a particular topic and include review articles, meta-analyses, and textbooks. Secondary scientific literature sometimes serves as a good place to start because it typically provides a broader context and usually contains references to key primary literature. Table 4-2 includes a list of prominent journals used in exercise science that may contain both primary and secondary types of research articles.

The main sources for searching both primary and secondary scientific literatures include online public bibliographic databases, private bibliographic databases, manual searches of cited references in articles, and expert guidance. Although the internet can also serve as a valuable source of information, it is sometimes difficult to distinguish between credible and questionable information; therefore, recommendations are provided later in this chapter to help identify quality research sources on the internet. It is also important to remember that a thorough search of the scientific literature is best achieved by incorporating more than one method (both manual and electronic) and may possibly be overlapping (2). The following section focuses on the most widely used public and private databases for finding both primary and secondary research and provides some tips for narrowing a search.

Table 4-2 Quality Journals Related to Exercise Science	
Medicine/Sports Medicine	*Medicine and Science in Sports and Exercise*
	Exercise and Sports Sciences Reviews
	Journal of Strength and Conditioning Research
	Research Quarterly for Exercise and Sport
	International Journal of Sports Medicine
	Journal of Sports Medicine and Physical Fitness
	American Journal of Sports Medicine
	British Journal of Sports Medicine
	Journal of Science and Medicine in Sport
	Sports Medicine
	Clinical Journal of Sports Medicine
	Journal of the American Medical Association
	New England Journal of Medicine
Physiology	*Journal of Applied Physiology*
	European Journal of Applied Physiology
	Annual Review of Physiology
	Journal of Physiology
	Physiological Reviews
Nutrition	*Amino Acids*
	International Journal of Sport Nutrition and Exercise Metabolism
	Journal of the International Society of Sports Nutrition
	Journal of the Academy of Nutrition and Dietetics (formerly *Journal of the American Dietetic Association*)
	American Journal of Clinical Nutrition
	Nutrition Reviews
	Annual Review of Nutrition
	Nutrition Research
	Nutrition Journal
	Journal of Nutrition
Biomechanics/Motor Learning	*Perceptual and Motor Skills*
	International Journal of Sports Biomechanics
	Journal of Biomechanics
	Journal of Motor Behavior

Online Public Bibliographic Databases

MEDLINE/PubMed. The U.S National Library of Medicine (NLM) and the National Institutes of Health (NIH) maintains the bibliographic database MEDLINE, which contains journal citations and abstracts from over 5,400 biomedical journals and is one of the most popular database systems used by clinicians and researchers in the fields of medicine, pre-clinical sciences, nursing, dentistry, veterinary medicine, and healthcare systems (4). MEDLINE was created in the 1960s and currently provides over 20 million references to biomedical and life science journals dating back to 1946. Like MEDLINE, PubMed is a free resource developed and maintained by the National Center for Biotechnology Information (NCBI) at the NLM, which provides access to the MEDLINE database and links to full-text articles found at publisher websites and to PubMed Central (PMC), which is a free archive for full-text biomedical and life sciences journals. A distinct feature of MEDLINE and PubMed compared to other electronic databases is that the records are indexed with Medical Subject Headings (MeSH) as opposed to subject headings (SU) or descriptors. This is discussed in more detail later in the chapter.

Google Scholar. Google is a widely used search engine, accounting for about 67% of all internet searches worldwide (6). Google Scholar is a subset of the Google search engine for a wide range of academic fields and is simple, fast, and provides broad coverage. It searches for scholarly publications including articles in peer-reviewed journals, theses, dissertations, books, and abstracts from academic publishers, professional organizations, and universities. Within one year of its introduction as a beta version in 2004, Google Scholar surpassed PubMed in the number of referrals to many online biomedical journals (1). A password or subscription may be required to access full-text articles if the search is being performed using the internet from home or another private location that does not have a subscription to the scientific journal of interest. Google Scholar has come under some criticism for the limited advanced search features, an unclear definition of its database content, insufficient indexing, and a concealed search algorithm. It also appears to have only indirect, partial access to MEDLINE; therefore, it may lack the most recent MEDLINE publications.

There is an ongoing debate between clinicians and researchers about the clinical relevance of using Google Scholar (4). However, despite its limitations, Google Scholar may offer unique options in the scientific community by providing free full-text articles from various websites. In some cases, the ability of Google Scholar for retrieving information is superior to PubMed. For example, a search of PubMed using the search terms "bee pollen and supplementation" produced 26 results. In contrast, the same search terms using Google Scholar produced approximately 18,000 results, although not all were relevant or highly vetted. The point here, however, is that a search using Google Scholar for some information may be more rapid and efficient than a PubMed query. Because PubMed and Google Scholar are the most frequently used public bibliographic databases, an example of how to get started using both is presented in this chapter.

Searching PubMed. You can find a full tutorial with detailed information about how to conduct a PubMed search at the NLM website. To access the PubMed homepage, go to http://www.ncbi.nlm.nih.gov/pubmed and select PubMed from the list of other databases maintained by the NCBI (Fig. 4-1).

Like all other electronic databases, PubMed has a search box to enter key words (*i.e.*, MeSH) with an advanced search option (Fig. 4-2).

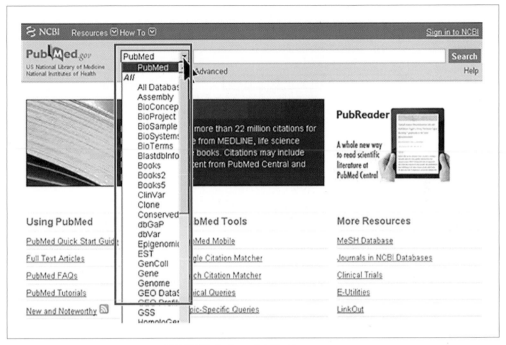

FIGURE 4-1: PubMed homepage.

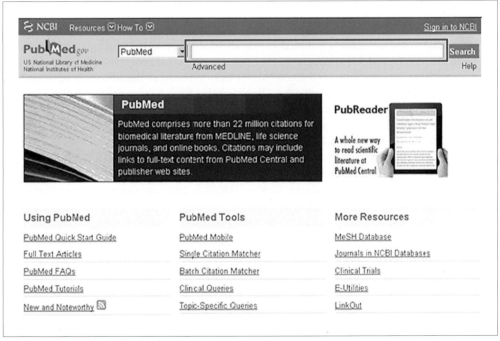

FIGURE 4-2: Search box for entering key words.

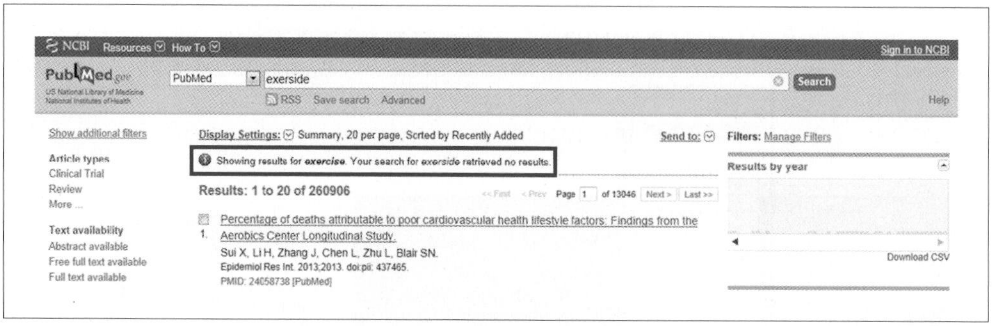

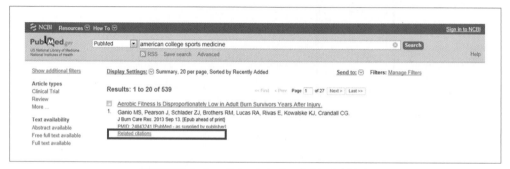

FIGURE 4-3:   Search term spellcheck in PubMed.

FIGURE 4-4:   Related citations link in PubMed.

MeSH is the controlled vocabulary thesaurus for the NLM; therefore, familiarity with MeSH may make a PubMed search a smoother process. For a more comprehensive explanation of MeSH vocabulary, an 11-minute video that provides an introduction to the development, structure, and use of MeSH can be found at the following website: http://www.nlm.nih.gov/bsd/disted/video/. PubMed also has a feature called "spellcheck," which suggests alternative spellings for search terms that include misspellings. If the term is misspelled, the closest common word will display and, in some cases, a link to an alternative spelling is provided (Fig. 4-3).

Another important feature of PubMed is the "Related Citations" link, which compares words from the title, abstract, and the assigned MeSH to other articles related to your search (Fig. 4-4). Many other databases, such as Web of Science and Google Scholar, also include this feature.

PubMed also provides a number of filters to narrow search results. You can easily deselect these filters if you decide not to use a specific filter (Fig. 4-5).

Searching Google Scholar. Google Scholar can be accessed at http://scholar.google.com/. Google Scholar accepts up to 32 search terms; therefore, choose as many as possible because choosing too few may give poor results. Another useful strategy is to select nouns to avoid stop words (*i.e.*, "a," "about," "the," "for," "has," etc.). If you want to customize your search, explore the search settings to set your Google Scholar preferences (Fig. 4-6).

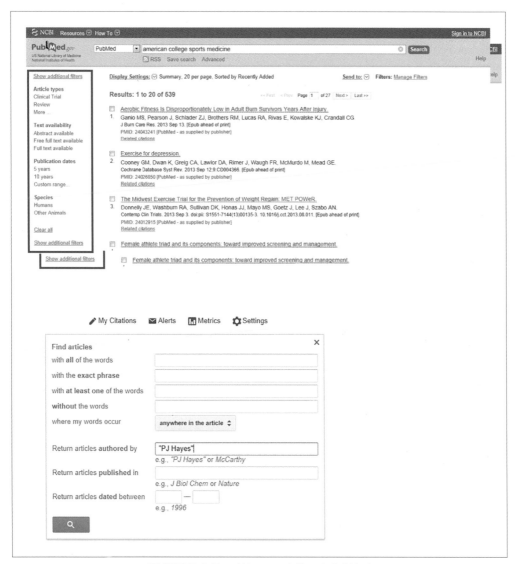

FIGURE 4-5: Using search filters in PubMed.

You can also change your results settings, preferred language, and library links (Fig. 4-7).

The library link setting allows you to connect to your institution's library so you can access full-text articles. Make sure you click the save button to save all your settings. Your next step will be the search itself (Fig. 4-8).

If you want to make your search more precise, Google Scholar allows for the use of multiple operators, which are shown in Table 4-3. If you don't prefer using these operators, use the advanced scholar search (Fig. 4-9).

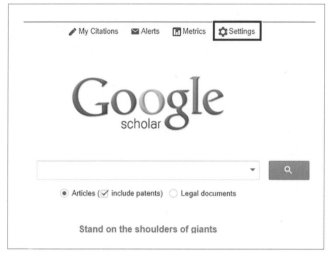

FIGURE 4-6:   Exploring search settings in Google Scholar.

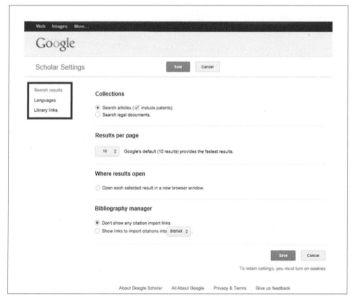

FIGURE 4-7:   Results settings in Google Scholar.

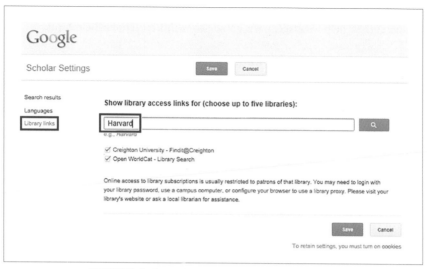

FIGURE 4-8: Library link setting in Google Scholar.

Table 4-3 Common Operators to Search Google Scholar

Operator	Description	Example
""	Exact phrase search	"endurance exercise"
+	Add words in the results	"endurance exercise" + strength
−	Exclude words in the results	"endurance exercise" − altitude
Site:	Restrict search to a particular website	Sports medicine site:edu

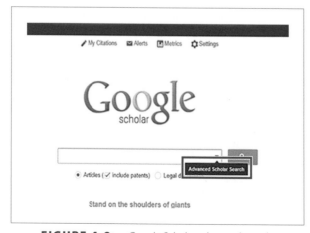

FIGURE 4-9: Google Scholar advanced search.

More detailed information about conducting searches using Google Scholar can be found at their help webpage: www.google.com/intl/en/scholar/help.html.

Online Private Bibliographic Databases

Private bibliographic databases are maintained by private entities such as EBSCO and are available only by subscription. Most universities hold subscriptions to a wide variety of private bibliographic databases that are only available to enrolled students. A few of the commonly used private bibliographic databases in exercise science include SPORTDiscus, EMBASE, Web of Science, Annual Reviews, ScienceDirect, and Academic Search Premier. The Cochrane Library is another excellent resource that consists of a collection of databases in the health sciences including the Cochrane Database of Systematic Reviews, which includes review articles and meta-analyses, and the Cochrane Central Register of Controlled Trials. The Cochrane Library listed in Table 4-1 is a primary resource in evidence-based medicine to make informed decisions regarding healthcare (3).

Before discussing other resources for conducting a scientific search, the following section provides information about selecting key words to use in the search and tips for narrowing your search results when using both public and private bibliographic databases.

Identifying Key Words

Identifying key words is the foundation for conducting an effective search of the scientific literature. **Key words** are also referred to as "descriptors," "identifiers," and "search terms" and represent the major concepts included in the search because they are what will pull up the most relevant articles related to your topic (8). Although searching the scientific literature usually occurs after a specific research question or topic of interest has been developed, selecting a research topic itself can be difficult; therefore, starting with a broad, comprehensive search of the literature may help students identify a specific topic of interest and identify key words or help determine whether or not there is enough published research to complete the assigned project. For example, selecting the key words "creatine" and "supplementation" using a database such as SPORTDiscus results in over 900 citations, which is too broad and an unmanageable number of resources to sort through, but this initial search may be used to identify other key words to help limit subsequent searches and narrow down the research question. On the other hand, a search of the key words "bee pollen" and "supplementation" using the same database results in the message, "No results were found," which suggests that there may be a limited number of resources, and therefore, this may not be a practical topic (Fig. 4-10).

When first beginning a comprehensive search, using a database's thesaurus can be valuable for identifying subject terms and key words, particularly if the search does not yield many results. A **thesaurus** includes different terms that are related to each other that describe the same concept and results in a list of subject terms that can be used in the search. You can then select one of those subject terms, and the database will perform a search on that term. In addition, most thesauruses also include an "Explode" option to search many related terms at the same time. In the example in Figure 4-11, using the thesaurus in the database SPORTDiscus, the search term "creatine" displays other related terms that could also be used in a search.

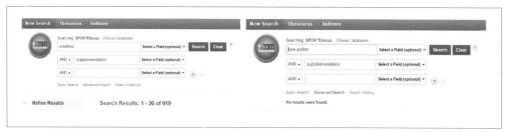

FIGURE 4-10: An example of an unsuccessful search strategy in SPORTDiscus.

Once you have identified a few key words, you can also begin narrowing your search by using delimiters such as publication type (*e.g.*, journal article, monograph or government document, book review), language (*e.g.*, English, Spanish), range of publication dates, etc. Searches can also be limited by using specific authors, titles of articles or words from a title, and by publication name. In the example in Figure 4-12 using the database Academic Search Premier, entering the search terms "creatine AND supplementation" without using any delimiters produced 646 results. The second search, which narrowed the range of publication date and used only those articles with references, produced 72 results, which is a much more manageable number of resources to review. Selecting the "Advanced Search" option versus "Basic Search" also provides a larger number of options to delimit the search.

The results for the search terms "creatine" and "supplementation" using the two different databases described earlier (SPORTDiscus and Academic Search Premier) also demonstrates the importance of using more than one database to conduct a scientific search of the literature. SPORTDiscus yielded over 300 more results than did Academic Search Premier

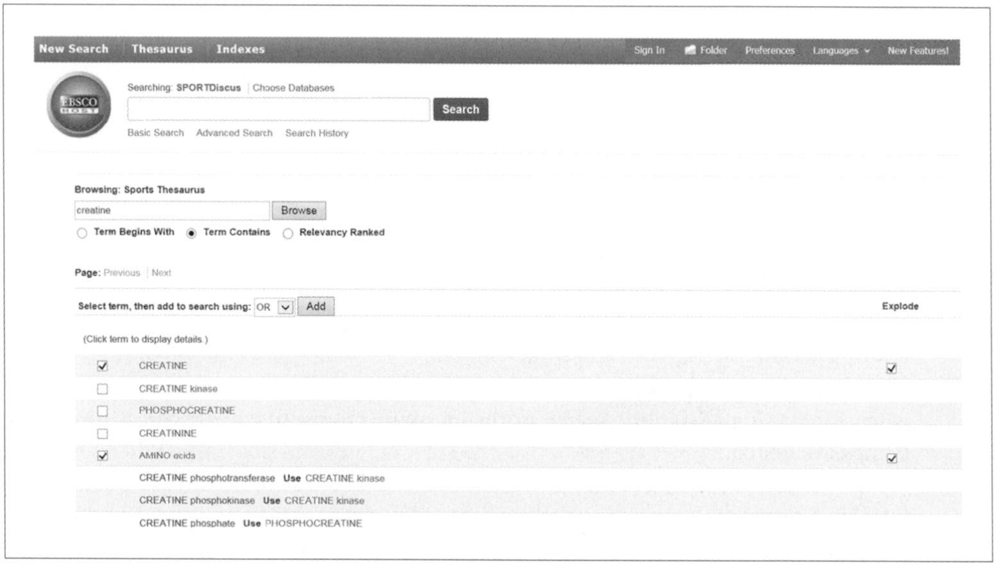

FIGURE 4-11: Using the thesaurus and explode option in SPORTDiscus.

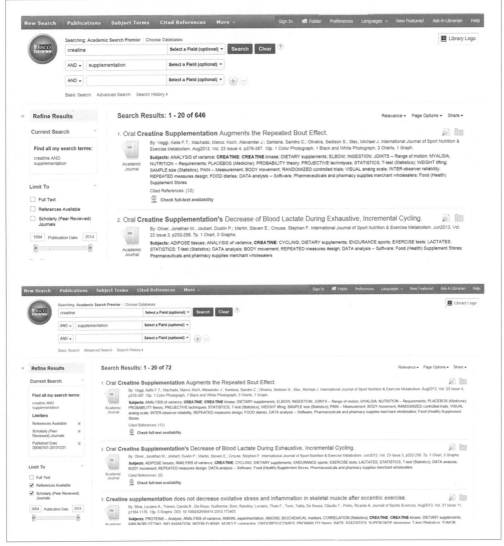

FIGURE 4-12:   Using delimiters to narrow a search.

when using identical subject terms. Therefore, it is important to use overlapping databases when conducting a scientific search of the literature to ensure you are conducting a comprehensive search.

In Academic Search Premier and many other databases, the default for searching is set to subject terms (SU), which is the same as a descriptor; however, using the drop-down menu allows you to search by author (AU), title (TI), and source (SO), just to name a few. Most other databases, including SPORTDiscus, have a similar feature (Fig. 4-13).

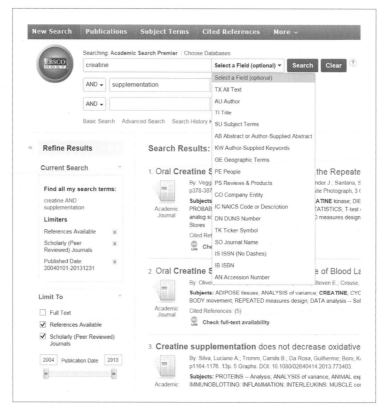

FIGURE 4-13:   Searching by fields.

Searching with the **Boolean operators** "AND," "OR," and "NOT" are also useful for limiting or expanding a search. For example, "creatine" AND "supplementation" retrieves a set of citations that includes both search terms and can occur in any order, whereas "creatine" OR "phosphocreatine" retrieves a set of citations that includes one of the search terms and usually results in a much larger yield of resources. To exclude terms, the Boolean operator "NOT" is used (*i.e.*, "creatine" NOT "women" excludes the key word, "women," from the search).

Using wildcard and truncation symbols creates searches where there are unknown characters, multiple spellings (*i.e.*, pediatric vs. paediatric), or different endings. Neither the wildcard and truncation symbol can be used at the start of a word. The wildcard is usually represented by the pound sign (#) or a question mark (?). To use the "?" wildcard, replace each unknown character with a "?," and the database finds all citations of that word with the "?" replaced by a letter. For example, "Ta?k" finds all citations containing words such as talk, task, tack, and tank. Adding the "#" wildcard in places where an alternate spelling may contain an extra character results in all citations of the word that appear with or without the extra character. Typing "orthop#edic" finds all citations containing orthopedic or orthopaedic. Truncation involves searching the root of a word by replacing the end of the word with a symbol, such as an asterisk (*) to find all forms of that word. For example, "nutr*" results in records

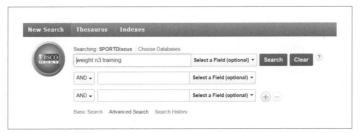

FIGURE 4-14:   Example of a proximity search in SPORTDiscus.

containing words such as nutrition, nutritious, nutrient, nutritional, etc. Different databases use different symbols, so use the "Help" menu to find the appropriate symbol for both truncation and wildcards as well as for other tips to help you search.

Proximity searches are also useful for searching for two or more words that appear within a specified number of words of each other, and these can be used with either a keyword or Boolean search. The most common proximity operators are the letters "N" (near) and "W" (within) and are placed between the words included in the search. For example, using the near operator with the key words "weight" and "training" (weight N3 training) finds the two words if they are within three words of each other, no matter what the order, and it would find results such as weight training, training using body weight, train with body weight, weight-bearing training, etc. (Fig. 4-14). However, using the within operator in the same example (weight W3 training) will find words if they are within three words of each other and in the order in which they were entered.

In addition, multiple key words can be used on either side of the near or within operators and may also include Boolean operators within parentheses (*i.e.*, weight W2 [lifting OR training]).

Because each database is different, it is recommended to use the "Help" button (or similar buttons, such as "Ask-a-Librarian") to learn how to navigate the database and conduct a more efficient search. Many databases also include "Frequently Asked Questions" sections, which can provide useful tips.

Other Resources for Finding Relevant Research

Browsing Reference Lists of Relevant Studies. Once key primary and secondary literature studies relevant to the research topic have been identified, a good place to find other related studies is in the reference list of the article. In some cases, the citation in the reference list may be linked to the corresponding journal or periodical.

Searching Trial Registers. A trial registry is an official catalog for registering a clinical trial and is useful for finding unpublished or ongoing trials. Clinical trials are usually registered by a funding sponsor, pharmaceutical or biotechnology company, hospital, foundation, or contract research organization. Many clinical trial registries are easily accessed on the internet and are searchable by drug name, condition, or location. Two major registries available on the internet include www.clinicaltrials.gov and www.who.int/trialsearch.

Topic Experts and Manufacturers. Research laboratories and experts in a particular discipline, as well as manufacturers, can serve as excellent resources of research and may be able to provide information about unpublished work or work in progress that would not be included on an electronic database. This method of searching is not recommended as a primary search strategy; however, topic experts can check lists of citations to determine if key resources are missing (2).

Professional Organizations. Information posted by professional organizations, such as the American College of Sports Medicine (ACSM; www.acsm.org) may also serve as a valuable source for research-related materials. Many organizations including the ACSM and the Academy of Nutrition and Dietetics (formerly known as the "American Dietetic Association") provide links to position papers published in their official journals as well as other educational materials. For example, the ACSM has position papers on exercise and hypertension and exercise and physical activity for older adults (see Chapter 2), which can be accessed on their website with links to the published article appearing in *Medicine and Science in Sports and Exercise.*

Citation Searching. Once several key journal articles have been found, searching for other papers that have cited those works can result in a number of other highly related articles. This technique is referred to as "citation searching" and is becoming more and more commonly included with search indexes such as Web of Science, PubMed, Google Scholar, CINAHL, and PsycINFO (2).

Unpublished Literature. Unpublished literature may include grant reports from funding organizations, government documents, and dissertations and master's theses. ProQuest Dissertations and Theses (PQDT) database is the most comprehensive collection of dissertations and theses, and it serves as the official digital dissertation archive for the Library of Congress. Because it is estimated that 95%–98% of doctoral dissertations in the United States are included in the PQDT database, it is considered the database of record for graduate research. The bibliographic database without full-text dissertations is known as "Dissertations Abstracts International," and citations include title, author name, degree granting university, and potentially the names of the dissertation advisor and committee members. Titles published since 1980 also include a 350-word abstract.

Using Internet Search Engines for Searching the Literature: A Warning. Internet search engines such as Google, Yahoo!, Bing, and Ask.com can be powerful tools for finding websites for a wide variety of information, including scientific research, but much of the information is not well substantiated and has little quality control (9). For example, Wikipedia is one of the top 10 most visited websites worldwide and is often used as a source of information; however, it may be filled with inaccuracies because anyone can make edits to the site. In addition, with the availability of free web server software, anyone with a computer can develop a website and publish any data they wish. Therefore, assessing the credibility of a publisher and the accuracy of resources retrieved from the internet can be problematic.

To help online users identify reliable and trustworthy information, the Health on the Net (HON) Foundation (www.healthonnet.org), a non-profit organization based in Geneva, Switzerland, developed the HON Code of Conduct (HONcode) in 1996 for medical- and health-related websites. The HON site also includes a search engine for health and medical information from HON accredited sites. To become accredited, a website must meet the eight ethical principles of the HONcode and requires publishers to provide the following information: (a) the authoritative body from which the information was derived;

(b) the purpose of the site; (c) the confidentiality policy; (d) the origin of the sources; (e) justification regarding benefits and performance of a specific treatment; (f) transparency of authorship; (g) the credibility of the health/medical-related data; and (h) transparency regarding sponsorship of the site and honesty in advertising. Currently, the HONcode has accredited approximately 5,000 sites representing 72 countries and includes MEDLINE and PubMed. When searching the HON site, a free "plug-in" service can be downloaded that will automatically indicate if a visited webpage has been accredited by HON (5).

Intute (www.intute.ac.uk) is another free online service that helps find the most credible websites for research in a variety of disciplines including the biologic sciences, nursing, and allied health. Intute also provides free internet tutorials as part of a Virtual Training Suite for education and research that have been developed by qualified professionals and librarians. A list of credible websites related to exercise science can be found in Table 4-4.

Mobile Apps for Searching the Scientific Literature. Mobile apps for accessing library resources are available if the mobile user is associated with the institution. Some apps are useful for searching, whereas others also allow access to abstracts and full text. For example, PubMed mobile allows for searching and abstract retrieval, whereas the American Chemical Society (ACS) mobile app provides full access to full-text articles (7). Although it is not recommended that handheld devices with mobile apps be used for conducting comprehensive searches, they may be convenient for looking up articles quickly while in a class or study group. Databases that are subscribed to by university libraries including ProQuest, EBSCO, and Elsevier will require authentication so that the user can be associated with the university. Check your university library's homepage or ask a reference librarian to determine which mobile apps may be available to you. The following includes a short list and description of apps to access scientific literature on your mobile device (7).

- PubMed mobile: free index to biomedical research with links to PMC for free full texts and links to publisher's websites
- Google Scholar app: free application that searches a wide variety of topics and allows access to full-text articles when available. If your institution has configured their Google

Table 4-4 Quality Websites Related to Exercise Science

Academy of Nutrition and Dietetics	www.eatright.org
American College of Sports Medicine	www.acsm.org
American Diabetes Association	www.diabetes.org
American Heart Association	www.amhrt.org
American Medical Association	www.ama-assn.org
American Physiological Society	www.the-aps.org
American Society of Biomechanics	www.asb-biomech.org
Centers for Disease Control and Prevention	www.cdc.gov
International Society of Sports Nutrition	www.sportsnutritionsociety.org
National Strength and Conditioning Association	www.nsca.com

Scholar library links and you are working on campus, the search results should link to the university library.

- EBSCOhost mobile: allows access to full-text articles and abstracts from library databases that use the EBSCO platform
- ACS mobile: an indexed list of more than 35,000 research articles published annually across 40 peer-reviewed ACS journals, complete with graphical and text abstracts

EVALUATING THE QUALITY OF ARTICLES AND OTHER RESOURCES

When evaluating both primary (*i.e.*, original journal articles) and secondary resources (*i.e.*, review articles and meta-analyses from journals) retrieved from a scientific search of the literature, it is important to assess their quality. Journal articles that are **peer reviewed** are considered high-quality resources because the review process by other experts in the field helps ensure that the information is accurate and up-to-date. Articles that are not peer reviewed may also be valuable, but it is important to consider the source of the document. For example, an article appearing in a magazine, such as *Men's Health*, *Sports Illustrated*, or another lay press publication would not be considered a high-quality resource, whereas an invited review appearing in a journal is considered high quality even though it may not have gone through rigorous peer review. Magazines have a different scope than do research publications.

When evaluating quality, it is also important to consider the research design of a study. Most studies are classified as either experimental or descriptive, as discussed in Chapter 1. **Experimental studies** are original research studies in which subjects (humans or animals) are placed into groups, an intervention (*i.e.*, treatment, procedure, or educational program) is applied for a period of time, and a result or outcome is then observed between the groups. Experimental studies that randomly assign participants to a group are considered the most robust and are referred to as "randomized controlled trials." The Cochrane Central Register of Controlled Trials, which is part of the Cochrane Library (see Table 4-1), is an excellent database to search if the primary studies of interest are randomized controlled trials.

Descriptive studies are sometimes referred to as "observational or correlational studies" and are those which collect data without manipulating the environment (*i.e.*, there is no intervention of any kind). A descriptive study can involve a one-time interaction with a group of subjects (*i.e.*, cross-sectional studies) or may track individuals over a long period of time (longitudinal studies), as in the case of a large epidemiologic study that tracks the health status of individuals over several years and then correlates death rates or disease states with risk factors such as hypertension, obesity, and smoking.

A **meta-analysis** is a type of systematic review that uses statistical methods to combine the results of several individual studies to help identify patterns among study results and assess whether treatment effects are consistent. For example, a meta-analysis to determine the effect of caffeine on anaerobic exercise performance may include several independent randomized controlled trials whose results are statistically combined to help gain a better understanding of whether or not it is effective and in what range of doses.

Searching public and private bibliographic databases, such as PubMed and SPORTDiscus, as well as those listed in Table 4-1, will typically provide high-quality resources. As previously mentioned, the internet can serve as a powerful tool when searching for scientific literature, but more scrutiny is necessary to ensure that the information is credible and valid. In addition to using the HONcode or Intute, other questions to ask yourself include who or what organization is sponsoring the site; when was the site last updated; and is the information in the site supported by peer-reviewed publications in respected journals, such as those listed in Table 4-3.

OBTAINING JOURNAL ARTICLES AND MANAGING RESOURCES

Once you find high-quality articles and abstracts related to your topic, you can save them to a folder on your personal computer and/or print a hard copy if the citation index has a link to full text in Portable Document Format (.pdf). Printing using PDF is recommended over HyperText Markup Language (HTML), which is the language used to create web pages, because the PDF file will look exactly like the article as it appears in the journal and is considerably shorter in length. If the article does not have a full-text link, you will need to determine if your library has either an electronic subscription to the journal or a hard copy of the periodical on the shelves. If they do not, you may need to access the material through inter-library loan, which may involve a small fee.

Most private and public bibliographic databases also include management software that allows you to register your own personal account where you can save and retrieve search histories, save references, organize your research into folders, create e-mail alerts and/or RSS feeds, and allows you to gain access to your saved research remotely. Figure 4-15

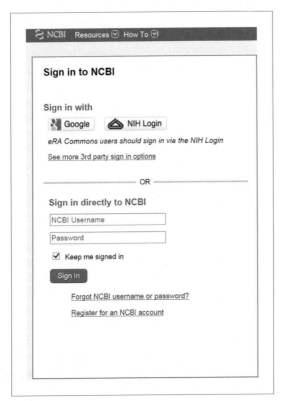

FIGURE 4-15:　Sign-in box to NCBI.

shows the sign-in box to My NCBI, which retains user information for most NCBI databases including PubMed.

Using other bibliographic research management tools such as EndNote, RefWorks, or ProCite also allows you to record and manage references to help document the process and will automatically generate the reference list for assignments and reports. Many university libraries subscribe to one of the previously mentioned research management tools and are therefore free for students.

CONCLUSION

In summary, an effective search of the scientific literature is dependent on a clear research topic and the identification of several key words to determine which electronic bibliographic databases and other resources will be most relevant to the search. It is a time-consuming process, but a systematic approach that is also reproducible will result in high-quality scientific information to write a comprehensive review of the literature for an assignment or for developing a research question as part of a thesis. In addition, using the skills and resources described in this chapter are recommended over "surfing the net" for staying informed and answering everyday questions about topics in sports medicine.

GLOSSARY

Abstract: a brief description of a research article used to help the reader determine the purpose of the paper and the major findings

Boolean operators: words such as AND, OR, and NOT used to combine or exclude key words that help produce a more focused search

Descriptive studies: also referred to as observational or correlational studies; these types of studies report naturally occurring information about a particular group such as health status, behaviors, and attitudes

Experimental studies: studies that manipulate the environment to determine if an intervention had a causal effect on a group of subjects

Key words: also referred to as descriptors, identifiers, and search terms; words used in a search engine or database that serve as reference points for retrieving relevant information

Meta-analysis: a type of systematic review that uses statistical methods to analyze the results of several similar studies to integrate the findings and determine if treatment effects are consistent

Peer review: process in which experts in a discipline review a scholarly work to make sure that it meets standards for publication

Primary scientific literature: includes original, peer-reviewed research articles that include methods, results, and discussion sections; conference papers; technical reports; theses; and dissertations

Scientific database: electronic indexes that provide information about a particular source such as a subject, author, and title that are linked to journals, giving a full citation for each article and abstract in an electronic format

Scientific literature: collection of scholarly writings on a specific topic that can include original research articles, review articles, meta-analyses, books, conference proceedings, and abstracts

Secondary scientific literature: publications that synthesize the primary scientific literature and include review articles, meta-analyses, and textbooks

Thesaurus: a dictionary of terms related to each other that describe the same concept

REFERENCES

1. Anders ME, Evans DP. Comparison of PubMed and Google Scholar literature searches. *Respir Care*. 2010;55(5):578–583.
2. Centre for Reviews and Dissemination. *Systematic Reviews: CRD's Guidance for Undertaking Reviews in Healthcare*. York, England: University of York NHS Centre for Reviews & Dissemination; 2009. Available from: http://www.york.ac.uk/inst/crd/
3. Cochrane Librarry Web site [Internet]. London, United Kingdom: Cochrane; [cited 2015 May 24]. Available from: http://www.cochranelibrary.com/
4. Falagas ME, Pitsouni EI, Malietzis GA, Pappas G. Comparison of PubMed, Scopus, Web of Science, and Google Scholar: strengths and weaknesses. *FASEB J*. 2008;22(2):338–342.
5. Health on the Net Foundation Web site [Internet]. Geneva, Switzerland: Health on the Net Foundation; [cited 2013 Jun 10]. Available from: http://www.hon.ch
6. Jain V, Raut DK. Medical literature search dot com. *Indian J Dermatol Venerol Leprol*. 2011;77(2):135–140.
7. Swoger B. Mobile apps for searching the scientific literature. [cited 2013 Mar 26]. Available from: http://www.blogs.scientificamerican.com/information-culture/2013/03/26/mobile-apps-for-searching-the-scientific-literature/
8. Timmins F, McCabe C. How to conduct an effective literature search. *Nurs Stand*. 2005;20(11):41–47.
9. Wang L, Wang J, Wang M, et al. Using Internet search engines to obtain medical information: a comparative study. *J Med Internet Res*. 2012;14(3):e74.

CHAPTER 5

Fundamentals of Study Design

Brent A. Alvar, PhD, FACSM, Mark D. Peterson, PhD, MS, and Daniel J. Dodd, PhD, CSCS*D

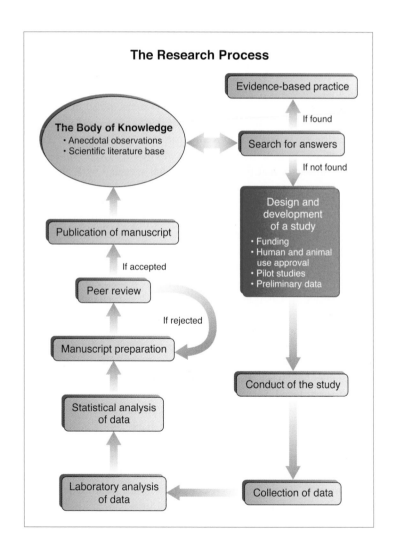

The Research Process

- Evidence-based practice
- If found
- The Body of Knowledge
  - Anecdotal observations
  - Scientific literature base
- Search for answers
- If not found
- Design and development of a study
  - Funding
  - Human and animal use approval
  - Pilot studies
  - Preliminary data
- Publication of manuscript
- If accepted
- Peer review
- If rejected
- Manuscript preparation
- Statistical analysis of data
- Conduct of the study
- Laboratory analysis of data
- Collection of data

INTRODUCTION

As health and exercise science professionals, we build our daily repertoire around an evidence-based practice. We do our best to answer questions that arise about various topics, such as: How much physical activity is necessary for health-related benefits? What is the optimal "dose" of resistance training in terms of frequency, intensity, and volume for a particular outcome (strength, hypertrophy, or power)? What type of flexibility training should be done prior to participating in a sporting activity? What is the best training modality for use with a group of structural firefighters? Are various supplements capable of increasing performance without negatively affecting health? Health and exercise science professionals ask these questions, all with the thought of finding the best possible outcomes for our health, physical activity, and exercise.

THE SCIENTIFIC METHOD APPROACH

As a review of the previous chapters, by using the scientific method (discussed in Chapter 1), you can proceed through the steps necessary to weigh the evidence to answer questions by developing a design necessary for an appropriate research process. As you learned in the first three chapters, you start by asking yourself what question or problem you wish to investigate. Never be afraid to ask the difficult question or even to question what might be considered as the norm. Such questioning can lead to a lifetime of purposeful and meaningful investigation. In fact, most of the aforementioned questions in the introduction are examples of quandaries that the author team has wrestled with and/or eventually carried out investigative studies to help resolve.

Once you've found your area of interest, you must frame your problem, narrowing the concept in a way that makes it a bit more manageable, as discussed in Chapter 3. One of the most common mistakes in research is trying to tackle too large of a problem at any given time. You need to make sure that you are framing the problem with the appropriate lens. The best approach to framing the problem is to narrow the focus and try to develop a clearer picture on a specific variable or grouping of variables.

As you learned in Chapter 3, after you have had a chance to ponder and frame the problem, you will construct your researchable hypothesis. In other words, you will now construct a plausible question that has the potential to clarify or solve a problem. The easiest way to consider your hypothesis is to begin to look at the variables that are involved in the problem. In other words, the explanatory values will affect the problem, and the response variables will measure and observe the effects. We will have a much more in-depth discussion of variables a bit later in this chapter.

Once you think you have a researchable hypothesis, it is time to conduct your literature search, which you learned how to do in Chapter 4. If a thorough literature review and synthesis does not lend itself to a clear and concise answer to the question, or the literature has too many gaps, then there may be a need to conduct original research. It is important to remember that one study cannot fill all of the gaps in the literature and thus you can be prone to doing too much in a study rather than focus on one or two primary hypotheses to be tested. Problems arise when our personal knowledge is lacking, and a search of the literature turns up no reasonable answer to the question that is being posed.

Table 5-1 National Heart, Lung, and Blood Institute Evidence Categories (7)

Category	Source of Evidence	Definition
A	Randomized controlled trials (RCTs; rich body of data)	Evidence is from well-designed RCTs that provide a consistent pattern of findings in the population for which the recommendation is made; requires substantial number of studies involving substantial number of participants
B	RCTs (limited body of data)	Evidence is from intervention studies that include only a limited number of RCTs, post-hoc or subgroup analysis of RCTs, or meta-analysis of RCTs; pertains when few randomized trials exist, they are small in size, and the results are somewhat inconsistent or were from a non-specific population
C	Non-randomized trials, observational studies	Evidence is from outcomes of uncontrolled trials or observations
D	Panel consensus judgment	Expert judgment is based on panel's synthesis of evidence from experimental research or the consensus of panel members based on clinical experience or knowledge that does not meet the earlier listed criteria.

Worse, there may be conflicting information in the literature. As such, a need for clarification or answers to a professional question often perpetuates our desire to conduct research to clarify why there is a conflict.

In Chapter 2, you learned how evidence-based practice is important, making it necessary to gauge and use the research literature to guide our professional practice. This can also help guide you in terms of accepting where a question is in terms of research as well as how you might want to proceed in the development of your research study. Use of the online search engines (PubMed, SPORTDiscus, Google Scholar, etc.) along with the National Heart, Lung, and Blood Institute (7) (Table 5-1) evidence categories are ways to evaluate the current literature on a particular topic or problem, and these can act as guides in the development of a study or your own research endeavors. An example using the evidence categories can be found in the American College of Sports Medicine (ACSM) Position Stand: Progression Models in Resistance Training for Health Adults (1). If you have a question or problem and a search of the literature only reveals that there is a limited or conflicting body of knowledge, then designing a well-controlled study would not only add to the literature but be an ideal way to help you resolve the question. But we are getting a bit ahead of ourselves; you are now at a critical point in the process. It is now time to test the hypothesis by conducting your own research, which for the purpose of this chapter, we will discuss in terms of study design.

APPLICATION OF THE SCIENTIFIC METHOD APPROACH: STUDY DESIGN

Study design should be considered the most important aspect of the overall research process. Many would conclude that data analysis is the top area in terms of importance, but if your design is flawed, then no matter how much analysis is done, the results will never reveal the true answer to the question posed. Therefore, it is imperative that the appropriate design is chosen prior to embarking on the research process.

As such, study design is the foundational framework on which all research is built. It is the point in the research process that allows us to find a way to try to answer the question that has been posed. The main point is to find the best way to answer the question and have an understanding of the possible results prior to delving into the study design. Remember there is no "right" way to answer such a question, and research is an evolving process. You are merely trying to add to a much larger body of knowledge by adding your own contribution.

THE IMPORTANCE OF UNDERSTANDING VARIABLES

Often, our personal and cultural beliefs influence our choices, behaviors, perceptions, and interpretation of information when establishing evidence-based research; however, it is through the use and adherence to the scientific method that helps minimize any influence of our belief systems. The ability to understand and correctly apply the principles and procedures of the scientific method is paramount in establishing valid scientific research and accurately contesting a given hypothesis.

One of the more common mistakes in research design is the failure to adequately understand, identify, and control variables that are present during the administration of the proposed research. It is important to establish an understanding of the types of variables that one uses or encounters in evidence-based research as it assists the researcher with the knowledge necessary to design more suitable conditions to answer the proposed research question. It is also advantageous to distinguish between those that aid, conflict, or interfere with the research design, as doing so strengthens the structure of the study design, increases the ability to foresee possible outcomes, provides countermeasures, and ultimately, but most importantly, maintains scientific control and integrity of the research.

Types of Variables

A variable includes any trait or characteristic with two or more categories. They exist in all forms of research, although with different scales of measurement or identification. In research, the term **variable** is used to identify any object, occurrence, condition or exposure that can be measured, controlled, and/or changed within an experimental application. Examples of variables found in exercise and health-related fields may include gender, height, weight, equipment type, protocol, environmental conditions, playing surface, physiologic responses to movement such as oxygen consumption or energy expenditure, the dosage for drug or supplement treatment, etc. The purpose of most empirical research, experimental or non-experimental, is to observe the interaction of one variable on another. To achieve this in experimental research designs and specifically answer a research question, variables are classified in two main categories: **explanatory** and **response variables**.

Explanatory variables (interchangeably referred to as "independent or predictor variable") are variables that the researcher manipulates or controls. The interaction that occurs between two or more variables can be *explained* or *predicted* by one or more of these explanatory variables. Response variables (often subscribed to as dependent or output variables) are variables measured by the researcher to identify the level of impact or *response* that has occurred when one or more explanatory variables have been introduced. For example, if a team of researchers was choosing to explore the effects of resistance training intensity on bone density, they would identify what is to be changed and what is to be observed. The explanatory variable that can be controlled and manipulated by the researcher would be the intensity of the resistance training. The response variable, that is measured and observed in *response* to the resistance training intensity, would be the bone density.

All variables, including explanatory and response variables, can be further sanctioned as either **quantitative** or **categorical variables**. Quantitative variables describe those variables that are measured numerically, such as height and weight, distance, velocity, heart rate, temperature, etc. Categorical variables are any variables that do not qualify as quantitative, or as numerical in nature, such as gender, race, level of experience, etc.

To present and analyze information, particularly for data collection purposes, both quantitative and categorical variables are often divided into four subcategories: **nominal**, **ordinal**, **interval**, and **ratio variables**. *Nominal variables* are those with two or more categories that do not contain any intrinsic order to the categories, or set level of distance between them, such as gender or race. Gender has two categories, and race has multiple. Each of these variables, gender and race, do not establish a specific order to their subsequent categories, and regardless of any order in which these categories are placed, the order does not affect the relationship they have to the other corresponding categories. There is also a non-specified level of separation from one to another. The categories male and female have no measurable distance between them that distinguishes one from the other. These categories are distinguishable from one another only by name.

Ordinal variables are similar to nominal variables in that they are categorical in nature. But ordinal variables have an establishment of order, such as by level or ranking, which gives them meaning. We see this in examples such as novice, amateur, and professional when referring to level of experience or skill in athletic populations, or novice, intermediate, advanced, or elite when referring to an individual's level of experience in resistance training. The spacing between each category may not be identical; however, there is an assumed order based on the structured definition provided to each variable. For example, according to the ACSM position stand on Progression Models in Resistance Training for Healthy Adults (1), individuals can be categorized or ranked as either novice, intermediate, or advanced according to their level of experience in resistance training. Novice individuals are categorized as untrained individuals with no resistance training experience or who have not trained for several years, intermediate individuals are those with approximately six months of consistent resistance training experience, and advanced are classed as individuals with many years of resistance training experience. There now becomes a clearly defined separation between each of these categories based on level of experience; however, there is a non-uniform level of difference separating the categories.

Interval variables follow similarly to ordinal variables, except the spacing between categories is uniform across all levels. It is also important to note that interval variables are not typically structured with reference to a zero point. An example of this is the use of the Borg Ratings of Perceived Exertion (RPE) scale, an approach to numerically quantify the perceived level of physical exertion (6) (Fig. 5-1). Scores range from 6 to 20 and equate to the progressive variation of exertion levels from no exertion at all (score = 6) to maximal exertion (score = 20).

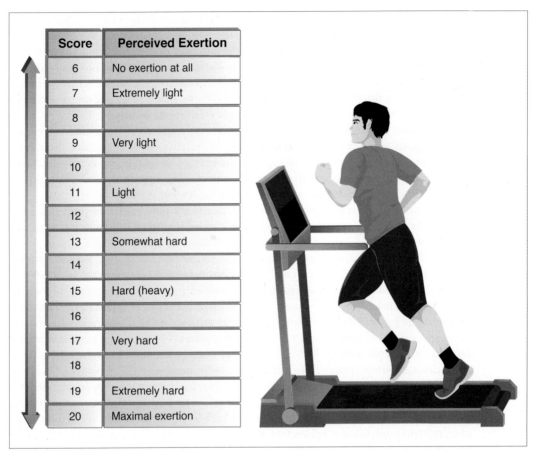

Score	Perceived Exertion
6	No exertion at all
7	Extremely light
8	
9	Very light
10	
11	Light
12	
13	Somewhat hard
14	
15	Hard (heavy)
16	
17	Very hard
18	
19	Extremely hard
20	Maximal exertion

FIGURE 5-1   Borg Ratings of Perceived Exertion scale.

In this example, as there is no reference to a zero point, a perceived exertion score of 17 ("very hard") is not categorically rated as twice the physical difficulty as a score of 9 ("very light").

In essence, *ratio variables* are interval variables; however, the values or categories have meaningful relationships between them, and zero can be used as a referencing point such as the percent of repetition maximum (RM) in resistance training. RM is often used to identify the level of resistance an individual can lift for a given number of repetitions. A 1RM would equate to a load or resistance that an individual can successfully complete one time, whereas a 5RM would equate to a load or resistance that can be successfully completed five times but no more. However, for exercise prescription purposes, RM can also be expressed as a percent RM (%RM). This is done to allow for individual differences and training adaptations that may occur as well as to maintain progression during training and over time. It can also be representative of the training zones conducive to specific muscle adaptations that can occur in various groups of individuals. It is suggested that the load required to increase maximal strength in untrained individuals equates to 45%–50% of 1RM or at least 80% of 1RM in experienced lifters (1). Meta-analytical data indicated that 60% of 1RM in novice individuals, 80% of 1RM in trained individuals, and 85% of 1RM in advanced individuals produced the largest effect sizes for strength increases (17). In these examples, the variable of intensity equates differently in a given population. For increases in muscular strength, a training load of 45%–60% RM is sufficient for untrained/novice individuals; however, it is 20%–25% too light for trained or advanced individuals.

It is not uncommon for categorical variables to be sanctioned as quantitative variables in research. This may be done to add meaning to the variable and thus establish a more quantifiable way to measure that variable in relation to others. The previously discussed Borg scale is an example of a categorical variable that can also be used as a quantitative variable. The RPE scale has been a valuable tool for the health professional, specifically for exercise prescription. It allows the monitoring of an individual's subjective response to exercise and quantifies that response for the purpose of evaluation, progression, and/or manipulation of the physical activity prescription.

Variable types that will be explored later in this text in reference to validity (Chapter 10) are **extraneous variables** (also called "confounding or intervening variable"). Extraneous variables are those that are not controlled or accounted for in the research design, and as a result, they may impair the ability to accurately conclude that the interactions that occurred within the study were due to the predictor variables and not due to chance. To some degree, all variables can be extraneous in nature, largely depending on the research question and subsequent study design. More common examples in health and fitness studies may be nutrition status (including supplementation), levels of fatigue, current fitness level, motivation for the test, experience, familiarity with the testing or training protocols, and possibly environmental or surface conditions, among others. Each of these variables are examples that, if not controlled or accounted for, may place doubt in the ability to rightfully conclude that the results observed were as a result of the given condition. For example, controlling for hydration status before testing a participant on his or her maximal oxygen consumption is vital for optimizing the resulting data. Control of various influences (called "confounding variables") such as nutrition, sleep, and time of day are all important for optimizing the quality of the data collected and reducing variance in the responses.

DIFFERENT TYPES OF RESEARCH

Research may be categorized in several ways, depending on the context and scope; however, a clear distinction is needed to delineate the various categories of research evidence, research purposes, study design options, and methods of data collection and analyses. Although the point of this chapter is to focus on the fundamentals of study design, it is imperative to also describe the context through which designing a study actually occurs. From a clinical perspective and as previously described, a hierarchy of evidence is often used for making decisions about interventions and/or proving causation about disease etiology (7). Such evidence hierarchies are also integral to evidence-based practices for exercise testing and prescription as well as for designing and conducting research in the exercise sciences. Thus, the amount and quality of evidence is fundamental for understanding the state of the science for a given research topic and should be used *a priori* for determining the purpose and design of studies.

For that reason, we have provided the contextual bases for differing purposes of research as well as the study design options through which a range of investigations are framed. In accordance with a recent ACSM position statement (10), we also refer to the hierarchy of evidence to categorize different study designs for the field of exercise science. Whereas a study **purpose** provides the context and rationale for pursuing an investigation, the research **design** provides the framework for a study plan of action, a strategy that indicates the methods for collecting and analyzing the needed information, and a general description on how the data will be collected. Conversely, the specific methods of data collection, such as gold standard versus proxy assessments, are outside the scope of this chapter, as are detailed analytical procedures that coincide with different study purposes and designs.

The Purpose of Research and Design Options

The underlying purpose of research is usually dictated by the amount *and* quality of available evidence for a given topic and the context or setting in which the study will occur. The purpose of research is to produce factual data on a topic under documented and specific conditions in order to understand and gain insights into the question at hand or the problem it addresses. Every research study is bounded by its **independent variables** and the results of the **dependent variables** are directly related to these specific conditions. Epidemiologists tend to focus on population-based disease exposures and outcomes, so research falls into two general categories: descriptive (*e.g.*, disease prevalence) and analytic (*i.e.*, causal relationships between exposure and disease). In this case, the definition of study design is based on the investigator's primary questions that are of interest to his or her study, including the following: How was the study population selected? What is the time relationship between exposure and disease/outcome (*i.e.*, does the exposure refer to a time before the occurrence of disease)? How was the data on exposure obtained (*i.e.*, observed or provided)? and How was the data on disease status obtained (*i.e.*, observed or tested)? to mention a few. Other questions could also be considered such as what type of exposure, how long was the exposure, etc. Clinical researchers, on the other hand, are not only concerned with threats to public health at large but also with directly studying translational, patient-oriented outcomes or disease etiology through observational research (*i.e.*, playing a passive role to observe a clinical phenomenon) and treatment studies (*e.g.*, randomized clinical trial). Although there is, of course, a reliance on both epidemiologic and clinical research designs and methods in the field of exercise science, our studies typically fall into one of three broad purpose categories, including descriptive, observational, and experimental research.

Descriptive Research

Descriptive research is conducted for a problem or theory that has not been clearly defined, and it is instrumental in the initial phases of research for generating hypotheses. As the name implies, descriptive research entails a method of gathering, synthesizing, and reporting general information about an individual or group of individuals with a given outcome of interest with respect to describing the development, process, and/or exposures related to that outcome. In using descriptive research designs, there is no attempt to identify a causal link between treatment or exposure and the outcome; rather, descriptive designs range from reporting case studies or case series, general descriptions of sample means and distributions, or correlations between variables. In the simplest form of descriptive research, a **case study** or **case report** is intended to report a phenomenon that is novel or rare but is difficult to investigate with a sample. Case studies may be qualitative in nature to describe, for example, the comprehensive details of a subject's experience during a major life event, in facing disease, encountering obstacles for changing behavior, etc. Case studies may also be quantitative and thus provide a compelling account from retrospective, information-oriented sampling, such as key cases (*i.e.*, highly interesting circumstances involved in a case) or outlier cases (*i.e.*, extreme or deviant cases). Conversely, longitudinal case studies may be used to report the prospective trajectory of changes after a novel intervention. **Case series** are an extension of clinical case reports that provide tracking of patients with a known condition who were given similar treatments, or in epidemiology, to describe the general characteristics and distribution of a homogeneous sample or the percentage/counts of exposures among disease cases.

Whereas case studies and case series provide valuable information in a clinical forum to describe a patient's or patient group's unusual symptoms or treatment responsiveness, they are not always employed in the exercise sciences. However, with the ever-evolving state of the literature to support the value of exercise interventions across special populations, there is certainly a demand for identifying and reporting individual patient accounts regarding the accessibility and feasibility of specific physical activity modalities and programs. Ultimately, if we want to continue supporting the notion that "exercise is medicine," then it is vital to better understand the unique aspects of exercise prescription for high-risk, unhealthy, or special populations, in which exercise may be an effective complementary intervention. Case studies and case series are also vital to our understanding of extreme pathologic responses to exercise and sports participation, as in the case of sickle cell trait and fatal rhabdomyolysis (3), sudden death in hypertrophic cardiomyopathy (14), diagnosis and management of sports-related concussions (21), or understanding heat intolerance or heat exhaustion (2). Indeed, although such adverse events could never be investigated formally or prospectively, the reporting of such case studies raises awareness about risk and provides a basis for conceptualizing future research to reduce risks through improved clinical screening, tailored exercise prescription, and technological advancements.

Despite the potential usefulness to describe rare or novel circumstances and formulate hypotheses, case studies and case series come with disadvantages. Specifically, because they are based on the experiences of one or a limited number of individuals, they do not necessarily reflect the general population. Moreover, in the absence of a control group, there is no way to determine the experience of exposure in non-cases, and thus the association between exposure or treatment and the outcome can only be assumed. As a consequence, the level of evidence for case studies and case series tends to be regarded as inferior as compared to other forms of research, and it is only considered stronger evidence than editorials or expert opinion.

Correlational studies are a type of descriptive research that extend beyond the limitations of case reports in that they provide the ability to simultaneously assess the strength and direction of association between exposures and disease or between predictive variables and biologic or physiologic outcomes. Correlational studies are likewise useful in describing the distribution, central tendency, and variation of measurements of interest, and they can be carried out on two levels of organization. Epidemiologic **cross-sectional studies** use data in which exposure and disease are assessed simultaneously in each individual at a given point or snapshot in time. Because this type of epidemiologic study is relatively inexpensive and the sample is generally representative of the greater population, they provide valuable insight about the potential risk factors for disease and are therefore useful for health planning and allocation of resources. Likewise, in the exercise sciences, cross-sectional research is heavily used to assess the association between modifiable behaviors or physiologic variables (*e.g.*, physical inactivity, muscular strength, etc.) and various health- and performance-related outcomes in individuals (*e.g.*, greater adiposity, functional impairment, etc.) (4,8). A recent study by Barbat-Artigas and colleagues (4) examined 1,462 women aged 75 years and older. They compared association between muscle mass and strength as well as self-reported functional performance to detect individuals at risk for functional impairments. The snapshot of only women of a particular age (75 years old and older) is a clear example of using the cross-sectional design. The older women are a cross-section of a society. Conversely, **ecologic studies** are correlational studies that rely on aggregate data from entire populations (usually geographically defined) to describe disease occurrence in relation to exposures. Although ecologic studies rely on similar correlation coefficients to describe the association between predictors and outcomes, they are inherently biased because exposures and disease status cannot be linked in particular individuals. Known as the "ecologic fallacy," this logical fallacy occurs when the interpretation of a correlation leads to inferences about the nature of individuals that have been deduced from inference for an aggregate population from which the individuals belong. Due to these limitations in cross-sectional and ecologic studies, they are generally considered to be only one step above case studies and case series for quality of evidence.

Although correlation does not necessarily imply cause and effect, this type of research is extremely valuable for generating hypotheses that underlie causal research designs. Moreover, because all correlational studies are subject to confounding factors that correlate (positively or negatively) with both the dependent variable and the independent variable, they are thus at risk for revealing spurious relationships (see Chapter 18). However, robust regression analyses are available, which can account for the mediating effect of these variables by testing interactions terms, and/or by controlling for covariates in the model. Although these methods still cannot provide inference for a cause-and-effect relationship, they greatly strengthen the ability to detect the true, independent association between a given predictor and outcome.

An additional limitation of cross-sectional research that is common in the exercise sciences is the blatant overinterpretation of results. Due to the nature of our field, we are often confined to small, sometimes homogeneous samples. In these circumstances, it may not be appropriate to explore a correlation between a predictor and outcome, as this may be subject to selection bias and therefore a likely distortion of the true association. Moreover, because behavior and physiologic processes occur gradually over time, it is often quite difficult to unravel the direction of causality when assessing a single snapshot in time, for example, the correlation between sedentary behavior and obesity. Indeed, whether excessive sedentary behavior "causes" obesity or obesity itself is a cause of increased sedentary behavior (*i.e.*, reverse causality) is an interesting and complex topic (18); however, cross-sectional research is inherently limited for answering such questions.

Observational Research

Descriptive research is useful for exploring the association between exposures and disease as well as for identifying predictors of health and functional outcomes, and it is often used in the initial stages of the research process. However, the goal of biomedical research in the broadest sense is to build a body of evidence that determines the causal relationships between exposures and diseases, uncovers biologic pathways and mechanisms, and ultimately leads to a refinement of clinical and behavioral interventions that cause positive adaptations in human health on a wide scale. **Observational research** draws inferences about the possible causal effect of an intervention or disease, where the assignment of subjects into a group is outside the control of the investigator. Thus, like correlational research, observational studies share the same limitation that interpretation of causal inference is potentially influenced by the misleading effects of unaccounted confounding variables. Observational research can be retrospective or prospective, but these studies are always longitudinal. In general, a prospective study is one in which a group or groups are followed over time to assess a specific study outcome. Conversely, a retrospective study is one in which a group or groups are examined back in time to evaluate changes that had occurred over a specific historical time frame in the past.

One type of observational study design is the **cohort study**, which involves following groups of subjects over time to describe the occurrence of outcomes and to analyze the association between predictors and those outcomes (12). Epidemiologists use cohort studies to determine relative risk (RR) ratios for disease (*i.e.*, the ratio of the cumulative incidence among those exposed compared with those not exposed or $RR = \frac{Risk\ in\ exposed}{Risk\ in\ nonexposed}$).

In prospective cohort studies, an investigator actively recruits subjects and measures certain characteristics that might be predictive of the subsequent outcomes. Because this type of research requires following the subjects over time and periodically collecting measurements on the outcomes, it is expensive and extremely time-intensive, but it is considered a robust method of assessing disease incidence (*i.e.*, the number of new cases in a specified time frame). Moreover, it is a powerful design because it allows an investigator to choose any potential predictor variables that are theoretically relevant—a huge design advantage over retrospective studies. For example, in a recent study to examine whether improvements in healthy behaviors (*e.g.*, increased physical activity) were associated with reduced risk of cardiovascular disease (CVD) among newly diagnosed diabetic patients, Long and colleagues (13) demonstrated that the RR for a primary CVD event among individuals who increased physical activity (*i.e.*, compared with those who did not change) was 0.53 (95% confidence interval [CI]: 0.21–0.78). Thus, because RR was less than 1, there was a risk for CVD events among the exposed (*i.e.*, people who increased physical activity; *Decreased risk* = $[(0.53-1) \times 100\%]$ = 47% decreased) that was significantly less than the risk for CVD among the nonexposed (*i.e.*, people who failed to increase physical activity; *Increased risk* = $\left[\frac{1}{0.53} \times 100\%\right]$ = 89% increased).

Retrospective cohort studies, on the other hand, have many of the same strengths as prospective studies but have the advantage of any secondary data analyses in that all data have already been collected. Despite this enormous economic advantage, the tradeoff in this design is complete lack of control over choosing predictor variables, ensuring the quality and accuracy of data collection procedures and in determining the approach to sampling the population. Cohort studies have been used extensively in the exercise science field for a wide range of study purposes from determining the effect of differing doses of physical activity on longevity (20) to determining the intrinsic predictors of injury risk in athletes (9) and to examining the effects of exposure to air pollution during exercise on the development of asthma in children (15).

Due to the various disadvantages of cohort studies, many researchers choose a different type of observational research: the **case-control study**. An extremely common design in epidemiology, participants are selected and compared on the basis of whether or not they have a condition or disease (these are the "cases") or do not have the condition or disease (these are the "controls"). Because participants are selected on the basis of having or not having a condition or disease, exposures for every participant are collected retrospectively on specific outcomes. The objective of this design is to look backward in time to identify differences in predictor variables, or exposures, which might explain the cause for cases having the disease or condition. Generally, the selection of controls in a case-control study should come from the same population as the cases, and selection should be independent of the exposures of interest. Theoretically then, controls should have had an equal risk for developing the disease and becoming a case. Although case-control studies are typically used to understand risk factors for a disease, it should be pointed out that the outcome need not be the presence or absence of disease, per se. Rather, and as is particularly useful in the exercise sciences, the case-control design may be used to investigate other outcomes such as the relationship between exercise as an exposure and secondary comorbidities among individuals with and without a given condition/disease.

For example, in a study designed to investigate whether physical exercise was associated with decreased risk of mild cognitive impairment (11), investigators from the Mayo Clinic recruited subjects on the basis of having or not having mild cognitive impairment and then tested whether the frequency or intensity of exercise was associated with reduced risk of impairment. Because study participants in case-control studies are selected on the basis of a disease status, prospective incidence of disease cannot be determined, and thus, RRs cannot be calculated. In a case-control study, we cannot examine the risk of developing disease, but instead, the "odds" of being exposed. In addition to the need for recall bias pertaining to the extent of exposure, this issue is usually considered a major limitation of all case-control studies. Rather, the association between exposures and disease or condition in a case-control study is calculated as an odds ratio (OR). In its simplest form, the OR in a case-control study reflects a ratio of the number of ways an event *can* occur, relative to the number of ways that an event *cannot* occur $\left(Exposure\ OR = \dfrac{Odds\ of\ exposure\ in\ disease}{Odds\ of\ exposure\ in\ non\text{-}disease} \right)$.

In the previous example, the researchers found that the ORs for any frequency of moderate exercise were 0.61–0.68 ($P < .05$) for midlife (age range, 50–65 years) and late life (older than 65 years), respectively (11). Thus, the odds of mild cognitive impairment among adults who engaged in moderate intensity exercise were significantly less (*Decreased odds* = $[(0.61 - 1) \times 100\%]$ = 39% lower for midlife; and *Decreased odds* = $[(0.68 - 1) \times 100\%]$ = 32% lower for late life) than those who did not exercise.

In the event that selection of controls in a case-control study do *not* have the potential to become cases (*i.e.*, they are not susceptible for the disease of interest), then caution is warranted to ensure the investigator elects to use more than one type of control. For example, in certain types of cancer or pediatric-onset neurologic disorders (*e.g.*, cerebral palsy), there may be no group similar enough to the cases group. In this situation, it is important to select controls on some other factor (*e.g.*, similar environment also known as "neighborhood control" or similar genetic makeup also known as "sibling control") to reduce the risk of biasing or inflating the association. Generally, there is a diminished return of statistical power after three to four matched controls. Conversely, controls may also be selected on the basis of matching for influential factors, which helps with reducing potential problems of residual confounding. For example, many factors that influence the adaptive response to exercise, such as gender, age, and body mass index, may also influence the outcome of interest. Therefore, it is imperative to either select controls based on matching for these factors or plan to adjust for them statistically in the analysis. There are several derivations of case-control designs that are outside the scope of this chapter but that have specific clinical or epidemiologic application and specific strengths and weaknesses. These include nested case-control studies, nested case-cohort studies, and case-crossover studies (12). Depending on the source, case-control studies and cohort studies are often considered to be of similar level of evidence; however, prospective cohort studies are sometimes considered superior in the hierarchy due to having more control.

Experimental Research

Experimental research entails a range of investigator-initiated studies intended to test hypotheses and in which the exposure is assigned or provided by the investigator. Experimental studies are informally regarded as causal research because there is a direct and deliberate change in the exposure which, in turn, has a direct and sometimes unpredictable effect on the outcome. Experimental research may be designed to test the acute effect of a treatment or the longitudinal effect of an intervention and can range from basic laboratory studies in animal models to large, multi-site clinical investigations in humans. Experimental research forms the foundation of our principles in exercise science, as there is a huge body of literature pertaining to the application of exercise to *cause* positive changes for health and fitness. Unfortunately, the exercise science community has long been criticized for low-quality evidence in support of our principles. Although experimental research is an effective means to demonstrate causality, only certain types of studies meet the criteria of "high-quality" evidence.

Randomized controlled trials (RCTs) have long been considered the apex of evidence in the hierarchy of research, and these are upon which the basis of many medical decisions are reached. RCTs comprise rigorous scientific experiments involving human subjects that are designed to evaluate the effects of a treatment or intervention for a particular disease or condition in order to reduce adverse events and elucidate the most appropriate care for future subjects. The process of randomization of eligible subjects is fundamental to this design, and it is explicitly intended to remove investigator bias, produce comparable groups, and to ultimately ensure validity of statistical evaluation. There is paucity in the sheer number of RCTs in the exercise sciences, primarily due to the challenges related to expenses, time commitments, and subject attrition. However, because the exposure of interest (*i.e.*, exercise) is a readily modifiable behavior in the context of a research investigation, the viability of conducting RCTs in our field is seemingly quite favorable. Although the process of randomization (see Chapter 8) and treatment and intervention is intuitive, several other factors pertaining to the design of RCTs is less evident. For example, because RCTs are designed to assess the effect of a treatment versus the effect of a control, there is often confusion about what constitutes an acceptable control (see Chapter 7). This issue is of particular relevance in the exercise sciences, as many researchers believe there is little perceived value to understanding the differences induced by exercise intervention against those of a nonintervention control. However, there is a dearth of quality evidence regarding the use of different exercise modalities and doses as a complementary means to target numerous disease processes. Therefore, RCTs offer a rigorous method to examine such effects against alternative interventions and/or a nonintervention control while enforcing strict control over subject eligibility and potential confounding factors. Typical comparison or control groups in RCTs consist of (a) placebo or sham therapy groups, (b) alternative interventions (*i.e.*, to possibly compare a new intervention to a best existing alternative), or (c) a "usual care" intervention. Although the details pertaining to advantages and disadvantages of each of these in exercise-related RCTs is out of the scope of this chapter, careful attention is warranted in the selection of controls to reduce the risk of bias. For additional detail, the Consolidated Standards of Reporting Trials (CONSORT) statement should be used as a guide in considering, designing, and reporting RCTs (19).

Intervention studies that do not include randomization of subjects or the inclusion of a comparison or control groups are generally considered to be of much lower quality of evidence. Non-randomized intervention studies are prevalent in exercise sciences and typically entail a pre-, post-, or longitudinal design in order to assess the effect of an exercise intervention within subjects of a given group. Although there is merit in understanding the effects of a single exercise intervention to elicit changes in clinically relevant outcomes, there is currently a dire need for more robust designs such as RCTs to bolster the support of exercise in the context of preventive medicine and public health.

Double-Blind Placebo Crossover Study Designs

A host of different topics examining the effect of a treatment, such as drug or nutritional supplement use, use the experimental design of a double-blind study in which both the participants and the investigators do not know which treatment is the actual compound being studied. Additionally, a placebo treatment is also used (*e.g.*, the proverbial sugar pill) that looks like the real thing but is not and addresses the effect of the participant just believing he or she is using the real compound. To strengthen the design, a crossover is used, allowing the participant to act as their own control and involves performing both treatments by waiting for a specific time frame to "wash out" or get rid of the effects of the first treatment and then start the other treatment under the same time course and conditions as the first. This design approach is aided by having half the participants start with one treatment while the other half starts with the other treatment and then crosses over after completion of the time frame for the study of the compound. This allows for a balanced design over time, reducing the effects of the time frame and seasonal effects confounding the findings. Addressed in more detail in Chapter 8, such study designs will allow for a less biased approach to such experimental questions.

Systematic Reviews and Meta-Analyses

A systematic review is a literature review that is focused on a specific research question with the intent to identify, appraise, select, and synthesize all research pertaining to that research question (see also Chapter 3). Systematic reviews may have a statistical combination of studies relevant to the question, but this is not required of them. Moreover, systematic reviews may or may not have strict inclusion criteria to synthesize studies of high quality (*e.g.*, only RCTs). The Preferred Reporting Items for Systematic Reviews and Meta-Analyses (PRISMA) statement (16) is similar in nature to the CONSORT statement in that it is an evidence-based minimum set of items for reporting in systematic reviews and meta-analyses. This statement incorporates the definitions of systematic review and meta-analysis used by the Cochrane Collaboration.

Often, a systematic review will be informally incorporated early in the research process to identify gaps in the literature or to determine effect sizes for subsequent power calculations. However, when conducted for the purpose of statistically pooling effect size data in a meta-analysis, this research design can be extremely robust. In fact, systematic reviews with meta-analyses of high-quality RCTs are crucial to evidence-based practices and are often considered the very highest level of quality of evidence. Meta-analyses incorporate the synthesis of effect size data from similar studies to better understand the effectiveness of an intervention in a much larger sample than would be possible with traditional research designs. However, the process of conducting meta-analyses has been heavily criticized, as there are many poorly conducted and published studies that pose a risk to confusing the state of the literature with "garbage in, garbage out" findings. Thus, strict adherence to the design and reporting guidelines of the PRISMA statement is generally encouraged to ensure that the systematic review and meta-analysis is not biased or flawed. Unfortunately, because there are few high-quality RCTs in the exercise science literature, it is difficult at best to synthesize the findings of exercise interventions for a broad range of clinically relevant outcomes. Although there is certainly a dire need for subsequent stringent RCTs, many of the non-randomized interventions published in our literature are of high quality and thus are still eligible for synthesizing in a systematic review. For alternative methods of high-quality meta-analyses, the reader is encouraged to consider the latest text by Borenstein and colleagues (5), which provides an extremely comprehensive overview of theoretical and statistical guidelines for designing, conducting, and reporting meta-analyses.

ERROR IN STUDY DESIGN

Once the overall design has been determined, it has to be recognized that it is rare to find a research design without error or impedance from one or more variables; however, research designs that provide stringent adherence to the scientific method, including variable control, minimizes debatable interpretation of the results and enhances applicability of the research. This signifies the importance of a literature review. As discussed earlier in this chapter, a well-conducted literature review considers all factors and provides information about similar study designs. More importantly, it identifies variables specific to the research question. The literature review identifies the types of variables that have been included or observed as well as variables that were unexpected during the design of the reviewed research. As researchers embark on the development of a proposed study, it is important that any variable, directly or indirectly, be identified and classified according to its properties. In return, this provides better study awareness, greater study control, and allows structure to the data collection and analysis process.

Research Error

Every study is prone to some form of research error. The goal of every researcher should be to minimize the type and level of research error and, in doing so, provide a greater chance that the information obtained in the research was a direct result of the interaction between the designated variables and not due to an outside entity or occurrence. By virtue, this raises the credibility of the study design and the established results. As a researcher, this is crucial in defining the applicability of the study and the results across similar treatment groups or populations. There are two main categories of error often viewed in research: random and systematic errors.

Random errors are often those that occur as a result of unknown, often unpredictable, or undefined deviations in the study. The appearance of these deviations can lead to a disruption in the integrity of the study and thus lower the level of confidence in the results or the interpretation of those results. Random errors occur as a result of many factors, more commonly the established setting for the research project, the equipment, the measurement, or the data collection tools. It is often difficult for researchers to specifically prepare for random error-related events; however, it is the ability of the researcher to foresee possible scenarios whereby random errors may occur and provide appropriate alternatives or adjustments to minimize or negate its impact. Examining previous research through a literature review and identifying the more common random errors or reaching out to experienced professionals familiar with equipment or use of measurement/data collection tools can facilitate better control of these possible errors.

Systematic errors often occur as a result of measurement error, whether through instrument error (failure to operate as designed or the data collection process) or the inability of a research technician to operate the measurement tool in accordance to the designated protocols or data collection parameters. Systematic errors are more commonly observed in research studies, as they are more commonly assimilated to human error. The failure to adequately purchase, prepare, maintain, and calibrate measurement tools often leads to delays or irregularities in the research design. The inability to adequately train and supervise experiment technicians on equipment, software, and research protocols largely leads to discrepancies between test conditions and data collection protocols. Lastly, if the research group does not adequately instruct and teach research participants on what the tests involve or how the tests are to be conducted, this can lead to more error-driven fluctuations in results. The failure to instruct a subject on correct lifting techniques may misrepresent muscular capabilities, or the failure to provide appropriate instructions on pre-test food and exercise habits may overestimate or underestimate body composition results. It is the responsibility of the research group to firstly recognize both forms of possible errors in the study design and secondly to make every effort to control what can be controlled and restrict those that cannot. All research is exposed to some form of error, but it is better to defend a tightly controlled study that has results reflective of the original study design and questions rather than explaining what may have occurred if error-related considerations were unaccounted for.

CONCLUSION

Once again, the research design process is the foundational component of any successful research endeavor. Following the scientific method is an initial step in beginning the process. Defining the variables is the next logical and necessary step in the process to answer a given question or problem related to our evolving evidence-based practice. Once the variables have been considered and defined, deciding if observational, descriptive, or experimental research; systematic review; or meta-analysis is the ideal approach to answering your question will set the stage for a successful foray into the realm of research. Finally, consideration and management of possible sources of research error will help ensure the highest quality in your research endeavors.

GLOSSARY

Case-control study: epidemiologic design in which participants are selected and compared on the basis of whether or not they have a condition or disease (these are the cases) or do not have the condition or disease (these are the controls)

Case series: an extension of clinical case reports that provides tracking of patients with a known condition who were given similar treatments, or in epidemiology, to describe the general characteristics and distribution of a homogeneous sample or the percentage/counts of exposures among disease cases

Case study or **case report:** intended to report a phenomenon that is novel or rare but is difficult to investigate with a sample and may be qualitative or quantitative in nature

Categorical variable: any variable that does not qualify as quantitative or as numerical in nature, such as gender, race, and level of experience

Cohort study: type of observational study design; involves following groups of subjects over time to describe the occurrence of outcomes and to analyze the association between predictors and those outcomes

Correlational study: type of descriptive research that extends beyond the limitations of case reports that provides the ability to simultaneously assess the strength and direction of association between exposures and disease or between predictive variables and biologic or physiologic outcomes

Cross-sectional studies: use data in which exposure and disease are assessed simultaneously in each individual at a given point or snapshot in time

Dependent variable: a variable that is measured/observed in response to the interaction with the independent variable

Descriptive research: a method of gathering, synthesizing, and reporting general information about an individual or group of individuals with a given outcome of interest with respect to describing the development, process, and/or exposures related to that outcome. It is conducted for a problem or theory that has not been clearly defined

Design: the framework for a study plan of action, a strategy that indicates the methods for collecting and analyzing the needed information, and a general description for how the data will be collected

Ecologic studies: correlational studies that rely on aggregate data from entire populations (usually geographically defined) to describe disease occurrence in relation to exposures

Experimental research: studies intended to test hypotheses in which the exposure is assigned or provided by the investigator. Experimental studies are informally regarded as causal research because there is a direct and deliberate change in the exposure which, in turn, has a direct and sometimes unpredictable effect on the outcome

Explanatory variable: any variable that the researcher manipulates or controls

Extraneous variables: also called confounding or intervening variables; variables that are not controlled or accounted for in the research design and, as a result, may impair the ability to accurately conclude that the interactions that occurred within the study were due to predictor variables and not due to chance

Independent variable: a variable that explains or predicts the interaction of two or more variables

Interval variable: any variable where the spacing between categories is uniform across all levels, such as time, temperature, or RPE scale (also referred to as "scaled variable")

Nominal variable: any variable with two or more categories that do not contain any intrinsic order to the categories, or set level of distance between them, such as gender or race

Observational research: draws inferences about the possible causal effect of an intervention or disease, where the assignment of subjects into a group is outside the control of the investigator

Ordinal variable: any categorical variable that establishes order, such as by level or ranking, that gives them meaning, such as college degree (BS, MS, PhD) or training status (trained, untrained, or elite). The difference between levels or ranks may not be the same

Purpose: provides the context and rationale for pursuing an investigation

Quantitative variable: any variable that is measured numerically, such as height and weight, distance, velocity, heart rate, temperature, etc.

Random errors: errors that occur as a result of unknown, often unpredictable or undefined deviations in the study

Randomized controlled trials: rigorous scientific experiments involving human subjects that are designed to evaluate the effects of a treatment or intervention for a particular disease or condition in order to reduce adverse events and elucidate the most appropriate care for future subjects

Ratio variable: interval variables that have values or categories with meaningful relationships ratios between them, and zero can be used as a referencing point such as the %RM in resistance training

Response variables: any variable that is used to identify the level of impact or response that has occurred when one or more explanatory variables have been introduced

Systematic errors: errors that occur as a result of measurement error, whether through instrument error (failure to operate as designed or the data collection process) or the inability of a research technician to operate the measurement tool in accordance to the designated protocols or data collection parameters

Variable: any object, occurrence, condition, or exposure that can be measured, controlled, and/or changed within an experimental application

REFERENCES

1. American College of Sports Medicine. American College of Sports Medicine position stand. Progression models in resistance training for healthy adults. *Med Sci Sports Exerc.* 2009;41:687–708.
2. Armstrong LE, Hubbard RW, Szlyk PC, Sils IV, Kraemer WJ. Heat intolerance, heat exhaustion monitored: a case report. *Aviat Space Environ Med.* 1988;59(3):262–266.
3. Anzalone ML, Green VS, Buja M, Sanchez LA, Harrykissoon RI, Eichner ER. Sickle cell trait and fatal rhabdomyolysis in football training: a case study. *Med Sci Sports Exerc.* 2010;42(1):3–7.
4. Barbat-Artigas S, Rolland Y, Cesari M, et al. Clinical relevance of different muscle strength indexes and functional impairment in women aged 75 years and older. *J Gerontol A Biol Sci Med Sci.* 2013;68(7):811–819.
5. Borenstein M, Hedges L, Higgins J, Rothstein HR. *Introduction to Meta-Analysis.* Hoboken (NJ): Wiley; 2009.
6. Borg G. *An Introduction to Borg' RPE Scale.* Ithaca (NY): Mouvement Publications; 1985.
7. Clinical Guidelines on the Identification, Evaluation, and Treatment of Overweight and Obesity in Adults—the Evidence Report. National Institutes of Health. *Obes Res.* 1998;6(suppl 2):51S–209S.
8. Du HD, Bennett D, Li LM, et al. Physical activity and sedentary leisure time and their associations with BMI, waist circumference, and percentage body fat in 0.5 million adults: the China Kadoorie Biobank study. *Am J Clin Nutr.* 2013;97(3):487–496.
9. Engebretsen AH, Myklebust G, Holme I, Engebretsen L, Bahr R. Intrinsic risk factors for hamstring injuries among male soccer players: a prospective cohort study. *Am J Sports Med.* 2010;38(6):1147–1153.
10. Garber CE, Blissmer B, Deschenes MR, et al. American College of Sports Medicine position stand. Quantity and quality of exercise for developing and maintaining cardiorespiratory, musculoskeletal, and neuromotor fitness in apparently healthy adults: guidance for prescribing exercise. *Med Sci Sports Exerc.* 2011;43(7):1334–1359.
11. Geda YE, Roberts RO, Knopman DS, et al. Physical exercise, aging, and mild cognitive impairment: a population-based study. *Arch Neurol.* 2010;67(1):80–86.
12. Hulley S, Cummings S, Browner W, Grady D, Newman T. *Designing Clinical Research.* Philadelphia (PA): Lippincott Williams & Wilkins; 2007.
13. Long GH, Cooper AJ, Wareham NJ, Griffin SJ, Simmons RK. Healthy behavior change and cardiovascular outcomes in newly diagnosed type 2 diabetic patients: a cohort analysis of the ADDITION-Cambridge study. *Diabetes Care.* 2014;37(6):1712–1720.
14. Maron BJ, Roberts WC, Epstein SE. Sudden death in hypertrophic cardiomyopathy: a profile of 78 patients. *Circulation.* 1982;35(7):1388–1394.
15. McConnell R, Berhane K, Gilliland F, et al. Asthma in exercising children exposed to ozone: a cohort study. *Lancet.* 2002;359(9304):386–391.
16. Moher D, Liberati A, Tetzlaff J, Altman DG. Preferred reporting items for systematic reviews and meta-analyses: the PRISMA statement. *Ann Intern Med.* 2009;151(4):264–269.
17. Peterson MD, Rhea MR, Alvar BA. Applications of the dose-response for muscular strength development: a review of meta-analytic efficacy and reliability for designing training prescription. *J Strength Cond Res.* 2005;19(4):950–958.
18. Pulsford RM, Stamatakis E, Britton AR, Brunner EJ, Hillsdon MJ. Sitting behavior and obesity: evidence from the Whitehall II study. *Am J Prev Med.* 2013;44(2):132–138.
19. Schulz KF, Altman DG, Moher D. CONSORT 2010 statement: updated guidelines for reporting parallel group randomised trials. *J Clin Epidemiol.* 2010;1(2):100–107.
20. Wen CP, Wai JP, Tsai MK, et al. Minimum amount of physical activity for reduced mortality and extended life expectancy: a prospective cohort study. *Lancet.* 2011;378(9798):1244–1253.
21. Zafonte R. Diagnosis and management of sports-related concussion: a 15-year-old athlete with a concussion. *JAMA.* 2011;306(1):79–86.

CHAPTER 6

Understanding Research: A Clinician's Perspective of Basic, Applied, and Clinical Investigations

Craig R. Denegar, PhD, PT, ATC, FNATA, and Courtney Jensen, PhD

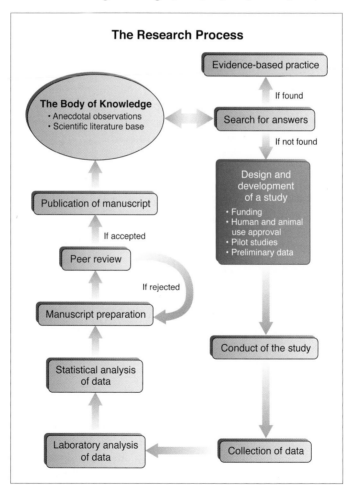

The Research Process

- Evidence-based practice
- The Body of Knowledge
  - Anecdotal observations
  - Scientific literature base
- Search for answers
- If found
- If not found
- Design and development of a study
  - Funding
  - Human and animal use approval
  - Pilot studies
  - Preliminary data
- Publication of manuscript
- If accepted
- Peer review
- If rejected
- Manuscript preparation
- Statistical analysis of data
- Conduct of the study
- Laboratory analysis of data
- Collection of data

INTRODUCTION: A BRIEF HISTORY OF THE DICHOTOMY

By the 4th century B.C., philosophers and theologians were already "researching" ways to improve personal and public health. Although primitive and ultimately discarded during the Renaissance, the principles of philosophy that advanced during the time of Aristotle influenced medieval scholarship and were a prerequisite for the development of the scientific method (1,5).

The first rudimentary statistical practices, known as "political arithmetic," appeared during the 17th century. This was a late Renaissance effort by Europeans to estimate the size and growth of their populations (as well as the life expectancies of those being summed). The increasingly complex analyses of these data, aimed at the creation of a healthier state, were coined "statistics" (4,10).

By the 20th century, the scientific method (and its statistics) had developed enough to begin supporting research as a career path in American and European universities (7). In response, *Science* editor James McKeen Cattell published the first directory of American researchers in 1906, entitled *American Men of Science: A Biographical Directory*. Stated in the preface: "There are included in the directory the records of more than four thousand men of science, and it is believed that the entries are tolerably complete for those in North America who have carried on research work in the natural and exact sciences" (12).

After World War I, American government and industry (and philanthropy to a lesser extent) joined the university system in the pursuit of research. It was at this time that the distinction between "basic" (or "pure") research and "applied research" was clearly delineated. Basic research was consigned to universities while its application became the goal of industry (10).

The dichotomy was further distinguished in the 1920s when Herbert Hoover, then secretary of commerce, began to champion "pure research" as "the raw material of applied science" (8). Hoover's promotion in this way is widely considered to be a major catalyst for the expansion of research and development programs throughout the United States. Between 1921 and 1940, the number of researchers employed by industrial firms grew from 2,775 to 27,777 (11).

Today, both basic and applied research have become feasible and desirable enough career paths that the number of postdoctoral fellows being trained in U.S. laboratories has reached an estimated 89,000 (13), making science a very competitive profession (3).

As today's postdocs begin to percolate into the latest directory of American researchers, they may find their careers quarantined within a single domain of research (*i.e.*, basic or applied). This directory is still being published but with the updated, gender-inclusive title of *American Men and Women of Science*. The latest edition (26th, 2009) is 9,100 pages and weighs just over 48 lb.

However, Hoover's 20th century dichotomy has expanded into a much broader gamut. It has evolved into a continuum that begins at bench science (animal models, human labs, etc.) and ends at the bedside (research aimed at informing clinical decisions). This continuum of translational research connects the work of an individual researcher to larger, often interdisciplinary research programs. The importance of accelerating the application of research findings to advance clinical care is well-recognized, and translational research has become a priority for funding agencies, organizations, and investigators. The National Institutes of Health, National Center for Advancing Translational Sciences was developed specifically to support programs dedicated to the translation of new knowledge to practice.

FROM BENCH TO BEDSIDE

To illustrate the scientific relationship between the bench and the bedside, consider these examples:

1. A physiologist examines the effect of a mechanical signal directed at cells in a culture as an effort to understand the relevant gene expression.
2. A physiologist and psychologist collaborate to evaluate the effect of athletic participation on physical and mental health among urban high school youth.
3. A physician investigates the most effective approach to reduce low-density lipoprotein (LDL) cholesterol to 100 mg/dL or lower among men with physically demanding jobs at high risk for repeated cardiac events.

Each line of work enhances our understanding of how we're affected by the world around us. However, the nature of each question may require a different research design. Each research design will yield a different type of data and require a different approach to analysis. The type of data and analyses performed affect the way findings are reported. Despite this, all three of these examples are interrelated on a fundamental level.

Although it is a long distance between characterizing a cell's behavior and demonstrating an effective treatment for a human pathology, a better understanding of cellular responses may facilitate a broader understanding of how a particular body system works. The downstream effect of this may be research into novel treatment options.

The researchers who examined the physical and mental effects of athletic participation among urban high school youth may discover novel information about the relationship between exercise and mental health leading to strategies to promote lifelong physical activity and reduce the risk of heart disease. In turn, this may influence the types of questions a physician is inclined to ask. For physicians who are principally concerned with medical outcomes, every patient presents with a unique biologic makeup and medical history. Thus, the most useful information will be the probability that a particular treatment approach will reduce the present patient's LDL cholesterol sufficiently against the probability that it will induce adverse side effects.

Although each of these examples occupies a different stage in the bench-to-bedside continuum, the respective researchers have a similar set of challenges to overcome. First, they must identify the purpose of their research (as well as the end user it proposes to affect). Only then can one properly decide how the data are to be collected. Once the data are collected, the nature of those data must guide the choice of statistical analysis. Statistics is really a process of coping with uncertainty. Thus, the consequences of that uncertainty must be considered. Researchers must weigh the potential of achieving a desired benefit against the risks of adverse events, selecting a statistical approach accordingly. Once the data have been analyzed, the results are to be interpreted and reported to the scientific, medical, and lay communities. At this stage, researchers must take particular care to avoid overinterpreting or under-reporting their findings, and they must present the information in a manner appropriate for the target audience.

This chapter addresses the major issues involved at each step of the research process, beginning with a review of how questions are developed, as discussed in Chapter 3.

FRAMING A QUESTION

Research studies are designed with specific questions or purposes in mind. A viable research question should clearly specify the population from which samples are drawn, any independent variable(s) to be manipulated or those that are thought to predict an outcome (see Chapters 5 and 7), and the outcomes of interest.

When the question of interest regards the efficacy of a treatment, the researcher will manipulate the independent variable so that the effect of that treatment can be isolated from other influences such as a placebo response (a perceived benefit to inactive agents) or the natural history of recovery from an injury or illness. When the research question concerns diagnostic accuracy or the occurrence of events, the independent factor (*e.g.*, administration of a novel therapy) is not manipulated. In such studies, one must ensure that the data of interest are acquired in an unbiased manner from samples drawn from a population or from an entire population.

Regardless of the purpose, it is important that a question be precisely (and often narrowly) framed. For example, a desire to learn more about coronary artery disease does not constitute a research question. When that desire to learn is distilled into a specific, directly answerable question (*e.g.*, Is cardiorespiratory function at age 50 years predictive of cardiac related death by age 80 years?), research may begin.

The pursuit of research is an endeavor that is inextricably tied to our nature. It is part of the human condition that our understanding of the world around us be continuously subjected to the scrutiny of a suspicious mind (it is at least in the nature of those inclined to read this chapter).

The beauty and curse of our inquisitive character is that the number of questions to be posed is endless. The beauty in this is not one that will expire with age. The ability to conduct research will *always* be in demand, and the process of truth-seeking will continue to connect people to a common cause. The curse, indissoluble from that beauty, is that there are also infinite questions we don't know *how* to answer. For example, how many anopheles mosquitoes currently carry malaria? Regardless of whether this is a useful line of inquiry, it is a simple question with a simple answer. However, despite its simplicity, we don't know how to design a research model that answers the question. In general, among the questions we *do* know how to answer, absolute certainty in those answers will remain a rare commodity.

Research is very much a building process. Step by step, knowledge is built on the foundation of previous work, as you learned in Chapter 4. If the question being asked is one that dates back to an Aristotelian line of inquiry, the present investigator will be standing on the shoulders of giants, who were themselves piggybacking on former giants. If the research is treading into relatively new territory, the investigator may be standing on the ground, readying his or her shoulders for future generations, but navigating with scientific tools that have taken centuries to develop.

THE HIERARCHY OF MEDICAL EVIDENCE

The scientific landscape is typically explored in a specific order, as discussed in Chapter 5. The different modes of exploration are often characterized by a "hierarchy of evidence." This hierarchy is depicted differently by different authors, but no matter how it is illustrated, it should never be construed as a hierarchy of *importance*. It is not a system of ranking by which research models at the base of the hierarchy are discounted relative to those at the top; rather, it should be thought of as a *sequential* depiction that begins with ideas, graduates to the bench, and ends at the bedside. The information illustrated by our hierarchy is intended to:

1. add perspective to the types of questions that can be asked (and the types of analyses with which they're associated),
2. help clinicians understand which levels of evidence may best support clinical decisions.

We have represented our hierarchy as a pyramid in Figure 6-1.

In the "cascade of knowledge," every pursuit begins with an idea and ends with a synthesis of the collected data. Once an idea has inspired a study, the pioneering investigation often begins at the bench with animal models, in vitro studies, and mechanisms research. In medicine (and particularly sports medicine), this type of research seeks an understanding of how external factors (*e.g.*, force, internal biologic events, etc.) alter subsequent physiologic events. For example, throughout the 1990s, a popular area of interest involved the relationship between hyperglycemia and the incidence of coronary artery disease. Such interest is often prompted by general observations among people; in this case, people with poor glycemic control seemed to be exhibiting an earlier onset of vascular complications. Initial testing of such observations typically begins with animal models, perhaps finding atherosclerotic development in mice based on the administration of chronic hyperglycemia. The research question might be "Is oxidative stress (which accelerates atherosclerosis) greater in hyperglycemic mice?" If the answer to that question is yes, those findings may be confirmed in large, non-randomized cohort studies. Following these studies, researchers may finally explore this relationship at the level of a randomized controlled clinical trial (RCT), testing how an intervention (*e.g.*, drugs, exercise programs, etc.) alters subsequent risk. Here, the question might be "Does a low-carbohydrate diet reduce the incidence of atherosclerosis in overweight, pre-diabetic patients?"

Although there are differences in how these two questions are answered (*e.g.*, how the data are gathered, which analyses are appropriate, the methods by which findings are reported, etc.), as well as the consequences of error, they are fundamentally linked. The answer to one question facilitates the design of the next research effort.

Between the base and apex of the pyramid are a variety of research modes. When a novel question is devised, the first human studies are generally accomplished by "epidemiologic surveillance." Epidemiologic surveillance is a form of observation that occupies four levels of the hierarchy: case studies, cross-sectional studies, case-control studies, and cohort studies.

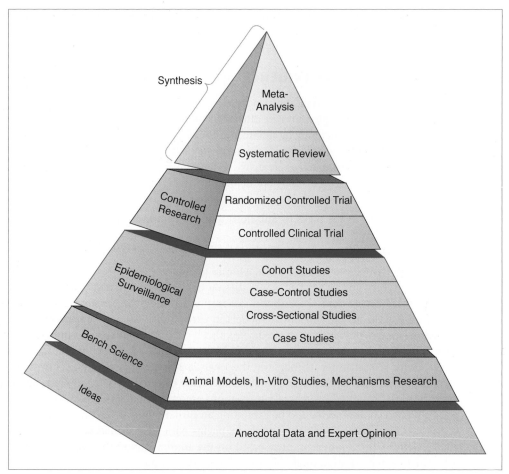

FIGURE 6-1: The hierarchy of clinical evidence, shown here as a pyramid, illustrates the diverse modes of quantitative research. It is more than a ranking system, grading the methodologic and statistical rigor of the various study types; it reveals the sequence by which research questions are answered. One must begin at the foundation and work toward the apex. In doing so, the results of one type of investigation should help guide the design of the next.

Continuing to review Chapter 5, a case study seeks to describe or explain phenomena by analyzing a person, a group of people, an institution, an event, etc., within a real-life context (18). Believed to be introduced to the social sciences in 1829 by Frederic Le Play (9), case study methods can be prospective, but they are typically retrospective. A retrospective clinical case study might be completed on a patient with tendinopathy who experienced an effective therapy. In this example, the report would provide a detailed description of the patient, the pathology, the treatment (both its components and its application), and the results. Such reports may function as the impetus for further research.

Earlier case studies are cross-sectional studies. A cross-sectional study is a snapshot of an entire population at a given time aimed at describing a specific feature of that population. For example, what is the current prevalence of diabetes among primary education teachers in Minnesota? A cross-sectional study could provide absolute and relative risks of diabetes among this population. Although cause-and-effect is lacking, these data help illustrate the magnitude of a problem and can provide incentive for further investigation.

Earlier cross-sectional studies are case-control studies. The case-control study is similar to the cross-sectional study, but the researchers identify two distinct groups (*e.g.*, smokers and non-smokers) and compare them in regard to a specific outcome variable (*e.g.*, prevalence of lung cancer). Case-control studies are practical in a variety of circumstances. In the present example, it would be unethical to recruit a sample of healthy, non-smoking adults, randomly assign 50% of them to a pack-a-day smoking intervention, and track incidence of lung cancer. However, the epidemiologic data already exist and can be evaluated with a case-control study, which may be the only means available to answer such questions.

Another advantage of the case-control study is the promptness with which results can be produced. If it were ethical to assign healthy adults to a smoking intervention, it would likely take decades to conduct the experiment. Contrarily, it may only require a period of months to collect and analyze the epidemiologic data. Lastly, the results of a case-control study can also be used to validate the need for a controlled experiment.

The last step between epidemiologic surveillance and controlled research is the cohort study. In a cohort study, the researcher identifies a risk factor (*e.g.*, obesity is a risk factor for type 2 diabetes) and follows a group of people who exhibit that risk (*i.e.*, a cohort) but do not yet have the illness or disease with which it is associated. After a period of observation, the researcher estimates the absolute risk of contracting the particular disease based on the presence of the identified risk. The use of longitudinal observation helps eliminate errors such as subject recall that may compromise the findings of a cross-sectional or retrospective case-control study.

Once a research question has been explored with regard to the potential of animal and observational models, the initial scientific cartography has probably been outlined. At this point, the researchers should know enough about the relevant terrain to begin asking questions that can be explored (safely and ethically) with controlled clinical trials. It is, however, prudent to begin clinical trials with one or more pilot studies to better establish the question and direction of the full clinical trial that follows.

In a controlled clinical trial, subjects are recruited according to specific criteria (inclusionary and exclusionary). If they meet the eligibility requirements, they are assigned to one of multiple interventions. Examples might be:

- Drug A versus drug B
- Drug A versus placebo
- Drug A versus drug B versus placebo
- Drug A versus drug B versus exercise versus control group

After group assignment, the conditions of the experiment are controlled such that extraneous effects are minimized in order to isolate the true effect of the treatment throughout the duration of the trial. Controlled clinical trials, if properly conducted, are the only type of experiment that can extrapolate cause and effect. The only known way to avoid bias generated by factors beyond the researchers' control in such trials is by incorporating randomization into group assignment.

Regarded as the "gold standard" of research methods, the RCT attempts to eliminate biases by employing randomization strategies designed to distribute the known (as well as unknown) subject features evenly throughout the groups. The data from these studies are least likely to be biased by factors and events beyond the control of the investigators. For this reason, one should be much more comfortable knowing, for example, that a medication has been shown to produce a beneficial effect in an RCT of human patients than a theorized benefit based on studies in mice or observational data. Despite this, a research question cannot begin with an RCT design. Research is a process, and that process requires a careful framing of each question. And this framing begins at the base of the hierarchy, hurdling upward only as propelled by findings.

The apex of the pyramid is the synthesis of prior clinical research through systematic review and meta-analysis of existing data. These are not experiments in themselves but summaries and summations, aggregates of multiple studies. In a meta-analysis, the researcher mathematically analyzes the pooled data from a collection of studies, comparing and contrasting their findings and sometimes finding relationships that only emerge in the context of the larger pool. Although the systematic review does not rely on the same quantitative techniques, it is not simply a review of the available literature. It is an effort to find and analyze existing data in a comprehensive, unbiased manner, conforming to best practices in research.

In both meta-analyses and reviews of the literature, unless the incorporated studies are flawed, such techniques provide the most precise estimates of the magnitude of a treatment effect. For the practicing clinician, evidence derived from systematic reviews and meta-analyses of RCTs offer the best information by which clinical decisions can be made. However, these syntheses cannot be conducted until enough data have been collected, validated, supported, and possibly overturned.

AIMING FOR THE CLINICIAN: THE BIOPSYCHOSOCIAL MODEL

When research is aimed at the clinician and the researcher focuses solely on human subjects, a **biopsychosocial model** of illness and injury offers a template by which questions may be framed (Fig. 6-2).

Any component of one's health and functioning is unlikely to be exclusively affected by biology, psychology, or social factors. Although the biomedical model of research relies on such reductionist principles, the biopsychosocial model presumes importance in evaluating these variables together.

For example, various forms of birth control may be 100% effective if used properly, but proper use depends on the diligence of the users. Therefore, if a particular mode of birth control demands greater user commitment, the Pearl Index (rate of effectiveness) might not reflect its biologic value (efficacy). Effectiveness in this case is based partly on user dependence, which cannot be accounted for with a strict assessment of biology. Conversely, a biopsychosocial model would be more inclusive of the factors influencing success rate. It is a more holistic evaluation of the phenomenon.

Within the context of sports medicine, use of the biopsychosocial model enables a broader evaluation of an illness or injury. If an athlete sustains a musculoskeletal injury, likely consequences are pain, possibly swelling, a loss of motion around the involved joint, and a loss of strength in one or more muscle groups. These impairments may result in functional limitations such as being unable to walk without an assistive device or raise an arm sufficiently to comb one's hair. In our example, the athlete is probably most concerned

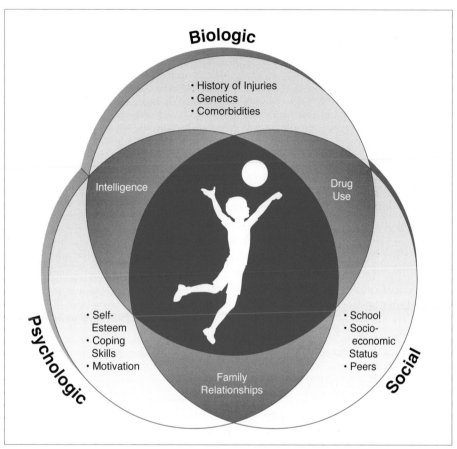

FIGURE 6-2: The biopsychosocial model of illness and injury shows how an athlete's recovery can be affected by biologic factors (*e.g.*, genetics), psychologic factors (*e.g.*, motivation), and social factors (*e.g.*, socioeconomic status) as well as the interplay between them.

with the inability to participate in his or her sport. For the sake of the example, our athlete will be a 16-year-old female volleyball player with patellofemoral pain syndrome. If an investigator wishes to study the most effective exercise treatment of this pathology, what are the data that should be collected?

Clinicians and other investigators may be interested in data generating a detailed biomechanical analysis, but the patient may only be interested in the likelihood that she will return to play given specific treatment options (*e.g.*, "You are twice as likely to return to play this season if you follow treatment option A."). In this sense, whether the athlete returns to play can be viewed as a dichotomous variable: "yes, she does" or "no, she doesn't." It is up to the researcher to figure out which data predict that outcome most accurately. This may involve demographic information (*e.g.*, age, gender, ethnicity, etc.), social and psychologic factors (*e.g.*, degree of motivation, injury-related depression, etc.), and physical variables (*e.g.*, history of injuries, severity of the present injury, etc.).

Another way of illustrating the biopsychosocial model as it applies to an injured athlete is represented in Figure 6-3.

Some of the variables that are important to an athlete's recovery may not be amenable to quantitative methods (*e.g.*, daily behaviors, certain psychosomatic phenomena, etc.) and would need to be explored by qualitative methods. Although typically employed by the social sciences, qualitative research is becoming more widely used in other disciplines, such as healthcare (17). In a qualitative approach, the investigator becomes the research instrument, observing the subjects without controlling or manipulating variables. The goal of this observation (which may also include interviews) is to learn about phenomena such as customs, motivations, and emotions in the subject's natural environment. Although the findings of qualitative research can be difficult to compare and contrast (or integrate in systematic reviews and meta-analyses), it offers data that may not be available through standard quantitative practices. Additionally, where possible, quantitative studies often trail qualitative pursuits in an attempt to provide empirical support for the conclusions drawn.

Regarding the physical variables that *are* readily quantifiable, information about pain, force development, and gait mechanics could advance understanding of the most effective treatment. However, increasing quadriceps muscle strength might not improve a patient's ability to ascend or descend stairs. Continuing forward, improved function might not translate to restoration of the ability to play competitive volleyball, which is not only the chief concern of the athlete but an important aspect of her quality of life. Before designing the study, the researcher must decide on what part of the puzzle he or she wishes to focus. This decision will dictate the question posed, which will define the methods used, which

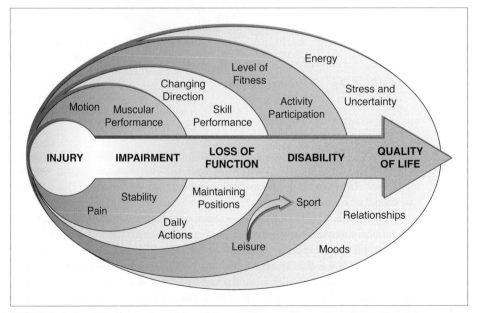

FIGURE 6-3:   The biopsychosocial model can be illustrated in a variety of ways. Here it is seen as a continuum, beginning with an injury and spanning the various consequences of that injury: the degree of pain and impairment, the loss of functioning and athleticism, the amount of disability, and, ultimately, how the quality of life is affected.

will alter the data generated, which will determine the appropriate analytic approach. In this case, if the researcher chooses to evaluate severity of pain, those data are likely to be managed differently from force data.

Once an investigator knows which data are to be collected, only then is it possible to design a study and articulate the precise methods needed to establish likelihood and odds ratios that are meaningful to the patient.

Although this would be an appropriate circumstance to employ the biopsychosocial model, its use is not limited to odds of patient recovery. Another practical use could be in testing responses to different resistance training programs. In this situation, the need to collect force data is obvious. However, if the training programs are intended for application in football linemen, then new questions emerge. Would an increase in force generating capacity measured on a dynamometer translate to improved function while running or during push-off? Furthermore, does improved push-off translate to better on-field performance? Each of these questions would require different methods to answer.

If you are reading this book, you likely value physical activity and sports. For us, physical activity is an important part of our lives and contributes strongly to our quality of life. Quality of life is an overarching theme in a biopsychosocial model, but it is a multifaceted construct. Consider the wheelchair-bound athlete. Despite impairments and losses of function, these athletes often compete at very high levels and lead quality lives. Thus, it becomes evident that the associations between impairments, losses of function, athletic participation, and quality of life are not linear. And each of these elements is worthy of independent study.

However, investigations across the whole span of a biopsychosocial model are likely to be limited by time, costs, and logistics. For this reason, it is important for us as researchers to remain humble when reporting our findings. We must maintain a sense of proportion as we allow our results to be mapped onto the bigger picture. How do our data concerning quadriceps strength or the severity of pain, for example, relate to what is known about other biologic, psychologic, and social predictors of a particular mode of therapy?

Furthermore, as consumers of research, we must be cautious not to interpret a "significant" change in one of these measures as sufficient evidence to predict an outcome. In this case, within the context of a particular study design, quadriceps strength may be a significant predictor of our volleyball player's recovery. However, there are many more variables that are likely to impact her physical functioning, athletic performance, or quality of life. Some of these variables we may already know; others we don't.

As we develop our scientific understanding, new findings must always be scaled with what is already known and what is still left to know.

DEFINING THE VARIABLE

The spectrum of questions of interest in research spanning bench to bedside yield multiple types of measurement and data. Within disciplines, the labeling of data can have important meaning. Biomechanists, for example, understand the differences between measuring kinetics and kinematics. There is a broader and convenient way to categorize data that has important and useful applications. To review Chapter 5, data can be labeled or categorized as "nominal," "ordinal," "interval," or "ratio." The type of data guides many of the decisions as to how the data are best analyzed.

Recall that nominal data are generated when investigators identify named groups by numbers. For example, one might code political affiliation by assigning a 1 to Democrats, a 2 to Republicans, and a 3 to Independents. Such coding allows for data to be analyzed using computer software but the values are of no importance. One could just as easily label Independents with a 0, Republicans with a 1, and Democrats with a 2 as long as they recalled the coding scheme. Ordinal data differ in that the assigned values convey some order. If one were to capture patient satisfaction data using a Likert scale code of 1 = strongly disagree, 2 = disagree, 3 = agree, and 4 = strongly agree, one would change the result if 3s were coded as 2s and vice versa.

Interval data are similar to ordinal data except that the magnitude of differences between values has meaning. The degree of conviction between "strongly disagree" and "agree" is unknown and may differ from that between "agree" and "strongly agree." However, if one were studying core body temperature, it is known that the difference between 98 and 100 degrees is of the same magnitude as that between 102 and 104 degrees. Ratio data are similar to interval data except that meaningful ratios can be formed because an absolute 0 exists.

One important distinction is that nominal and ordinal data are analyzed using nonparametric methods, whereas interval and ratio data are most commonly analyzed with parametric statistical procedures. The "parameters" in question are calculated mean scores and estimates of variance around those scores. Because the values assigned to nominal data are arbitrary, it is not possible to calculate a mean that can be interpreted. Ordinal data does not permit the calculation of variance estimates because the magnitude of difference between points is unknown.

The procedures used to analyze various types of data are discussed in greater detail in subsequent chapters, but there is an association between a biopsychosocial model and the types of data generated. Data related to impairments such as volume of swelling, strength loss, and joint motion are usually analyzed using parametric procedures assuming that data are fairly normally distributed and the variance around the mean in each group is similar. Function data may be ratio (time to climb 10 steps), ordinal (unable, with great difficulty, with difficulty, with little difficulty, without difficulty), or even nominal (can climb 10 stairs without assistance or not). The measurement and thus the analysis are determined after the purpose of the work is established. Measures of participation are much more likely to generate nominal and ordinal data. In many cases, these data are of greater interest to and more focused on the patient. The patient is likely to want to know his or her chances of returning to work or playing a sport at some future time. These outcomes may by dichotomous (nominal), where the probability or odds of an outcome are of great interest. The research consumer will encounter all types of data and multiple approaches to data analysis. It is important that the measurements used are appropriate for the question being asked and the data generated be analyzed and reported in a clear and meaningful manner.

DESIGN/APPROACH

The approach one takes in designing a study is affected by many considerations. In cases in which a considerable body of previously published data exists, investigators may seek clarity by conducting a systematic review of the literature and using meta-analytic methods to answer the research question. If few data exist to address the entirety of a question, then new data must be generated. The need for new data collection can be ascertained by considering whether (a) the specific population has been studied, (b) the specific intervention has been studied, and (c) the specific outcomes measures have been acquired. If the answer to one or more of these areas is "no," then research must develop new data to answer the question of interest.

Take, for example, the question, "Does transcutaneous electrical nerve stimulation (TENS) benefit patients with knee osteoarthritis?" The investigator must consider the population from which a sample might be drawn. For example, would a patient with grade IV knee osteoarthritis (OA) (severe) respond in the same manner as a patient with less severe joint degeneration? Or would a younger patient whose arthritis is linked to a traumatic knee injury respond in the same manner as an overweight 70-year-old? The investigator must also consider the specific treatment rendered and the outcome of interest. Might the specific parameters of TENS use affect outcome? Is the primary interest immediate pain relief or a more global assessment of knee function over time?

Assuming sufficient data are not available to permit meta-analysis of existing data, a new study must be developed. As noted earlier, an RCT is considered to provide stronger evidence than cohort and case series designs. In an RCT, the investigator has more opportunity to control for factors that threaten the validity of the data. Choosing to conduct an RCT, however, should not be done without careful consideration. In some cases, principles of ethics and equipoise preclude a randomized controlled design. One might, for example, ask, "Do statin medications increase the risk of musculoskeletal injury in people with physically demanding jobs?" Because these medications are known to protect against cardiovascular events in people with high cholesterol, it would not be possible to randomly assign some patients to receive a placebo medication. It would also not be reasonable to provide real and placebo medication to subjects who do not need to take statin medications solely to answer a question related to musculoskeletal injuries.

In this case, the question is best addressed through a study of cohorts. One might look at data retrospectively where the health records of workers taking statins are compared to peers not taking medication and matched to the greatest degree possible on factors such as gender, age, body composition, and job demands. Such data exist and thus an answer might emerge in a timely manner. When data are managed retrospectively, factors that affect the events of interest but are not recorded can bias the conclusions drawn from the analysis. An alternative is to work prospectively using a matching strategy while capturing complete records of factors associated with injury. The downside to such an approach of course is that the results will emerge over a long period of time.

Cohort designs may also yield greater external validity. Consider the study of TENS use in patients with knee OA. This intervention is likely one of several that a patient is exposed to in the management of his or her condition. Oral medications, injected medications, exercise programs, and bracing are also available options for the patient and his or her physician. Although it would be possible to study TENS in an RCT design and introduce a convincing placebo, it could be difficult to control for the effects of other treatments unless patients were carefully matched. Even if such a feat could be accomplished, an interaction between treatments (*e.g.*, TENS is most helpful in those patients who perform resistance or aquatic exercise three times per week) may still bias data used to answer the research question. In such a case, it might be better to perform a cohort study that compares patients "exposed to TENS" in their treatment to those who were not and use a Bayesian approach to data analysis. In a Bayesian approach, rather than exploring phenomena at the population level, analyses focus on the individual: What is the probability that an individual will achieve a particular result? In the present example, how likely is it that an individual patient will experience satisfactory pain management without gastrointestinal symptoms? These probabilities are compared between groups; which group gives patients the better likelihood of success? Such a study conducted in the course of routine clinical care might be more "ecologically sound" or have greater external validity.

In some cases, the best research strategy is to complete a case series. Seiger and Draper (16) studied the combination of therapeutic pulsed diathermy and joint mobilization on ankle range of motion in a series of patients with longstanding motion loss caused by fracture and/or dislocation. The use of pulsed diathermy in the presence of surgically implanted metal had not been extensively explored. This case series provided evidence of safety and the effectiveness of a new treatment for motion loss. Motion loss is of significant concern following such injuries, but the novelty of the intervention and the limited number of patients with the extent of motion loss treated precluded beginning with a larger study. Although an RCT could be used to compare actual and placebo intervention, it could take years to complete. Moreover, because the risk involved in the intervention was to some extent unknown, the case series limited the number of patients exposed while providing a foundation for wider study of a novel treatment (16).

Selecting a design for a study is more a process of compromise than is apparent on the surface. Investigators must weigh the availability of resources, access to population samples, and ethical principles among other factors in selecting a research study design. Although a systematic review or an RCT may yield stronger (least likely to be affected or biased by uncontrolled factors) data, such studies may not be possible or optimal. Investigators, however, should be expected to convey and defend the design decisions they make in a public reporting of results.

Before leaving the topic of study design, one more issue for consideration must be brought to light. We can be absolutely certain about very few aspects of life. Research in fact seeks to bring a sense of certainty by providing answers to important questions. However, the fact is that research is conducted on samples drawn from populations to make inferences about populations as well as the individuals making up those populations. We can neither be certain that a treatment associated with differences observed in a sample reflect population differences or that an individual from that population will respond like his or her peers. We must always be prepared to deal with uncertainty and the accompanying consequences.

UNCERTAINTY AND CONSEQUENCES

"In this world nothing can be said to be certain, except death and taxes" (a letter from Benjamin Franklin to Jean-Baptiste Leroy, 1789) (15). The passage of more than two centuries has not altered the truth in Franklin's words. Uncertainty is all around us, and it is the pursuit of "truth" or "proof" that drives research. Research yields data, but we are never sure that the data collected from a sample reflect the whole of the population from which the sample was drawn. This uncertainty led to the development of **inferential statistics** or analyses that permit researchers to estimate the probability that the data gathered are reflective of the population. To some extent, these processes manage the uncertainty inherent in research.

Uncertainty, however, is a messy subject. Consider cigarette smoking. The link between smoking and lung cancer is well known and widely accepted. More than 85% of lung cancer cases are attributable to smoking (19). However, fewer than 20% of people who smoke cigarettes develop lung cancer. In southwest England, the risk of dying from lung cancer among all lifetime smokers has been estimated to be 15.9% for men and 9% for women. If those lifetime smokers have spent their lives smoking more than 25 cigarettes a day, the risks rise to 24.4% for men and 18.5% for women (14). In Canada, lifetime risks for developing lung cancer among current smokers were 17.2% for men and 11.6% for women (20). At the population level, the link between smoking and an increased risk of developing lung cancer is approaching the certainty of death and taxes, but at the individual level, the fact that someone smokes does not assure the development of the disease.

In research, the issues of uncertainty and the consequences of being wrong can be considered from a number of perspectives. We have chosen three. First, we will discuss the **frequentist** approach to hypothesis testing. We then consider the magnitude of differences reported in our scientific literature, and finally, we address what research might mean to individual patients, athletes, clinicians, and coaches from a Bayesian point of view.

A frequentist approach to the uncertainties of research is founded in the work of R.A. Fisher (2). This perspective examines the frequency or probability that the results of an experiment would occur if the differences observed do not really exist in the population from which a sample was drawn. In this approach, an investigator will establish a **null hypothesis**. One might, for example, want to learn if the addition of a whirlpool bath before a program (*e.g.*, three times per week for 16 weeks) of cycling and resistance training is more effective at improving quadriceps muscle strength than the exercise program alone in patients with knee arthritis. The null hypothesis could read: strength gain following exercise + whirlpool = strength gain following exercise.

One would not expect the responses to be exactly equal, but the challenge is to determine if the differences observed can be attributed to the differences in treatment or the result of random events. Fisher recognized the need to repeat experiments before reaching conclusions. However, over time, investigators and consumers have focused on the results from single studies to make inferences about the effects of interventions. If we assume that the addition of the whirlpool bath was associated with greater strength gains, the question becomes do these differences reflect the results that would be obtained if all knee OA patients added a whirlpool bath to their exercise regimen? We attempt to answer this question through inferential statistical procedures (t tests, analysis of variance, etc.). Such analyses estimate the probability that the differences observed would occur if the addition of a whirlpool bath has no effect on strength gains. In this process, investigators choose the level of risk of being wrong about concluding that the differences observed can be attributed to the treatment. By convention, investigators generally accept the risk of being wrong five in 100 times, and we see indications of this when $\alpha = .05$ or $P = .05$ is written.

First, the established risk of being wrong is wholly arbitrary but should be driven by consideration of the consequences or error. If an intervention is costly or risky, greater certainty of benefit is required before making recommendations. In such a case, an investigator may only be willing to accept a risk of being wrong one in 100 times ($\alpha = .01$). On the surface, it would seem logical to minimize the risk of concluding that differences observed reflect "real" differences in error. However, by reducing this risk, which is known as making a type I error, a new risk emerges. If an investigator is not sufficiently certain that the differences observed are due to differences in treatment, they risk type II error. In this case, the null hypothesis is not rejected despite the fact that real differences would emerge if the entire population were studied. In this case, promising interventions may be dismissed denying advances in, for example, healthcare or performance training. One never knows if a type I or type II error has occurred until repeated experiments are completed that confirm or refute previous conclusions. This uncertainty and the associated consequences are unavoidable.

Magnitude of Effect

Not only is uncertainty not fully mitigated through inferential statistical analyses, it is often exacerbated. We attribute much of this problem to the use and misuse of the word "significant." It is not uncommon to read that investigators found "significant differences" between groups, suggesting a benefit of an intervention being studied or read about the "significant findings" of a study. The statistical meaning of significant is that the probability that a type I error has been committed is lower than the risk the investigators were willing to take. The word does not imply that the differences observed were of a magnitude worthy of attention. Reports of significant differences are typically accompanied by mean and standard deviation values as well as the mean difference found between groups. Although these data are valuable, two issues warrant consideration. These values are that of samples drawn from a population and in fact point estimates of a population phenomenon. If additional samples were drawn, each would differ in the calculated mean and standard deviation. Thus, we are never certain as to the precise magnitude of effect of the interventions studied. The reporting of confidence intervals can address this uncertainty, but before moving to that discussion, also consider that if the variation in the effect of a treatment between people is normally distributed, one-half of the population will experience less than average benefit. The importance of a finding cannot be conveyed through the rejection of a null hypothesis or significant differences.

Increasingly, the certainty or uncertainty of the magnitude of an effect is being conveyed through the reporting of **confidence intervals** (CIs). These statistics provide a range in which the population value is believed to lie at a given level of certainty. A 95% CI of mean differences provides knowledge (with 95% certainty) as to where a population mean difference may lie. Consider the CI depicted in Figure 6-4. The center line represents no difference between groups or a mean difference equal to 0. Line "A" lies to the right of center and does not include 0. Thus, there is 95% certainty that a mean difference exists. This is equivalent to rejecting a null hypothesis with a 5% risk of type I error. The line, however, suggests that the magnitude of difference is quite small and below a level considered "important." What is considered important is a qualitative judgment that is dependent on the nature of the measures used to acquire data and the consumer's view of what is important and/or values such as minimally clinically important differences. In any case, line A represents differences between group means that are "statistically significant" but *almost* certainly too small to be of importance. Line B also represents statistically significant differences, but there is now near certainty that the magnitude of the mean difference is of importance. Line C represents "non-significant" differences and near certainty that any real difference is too small to be of interest. Lines D and E introduce greater uncertainty. Because the CI represented by line D does not include 0, it corresponds to statistically significant differences. However, the broad CI reveals that the real population differences may be trivial in magnitude or rather important. More data (increased statistical power) are needed to narrow the estimate of the effect of the intervention studied. These findings are possibly important, and that is the strongest conclusion that should be drawn. Now, consider line E. The CI includes 0, and thus the results of an analysis would not permit rejection of the null hypothesis. However, is there any less certainty regarding the mean difference in the population conveyed in line E than line D? The upper range of differences portrayed in line E is also quite possibly important, and once again, additional data are needed.

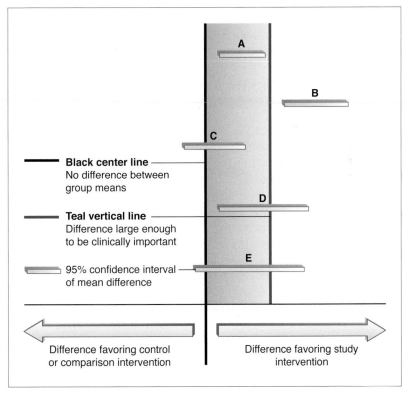

FIGURE 6-4: A CI is a range of possible values inside which the true mean is believed to lie and a level of certainty (or confidence) is statistically assigned to that belief. In this figure, group means following an intervention are shown. The *black vertical line* represents no difference between group means. The *teal vertical line* represents a clinically meaningful difference. Group A experienced a positive effect but not a meaningful one. Group B experienced a meaningful effect. Group C may have experienced a non-meaningful effect or they may have gotten worse. Group D experienced a positive effect, which may have been meaningful. And group E possibly got worse, possibly experienced nothing, and possibly experienced a meaningful effect.

Consider now how the scenarios depicted in lines D and E have been managed through a frequentist perspective and affected the sports medicine literature. Papers reporting significant differences have failed to address the magnitude of these differences and significance equated to importance. We have gotten excited about small, likely unimportant differences. Conversely, the failure to reject a null and report significant differences in findings has often caused those findings to be excluded from publication. Thus, efforts to be more certain about our sports medicine world may have actually misled rather than promoted certainty about our actions and beliefs.

INDIVIDUAL DECISIONS

The last element of uncertainty relates to individual responses. As noted previously, if mean differences or treatment effects are normally distributed, one-half of individuals will receive less than an average benefit. Moreover, many of the measurements performed in research yield data that is of little interest to an individual. Consider an avid tennis player with arthritis in a hip. This individual is not likely to be interested in the "average" pain relief obtained with a medication or range of motion gained with a therapeutic regimen. His focus is on whether he can resume tennis or not. The things that most interest individuals, especially individual patients, are outcomes of care that can often be simplified into either success or failure. The real clinical question is whether a particular plan of care improves the probability or odds of a successful outcome in comparison to an alternative intervention. Answering questions in this manner is associated with the teaching of **Thomas Bayes** and application of **Bayesian statistics**. Uncertainty is expressed on an individual level. Such an approach to research forces investigators to consider the outcome of intervention from the perspective of the individual client or patient. Issues of participation rather than impairment become the focus. A football player may be given 4:1 odds of returning to play after a particular surgery (80% probability). Conversely, without the surgery, the odds of returning to play may be 1:4 (20% probability). Uncertainty and consequences are placed on a personal level. If the athlete chooses the surgical option, only one in five do not achieve the desired outcome. Although there is no certainty that any individual would be destined for the success group, it is clear that the odds favor success if the surgical course of care is selected.

Research and data should inform decisions and make us feel more certain about the events in our lives. However, no single study will provide proof or certainty. Careful consideration of how data are analyzed and reported is necessary before allowing what we read and learn to dictate our decisions. Moreover, certainty is fleeting, and yesterday's fact is tomorrow's fallacy. Continued critical appraisal of the literature in our scope of work or practice is necessary to stay abreast of the changing understanding of truth.

ANALYSES AND REPORTING

The type of analysis depends on the nature of the data collected and the question being asked. If the data are qualitative, the results will be reported through descriptions using natural language. If the data are quantitative, they are reported numerically, but the specific analysis employed, and the subsequent reporting of one's findings, must reflect the type of data (*i.e.*, nominal, ordinal, interval, or ratio).

Descriptive Statistics

As the nomenclature implies, **descriptive statistics** describe one's data, characterizing whole datasets. Measures of central tendency (*e.g.*, mean, median) and dispersion (*e.g.*, standard deviation, range) should be reported for continuous (ratio and interval) and ordinal data, respectively. When reporting nominal data, the mode and frequency distributions should be reported.

The reporting of descriptive statistics should be consistent with the reporting of the results of the statistics of inference. For example, if the mean and standard deviation are reported, one would expect to see the results of t tests, or **analysis of variance** (ANOVA), ideally supported by CI. If such parametric procedures are not used because of violations of the assumptions prerequisite to these analyses, then it is appropriate to report median and range as measures of central tendency and dispersion. In these cases, **skewness** and/or **kurtosis** can be presented graphically.

When the purpose of research is to examine the relationships or correlations between variables, descriptive statistics should be used in conjunction with analyses that estimate the strength of the relationships.

For example, a strength coach wants to know which of two exercise programs will generate the largest improvement in vertical jump among high school basketball and volleyball athletes. He conducts an RCT that compares program A, which incorporates squat and dead lift exercises twice per week and plyometrics twice per week, with program B, in which the resistance exercises are only performed once each week. When writing the results, the following descriptive statistics would be important to the reader:

- How many athletes were assigned to each exercise program?
- What is the gender distribution of each group?
- What are the average age, body mass, and height of the athletes in each group?

These data (and any other relevant descriptive statistics) should be reported either in the methods section or in the results section of the paper.

Comparing Group Means

By comparing group means, a researcher can identify important differences in the outcomes of distinct groups. Continuing with the earlier example (the strength coach's evaluation of two different exercise programs), it is important for that coach to know the following information: (a) how the groups performed at baseline, (b) how the groups performed at the end of the study, (c) whether there were differences in improvement between groups, and (d) what, if any, moderating variables contributed to those differences (*e.g.*, Did males and females respond differently to either protocol?).

Because the jump height data are ratio, the measure of central tendency and dispersion for baseline, follow-up, and change are reported as mean $+/-$ standard deviation. To make inferences about the effect of the two programs on jump height performance in young basketball and volleyball players, ANOVA would be used for analysis, assuming the distribution of the data met the prerequisite assumptions for parametric analysis (chiefly that the values are random samples drawn from a normal distribution and that they have homogeneous variances).

The type of analysis that is appropriate for ordinal data is different from ratio, as ordinal data can be counted and ordered but otherwise have no objective numeric basis. As we stated earlier, variance estimates cannot be calculated because the magnitude of difference between points is unknown. As an example of ordinal statistics, the strength coach might develop a questionnaire that asks his athletes how satisfied they are with the exercise program to which they were assigned. Possible responses include very satisfied, somewhat satisfied, not satisfied, and very unsatisfied. In presenting the findings of such data, central tendency would be evaluated using mode (most common response) and range (difference between extremes; the lowest value subtracted from the highest value). Also, because these data are ordered, the 50th percentile (median) could be calculated.

With nominal data, a median cannot be calculated, as there is no order of responses. An example of nominal data involves the types of injuries that can be expected in the coming year. To investigate this, the strength coach may give a questionnaire to his athletes, asking for injury histories with checkable boxes next to options such as traumatic knee injury, ankle sprain, stress fracture, concussion, heat exhaustion/stroke, etc. When all data are collected, the mode, frequency (total number of each response), and relative frequency (proportion of responses corresponding to each injury) should be reported. These data can also be displayed graphically with a bar chart or a pie chart, but parametric statistics cannot be conducted.

In the place of parametric analyses, there are non-parametric methods that can be used to test group differences. Group median values can be compared with one of several statistical tests, which correspond to methods used to analyze continuous data. The comparison of medians from independent groups can be completed with a Mann-Whitney U, whereas a researcher testing more than two groups would likely select a Kruskal-Wallis one-way ANOVA. Repeated measures can be analyzed using a Friedman two-way analysis by ranks. Detailed explanations of these statistical procedures are provided in statistical texts. One of our favorites is *Biostatistics: A Foundation for Analysis in the Health Sciences* (10th edition) by Daniel and Cross (6).

One limitation in the analysis of ordinal data is the lack of a "mixed" model where differences between groups can be analyzed over repeated measures. Thus, it is not uncommon to see some data which are technically ordinal (*e.g.*, pain measured on a 0–10 visual analog scale) analyzed with parametric procedures. This is a topic beyond the scope of this chapter but worth noting. First, the reader should not be alarmed when this situation is encountered in the literature, and second, it should be appreciated that, despite appearing prescriptive and perhaps rigid, statistics is a discipline in which absolutes are uncommon.

Chi-square is a non-parametric test which can be used to compare differences between two groups of ordinal or nominal data. Instead of comparing differences between the group means (only possible in parametric tests), chi-square determines whether the sample *proportions* of those two groups differ significantly. The researcher typically displays the raw values in a "contingency table" and tests the null hypothesis (that the proportions of the groups do not differ significantly). Significance in a chi-square test implies that the observed difference in proportions of responses between the groups is greater than would be expected if those groups were drawn from the same population. Just like parametric tests, the validity of a chi-square is based on specific assumptions being met (chiefly that samples are randomly drawn, the measured variables are independent, categories used in the analysis are mutually exclusive, and frequencies are sufficient in size).

Bayesian Approach

Categorizing success and failure can yield important nominal data. Success at returning to sport or work following injury, or reporting substantial or complete relief following a treatment, provides valuable information to guide healthcare. Such nominal data could be analyzed using a non-parametric test (chi-square) to examine the association between an outcome and an intervention. For example, one might find that performing eccentric rather than concentric calf exercise is "significantly" associated with recovery from Achilles tendinopathy. Such information is useful at the population level, but not all athletes suffering from Achilles tendinopathy recover following a regimen of eccentric calf exercises, and some who do not perform these exercises have full resolution of their symptoms. A **Bayesian approach** to data analysis is principally concerned with the probability that an *individual* will respond to treatment rather than being concerned with a population phenomenon. Rather than using non-parametric tests to analyze proportional differences between samples, risk or odds ratios are generated.

Probability and Odds

Probability (*i.e.*, the fractional likelihood of an event occurring) is a ratio calculated by the number of favorable outcomes divided by the total number of possible outcomes. For example, if someone were to flip a coin twice with the goal of getting heads on both flips, the probability would be the number of favorable outcomes (one: heads-heads) divided by the total number of possible outcomes (four: heads-heads, heads-tails, tails-heads, and tails-tails). The probability is thus 1/4 or a 25% chance. If there are multiple favorable outcomes, the numerator must be adjusted to reflect that. For example, the probability of randomly selecting an ace out of a full deck of cards is 4/52 or 1/13.

Odds is a ratio between probabilities. The odds in favor of an event occurring are calculated by the probability that the specified event will occur divided by the probability that it will not occur. For example, the odds that two flips of a coin will yield two consecutive heads are 1/4 against 3/4 or 1:3. The odds that an ace is drawn randomly out of a 52-card deck is 4/52 against 48/52 (*i.e.*, 4 against 48) or 1:12.

The risk ratio (probability/probability, also called "relative risk") provides an estimation of risk relative to exposure. For example, what is the relative risk of developing lung cancer among current smokers? The risk ratio would be calculated by dividing the probability of cancer among smokers by the probability of cancer among non-smokers. Another example would be risk of injury: What is an athlete's risk of injury relative to a non-athlete's? The risk ratio would be calculated by dividing the probability of an athlete sustaining an injury by the probability of a non-athlete sustaining an injury. Using our earlier example of the questionnaire that assessed risk of various injuries among high school athletes, if the same questionnaire was completed by non-athletes (control group), we could calculate a risk ratio. Let's assume the questionnaire was completed by 200 students (100 athletes and

100 non-athletes), and the probability of injury among athletes was 12 out of 100, whereas the probability of injury among non-athletes was 3 out of 100. The risk ratio would be 12/3 or 4.0. Although probability yields a number between 0 and 1, risk ratio is interpreted relative to a value of 1, with numbers greater than 1 implying a higher likelihood compared to the control group. In the present example, athletes are at a higher risk of injury (four times greater) compared to non-athletes.

An odds ratio (odds/odds) estimates one group's odds relative to another. To calculate an odds ratio, one divides the odds of the interest group by the odds of a comparison group. In the previous example (athletes compared to non-athletes), the odds ratio would be 12:88 divided by 3:97, or 4.4:1.

Risk and odds ratios could also be conducted to compare men to women. Let's say 50 of the questionnaires were completed by males and 50 by females, male probability was 8/50 (odds of 8:42) and female probability was 4/50 (odds of 4:46). The risk ratio, comparing males to females, would be 4/1, whereas the odds ratio would be about 2.2:1. Among rare events, odds ratios provide an approximation of relative risk, but among common events, odds ratios can exaggerate discrepancies.

Before differences in risk and odds ratios can be asserted with confidence however, CI should be calculated. If the resulting CI includes the value of 1, then the differing probability or odds may just be the result of sampling error.

Measures of Association

Measures of association examine the relationships between variables rather than the differences between group means or medians. The most common measure of association is simple **linear regression** (also referred to as a "Pearson product moment correlation"). Here, a single explanatory variable is associated with a dependent or criterion variable. The statistical calculation is a "least squares estimator" in which a straight line is fit to the entire set of observations. The fitting of the line is based on minimizing the sum of squared residuals (*i.e.*, minimizing the vertical distances between all data points and the fitted line). The line's slope is the result of the correlation between the two variables, corrected by their ratio of standard deviations (Fig. 6-5).

Although learning about the relationship between a predictor (*e.g.*, quadriceps strength of community dwelling seniors) and a criterion measure (*e.g.*, time required to ascend 10 steps) is informative, it is important to recognize that measures of association do not establish cause and effect. It is also important to recognize that linear models underestimate the strengths of relationships when these relationships are nonlinear. For this reason, it is prudent for researchers to look at a scatter plot to help identify whether a curvature exists in the relationship.

When more than one predictor variable is included in an analysis, the process is called **multiple regression**. In a multiple regression, the relationship between several independent variables and a dependent variable is evaluated, and the results help substantiate one's answer to the question "what is the best predictor of . . . ?" For example, a researcher may be interested in figuring out what qualities of athleticism predict field goal percentage (FG%) among high school basketball players. Collected data may include bodyweight, age, sprint speed, mile time, bench press, vertical jump, reaction time, and a measurement of hand-eye

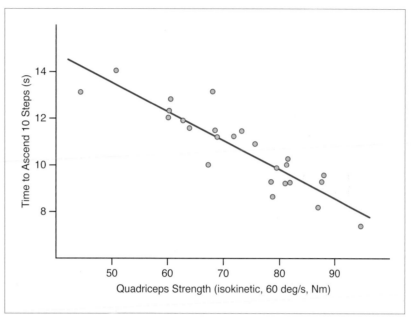

FIGURE 6-5:   In a hypothetical study among community dwelling elders, two variables were measured: quadriceps strength (independent variable) and time it takes to ascend a flight of stairs (dependent variable). A linear regression was conducted, fitting a line through 25 observations. The slope of the line indicates that stronger quadriceps strength predicts a faster time of assertion.

coordination. Once all of these data have been compiled for numerous athletes, one can calculate how well each of those variables associates with FG%, and graphs can be constructed displaying expected FG%, as it compares to observed FG%. Based on these data, the researcher may learn that vertical jump and endurance measures are better predictors than reaction time and coordination, or vice versa. In turn, such results may help a coach make statistically sound judgments about what training methods should be incorporated into practices. One important aspect of multiple regression is the ability to incorporate continuous, ordinal, and nominal data into a single analysis. Like other analyses, however, regression models require certain assumptions to be met. The assumption of normality requires the residuals to follow a normal distribution, whereas the assumption of linearity assumes the relationship between variables is in fact linear.

When measuring association non-parametrically, common statistical methods include Spearman rank correlation coefficient (or Spearman rho) and Cramér's V. Spearman rho, which measures statistical dependence (*i.e.*, relationship) between two variables (either continuous or discrete), evaluates how well that relationship can be described via monotonic function. In other words, the observations in each of the two samples are ranked in ascending order with duplicates being assigned an average value of their position. For example, if there is a tie for third and fourth places, each observation would be assigned a rank of 3.5. These two samples, now represented as ordered sets, are then compared to each other, testing to see if the relationship between their orders is preserved. The statistic generated (Spearman correlation coefficient) is based on what the dependent variable does in response to the increasing values of the independent variable. If it increases along with the independent variable, the correlation coefficient is positive. If it decreases as the independent variable increases, the correlation coefficient is negative. If it neither increases nor decreases, the correlation coefficient is 0. A coefficient of 1 implies a perfect monotonic relationship.

Lastly, Cramér's V is non-parametric method of measuring association; in this case, the association is between two nominal variables. It is calculated by dividing the square root of the chi-squared statistic by the total number of observations multiplied by the length of the minimum dimension (*i.e.*, number of rows or columns, whichever is smallest). A value of 0 implies no association between the variables, whereas a value of 1 corresponds to perfect association.

$$\text{Cramér's V} = \sqrt{\frac{\chi^2}{n \cdot \min{(K-1)}}}$$

SUMMARY

In the 17th century, the scientific method first reared its statistical head with a rudimentary practice known as "political arithmetic." This was a late Renaissance attempt to characterize demographic and economic data throughout Europe. After World War I, championed in part by Herbert Hoover, the distinction between basic and applied research was first made. Since then, the practice of research methods and the language of statistics have continued to mature, allowing Hoover's dichotomy to expand into a full continuum of practices that begins at the bench and ends at the bedside.

Today, research questions are often sparked by anecdotal data and expert opinions, after which, those ideas enter experimental methods at the level of animal models, in vitro studies, and mechanisms research. Investigations involving human subjects typically begin with empirical methods (*i.e.*, epidemiologic surveillance) before being tested by controlled research that systematically manipulates variables in an attempt to identify cause and effect. All of these levels of research fit into the larger picture known as the "hierarchy of evidence," and each level contributes uniquely to our understanding of the world around us.

No matter what type of investigation is being conducted, the researcher is faced with a similar set of challenges. First, a research question must be identified (with a specific purpose and end user in mind). This is a precise process which ultimately dictates the type of data that will need to be collected in order to pursue its answer. The nature of those data in turn determines the choice of statistical analysis. Once the analyses are complete, the interpretation of the results must be unbiased and their reporting must take into consideration the end user, communicating findings in a language that's appropriate to that audience.

When the research question is aiming for a clinical impact, the biopsychosocial model offers a useful template for study design, enabling illnesses and injury to be evaluated in a broader context. Any component of health and functioning is likely to be affected by a combination of biologic, psychologic, and social factors. The biopsychosocial model helps researchers assess these variables together, scaling single-study findings with the larger picture.

The data collected in pursuit of such a study can be categorized as nominal, ordinal, interval, or ratio. Nominal data are numeric labels for groups (*e.g.*, which sport is played). Ordinal data have similar numeric labels, but convey an order (*e.g.*, Likert scales). Interval data are also ordered but have quantifiable distances between values (*e.g.*, temperature). Ratio data are similar to interval data but for the existence of an absolute zero, which enables the formation of meaningful ratios.

The types of analyses conducted depend on the type of data collected. Interval and ratio data are most often analyzed with parametric methods, whereas nominal and ordinal data are analyzed using non-parametric methods. The parameters unavailable in analyses of nominal and ordinal data are mean scores and estimates of variance.

The type of data collected depends on the questions being asked, the overall purpose of the research, and the availability of existing data. If sufficient data are available, a meta-analysis might be warranted. If few or no data exist, a new investigation is needed. A number of considerations emerge to guide the design of new studies. Research may focus on one or more elements of the biopsychosocial continuum. The costs, risks, and availability of patients or subjects must be considered. An RCT is considered the strongest design, but the principles of ethics and equipoise, resource availability, and the desire to reflect real-world practice (as opposed to controlled laboratory environments) may preclude conducting an RCT. In other words, when selecting a study design, the researcher must also consider the availability of resources, access to the target population, and the desired balance of internal and external validity.

Even an RCT employing a strong methodology to minimize bias of the data (strong internal validity) does not inoculate research against uncertainty. One can never be completely sure the data collected from a single sample are an accurate representation of the population from which they were drawn. To cope with this uncertainty, we apply inferential statistics, which estimate the *probability* that the data collected accurately reflect the larger population.

Two philosophies to address uncertainty emerged separately over the past three centuries. These are labeled as frequentist (based on the work of R.A. Fisher) and Bayesian (based on the teaching Thomas Bayes). Frequentist statistics examine the probability that any differences observed in a dataset are simply the result of random chance. Although this offers information at the population level, it doesn't speak to individual probabilities. The Bayesian approach is more concerned with the individual's likelihood of experiencing a treatment effect or experiencing an event, relying on risk or odds ratios to communicate that information.

Clearly, there are a variety of ways in which data can be analyzed and outcomes reported. The optimal approach should be based on purpose of the work and the questions posed. Methodologic decisions must be based on the nature of the data, and the reporting of one's findings should reflect those decisions while also being mindful of one's audience or end user. Reporting "a significant improvement in an athlete's ability to return to play ($P < .01$)" is likely to be meaningless to the sidelined athlete and scarcely meaningful to the clinician. Odds and risk ratios, CIs, and other descriptions of effect size are likely to communicate the relevant information in a much more meaningful way. This chapter has provided a broad perspective of research in sports medicine. More detailed explorations of these issues are found in subsequent chapters and advance understanding of these often complex concepts.

GLOSSARY

Analysis of variance: a method of analyzing differences between group means. In statistics, "variance" describes the spread of a dataset (if the variance is zero, all data points are identical)

Bayesian statistics: a subset of statistics based on "Bayesian probability." Bayesian probability is a mode of evaluating propositions that makes room for belief and reasoning, not just frequency of the phenomenon occurring

Biopsychosocial model: a framework by which human health and disease is evaluated in terms of biologic, psychologic, and social factors (and the interplay between each)

Confidence interval: in statistics, a CI estimates a population parameter. After measuring a variable in a sample of that population and calculating the mean, one can create a range in which the true mean of the population is likely to fall. This range is the CI. Are you 99% confident the true population mean lies within a particular range? That's a 99% CI. Are you 90% confident? That's a 90% CI (which is likely to span a much broader range)

Descriptive statistics: a quantitative characterization of a particular set of information. Unlike inferential statistics, it does not seek to make inferences based on probability but merely to describe or summarize what exists (quantitatively)

Frequentist: the inferential alternative to Bayesian statistics; the framework that allows for the testing of a null hypothesis and the calculation of CIs

Inferential statistics: unlike descriptive statistics, which summarize and characterize information, inferential statistics make inferences about collections of data, testing predictions about the larger population based on the distribution of the collected sample

Kurtosis: when data are collected, the variance typically constitutes a bell-shaped distribution around a central mean. Kurtosis describes a quality of that curve: its peakedness (how wide or tall a particular peak is characteristic of the kurtosis)

Linear regression: a mathematical technique that determines the line that best represents the relationships between two variables (i.e., the line of best fit), plotted as data points on a scatter graph

Multiple regression: in statistics, a regression analysis estimates the relationship between variables (a dependent variable and one or more independent or explanatory variables). Typically, a single independent variable is manipulated to see how the dependent variable is affected. In a linear regression, there is only one independent variable; in a multiple regression analysis, there are multiple

Null hypothesis: a statistical starting point for most scientific investigations, stating that there is no difference between two measurable phenomena. Researchers then collect and analyze data so that they can either confirm or reject this hypothesis

Skewness: when data are collected, there is typically a bell-shaped distribution. If this distribution is asymmetric, that asymmetry is its skewness. The skew is generally either positive (tail on the right is larger than the left) or negative (tail on the left is larger than the right)

REFERENCES

1. Ackrill JL. *Aristotle the Philosopher.* Oxford, United Kingdom: Oxford University Press; 1981. 167 p.
2. Aldrich J. R.A. Fisher and the making of maximum likelihood 1912–1922. *Stat Sci.* 1997;12(3):162–176.
3. Benderly BL. Does the U.S. produce too many scientists? [cited 2010 Feb 22]. Available from: http://www.scientificamerican.com/article.cfm?id=does-the-us-produce-too-m
4. Best J. *Damned Lies and Statistics: Untangling Numbers from the Media, Politicians, and Activists.* Oakland (CA): University of California Press; 2001. 190 p.
5. Brotton J. *The Renaissance: A Very Short Introduction.* Oxford, United Kingdom: Oxford University Press; 2006. 160 p.
6. Daniel WW, Cross CL. *Biostatistics: A Foundation for Analysis in the Health Sciences.* 10th ed. Hoboken (NJ): Wiley; 2013.
7. Godin B. Measuring science: is there basic research without statistics? *Soc Sci Inform.* 2003;42(1):57–90.
8. Hart DM. *Forged Consensus: Science, Technology, and Economic Policy in the United States, 1921–1953.* Princeton (NJ): Princeton University Press; 1998. 286 p.
9. Healy ME. Le Play's contribution to sociology: his method. *Am Cath Soc Rev.* 1947;8(2):97–110.
10. Hogben L. (2003). *Political Arithmetic: A Symposium of Population Studies.* Vol 5. New York (NY): Routledge; 2003. 539 p.
11. Lazonick W. *American Corporate Economy: Critical Perspectives on Business and Management.* 1st ed. New York (NY): Routledge; 2002. 1648 p.
12. McKeen Cattell J. *American Men of Science: A Biographical Directory.* New York (NY): The Science Press; 1906. Available from: http://archive.org/stream/americanmenofsci01catt/americanmenofsci01catt_djvu.txt
13. National Science Foundation Web site [Internet]. Science and engineering indicators, 2008; [cited 2013 Aug 1]. Available from: http://www.nsf.gov/statistics/seind08/pdfstart.htm
14. Peto R, Darby S, Deo H, Silcocks P, Whitley E, Doll R. Smoking, smoking cessation, and lung cancer in the UK since 1950: combination of national statistics with two case-control studies. *BMJ.* 2000;321:323–329.
15. The Phrase Finder Web site [Internet]. Nothing is certain but death and taxes; [cited 2013 Aug 1]. Available from: http://www.phrases.org.uk/meanings/death-and-taxes.html
16. Seiger C, Draper DO. Use of pulsed shortwave diathermy and joint mobilization to increase ankle range of motion in the presence of surgical implanted metal: a case series. *J Orthop Sports Phys Ther.* 2006;36(9):669–677.
17. Souza PL, Romão AS, Rosa-e-Silva JC, dos Reis FC, Nogueira AA, Poli-Neto OB. Qualitative research as the basis for a biopsychosocial approach to women with chronic pelvic pain. *J Psychosom Obstet Gynaecol.* 2011;32(4):165–172.
18. Thomas G. A typology for the case study in social science following a review of definition, discourse, and structure. *Qual Inq.* 2011;17(6):511–521.
19. U.S. Department of Health and Human Services. *2010 Surgeon General's Report—How Tobacco Smoke Causes Disease: The Biology and Behavioral Basis for Smoking-Attributable Disease.* Atlanta, GA: Centers for Disease Control and Prevention; 2010. 704 p. Available from: http://www.cdc.gov/tobacco/data_statistics/sgr/2010/index.htm
20. Villeneuve PJ, Mao Y. Lifetime probability of developing lung cancer, by smoking status, Canada. *Can J Public Health.* 1994;85(6):385–388.

Experimental Design I— Independent Variables

Melinda L. Millard-Stafford, PhD, FACSM, Teresa K. Snow, PhD, and Gordon L. Warren, PhD

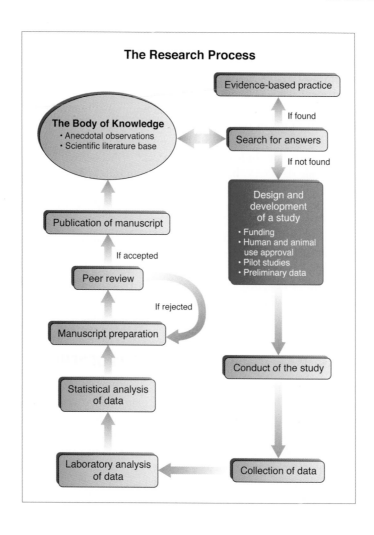

PLANNING THE RESEARCH DESIGN

Several noted historical figures (Benjamin Franklin and Winston Churchill) are credited with the quote, "If you fail to plan, you plan to fail." To "fail" in the domain of experimental research is to fall short of the intended objective of producing a study that adds to the body of existing knowledge on a topic. Research design is the process by which investigators determine how to answer their research question(s). Research is also often influenced by the investigator's knowledge of statistics. Countless well-intentioned studies are rejected outright by reviewers (and thus are never published in the public arena) for "fatal" fundamental flaws in research design. Flaws in the research design typically cannot be overcome with extensive editing or additional statistical analyses. As you learned in Chapter 6, statistics can help guide the ultimate decision of whether to accept or reject the null hypothesis; however, statistics cannot compensate for a bad design. The "file drawer" may be the ultimate outcome for research studies suffering from design flaws. Therefore, the importance of allocating the necessary time up front to develop a tightly focused research design is equally as important as the actual execution of the experiment itself.

Deliberate steps in planning the **research design** are encouraged for novice and experienced investigators alike. A well-designed plan will enhance the data analysis step of the experiment. The design should be as simple as practical. Although a simple design may limit the ability to generalize the research findings, it may increase the relevancy and focus the specific aims of the study. In many experimental studies within the exercise science field, the use of relatively small sample sizes (groups of 10 or less) is prevalent and often necessary for student projects as part of his or her degree program. In general, small sample sizes (*e.g.*, human subjects) require a more simplistic design in order to answer the research question. An essential part of identifying the most appropriate research design is to understand the "variables" and distinguish between those that are "independent" and "dependent."

By the end of this chapter, students should be able to distinguish between independent and dependent variables and identify extraneous variables that potentially impact research in exercise science. The need for specificity when defining key independent variables and how they might be designed through levels and types (within- vs. between-subjects) is presented. Finally, the difference between experimental research and other types (*i.e.*, quasi-experimental or non-experimental research) is also discussed.

IDENTIFYING VARIABLES: INDEPENDENT VERSUS DEPENDENT

The definition of a **variable** in research is some characteristic or factor that can have different values and is either subject to change or can be manipulated as a **treatment/intervention**. For experimental studies in exercise science, a researcher will often introduce a variable or factor into his or her design in order to elicit a change in another variable. Nearly any factor that can be measured in the laboratory or queried in a survey is a variable. The factor which is intentionally controlled or manipulated is termed the **independent variable**, whereas the outcome measure or attribute for which the researcher hopes to elicit an effect is termed the **dependent variable**. The independent variable can be a treatment (such as a nutritional supplement) or an intervention (such as an exercise training regimen) that the researcher imposes. For our purposes, we will use the terms "treatment" and "intervention" interchangeably in this chapter despite the classical definition that treatment stems from clinical studies examining the effects of a drug. There can be multiple levels (two or more) for an independent variable. The independent variable can also be a group classification that the researcher uses to evaluate a hypothesized difference (*e.g.*, to categorize based on sex, stratify by age ranges, etc.).

In contrast, the dependent variable is the presumed effect that is "dependent" on the differences in the levels of the independent variable. The dependent variable is the outcome or "what is measured" in the study. A known factor (independent) is thus controlled in order to examine the potential effects on the unknown (dependent variable). For example, to answer the research question, "Does carbohydrate ingestion improve endurance performance in elite cyclists," the investigator would implement a dietary treatment (carbohydrate and a placebo control) to determine if there is an effect on the dependent variable—endurance performance. However, there are other variables which also must be considered that could influence the dependent variable (endurance performance). These factors can be purposely controlled by making them a **constant**—a characteristic that has only one value in a study (such as gender or training status of subjects). Otherwise, the lack of control for such factors limits the interpretation of the results.

As a rule, the titles of published papers reflect the primary independent and dependent variables of an experimental study. Table 7-1 reflects selected examples. The independent variables are italicized, whereas dependent variables are in bold font. As suggested by these titles, there may be multiple independent and/or dependent variables. A single variable research design has a single independent variable, whereas a factorial design can accommodate more than one independent variable. Similarly, designs can be **univariate**, where only a single dependent outcome is measured, or **multivariate**, in which multiple dependent outcomes are examined simultaneously.

As listed in Table 7-1, researchers examined the effects of a catechin (green tea extract)-supplemented diet versus control diet on muscle inflammation and performance recovery in male mice (7). The independent variable has two levels of the treatment: catechin-supplemented diet versus control diet. There are several dependent variables: muscle inflammatory factors and measures of exercise performance. By keeping the diet constant in the two groups of mice (except for the addition of catechin in one group),

Table 7-1 Titles from Published Papers Reflecting Independent and Dependent Variables

Title	Reference
Effects of *ultrasound* and *stretch* on **knee ligament extensibility**	Reed et al. (2000) (12)
Metabolic and muscle damage profiles of *concentric vs. repeated eccentric cycling*	Penaililo et al. (2013) (11)
Catechins suppress **muscle inflammation** and hasten **performance recovery** after exercise	Haramizu et al. (2013) (7)

Independent variables are indicated in italics, and dependent variables are indicated in bold.

the experiment examines catechin's protective effect on tissue markers of muscle injury and run performance. Muscle injury is a conceptual dependent variable, which is concluded from measurements made on specific operational dependent variables (*e.g.*, changes in muscle enzymes in the blood and inflammatory measures extracted from the muscle).

Independent Variables: Levels and Types

Experimental designs can become more complex by adding independent variables or using multiple levels of a single independent variable (also known as a "factor"). For example, the previous study (7) might have further subdivided the independent variable (catechin supplement) into different doses of catechins or used male and female mice. If independent variable one (factor A) is treatment dose, multiple levels (*e.g.*, level 1—control, level 2—low dose, level 3—high dose) allow for the determination of a dose-response effect on the dependent variable. If factor B is sex (*e.g.*, two levels: male and female), whether catechin treatment

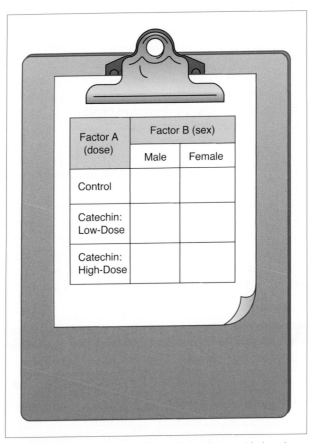

FIGURE 7-1:   Schematic of a two-factor design with three levels of factor A (dose of catechin) and two levels for the between factor B of sex (male or female).

and the sex of the mouse interact can be determined (*i.e.*, if the effect is different for male and female mice). Combining both of these independent variables yields a 3 × 2 factorial design to examine the interaction among the independent variables of catechin dose and sex. In Figure 7-1, each number indicates a factor (an independent variable) in the design and the number itself indicates the number of levels of that factor (catechin = 3; sex = 2).

If the change in response to catechins is the same for male and female mice, then there is no sex by treatment interaction, meaning both groups respond similarly. An interaction suggests the two groups do not respond in the same way. Statistics can also tease out if there is a main effect based on gender (*e.g.*, if across all levels of catechin dose, male mice responded higher or lower than female mice). Therefore, the effects can be analyzed for factor A (dose) across all mice and for male compared to female mice across all dosages. Finally, because the key independent variable is the level of catechin supplement versus control, if a significant difference is found, then the two dosages of catechin can be compared to control to determine if there is a dose-response effect (better run performance on higher dose than lower dose). The use of multiple levels within the independent variable provides additional insight into the findings of a study.

Between-Group or Within-Subjects Independent Variable

In addition to introducing multiple levels of an independent variable or multiple independent variables in designing a study, there are also different types of independent variables:

- **Between-group (or between-subjects) independent variable**: an independent variable in which a different group of subjects is used for each level of the variable
- **Within-group (or within-subject) independent variable**: an independent variable that is manipulated by testing each subject at each level of the variable

In the case of the latter (within-subject design), each subject serves as their own control group. This is known as a "repeated measures design," requiring more demands on the participant (performing all levels of the factor), but this yields in a powerful statistical design. Using the within-subject design reduces (a) the need to randomize subjects into groups (control vs. treatment) and (b) the sample size required to find an effect if one is present. To help further differentiate between "within" and "between" subjects, remember sex as an independent variable is always a "between-subjects" design. Table 7-2 represents how research might be designed with either a between-subjects or within-subject independent variable.

Table 7-2 Between-Subjects or Within-Subjects Independent Variable Research Design

Design	Independent Variable	Dependent Variable
Between-Subjects (2 groups × 8 subjects)	Catechin group (n = 8 subjects)	Run performance (minutes)
	Placebo group (n = 8 subjects)	Run performance (minutes)
Within-Subjects (8 subjects × 2 trials)	Catechin trial (n = 8 subjects)	Run performance (minutes)
	Placebo trial (n = same 8 subjects)	Run performance (minutes)

How does the researcher decide whether to use a within- or between-subjects design? There are advantages and disadvantages for each design to carefully consider. If multiple independent variables are used, it makes sense to design either the most important or the "noisier" variable (factor with greater variability in response) as within subjects. By doing so, the random variation due to subject variability should remain relatively stable across treatments. In the within-subjects example earlier, the total test time (number of trials conducted) would not differ, but the number of participants needed to meet eligibility would be less. Although the within-subjects design requires fewer subjects, it also takes place longitudinally such that the longer time period needed for a subject to complete the study, the greater the potential for other extraneous factors to influence the response. Moreover, the minimum time allowed between each level of treatment can also influence the results if there is potential for a residual effect from the previous treatment. For example, due to the "repeated bout protective effect," muscle damage might not occur to the same degree over time using a repeated measures design in a resistance training study. Therefore, if unclear whether residual treatment effects will "wash out over time" and return to baseline, a repeated measures design may not be appropriate. Alternatively, a factorial design with between-subjects factors may then be warranted (with appropriate subject selection techniques). Animal studies, like the one with mice previously discussed, frequently use between-subjects designs because genetically similar animals can be obtained and the environmental influences controlled.

Specific strategies can be implemented to prevent a treatment order effect (*i.e.*, differences occurring as a result of the timing of treatment administration rather than the treatment itself) when using a repeated measures design. A crossover design can be easily implemented when there are only two levels of the independent variable (half of the subjects receive one treatment first, and the other half get the second treatment first). As the number of levels in the independent variable increases in the within-subjects design, the order effect must be dealt with using other strategies (*e.g.*, **counterbalanced** or randomized order). In counterbalancing, the order of administrating A, B, and placebo (PLA) trials could be rotated across the subjects such that the presentation of trials has an equal number of times in the first, second, or third position, as illustrated in Table 7-3. However, depending on the number of subjects and trials, an equal "balancing" for order may not be possible. In that case, randomized order (*i.e.*, "drawing out of a hat") might be implemented to determine the trial order presented to subjects.

If using a between-subjects design, alternate approaches should be employed to ensure groups are similar. Random assignment to groups can reduce within group variability if the sample size is sufficiently powered. In the previous 3×2 design, this means six groups are required: (GRP1 = male/placebo, GRP2 = male/low dose, GRP3 = male/high

Table 7-3 Rotating Independent Variable Levels	
A first, B second, PLA, third	A first, PLA second, B third
B first, PLA second, A third	PLA first, B second, A third
PLA first, A second, B third	B first, A second, PLA third

PLA, placebo.

dose, GRP4 = female/placebo, GRP5 = female/low dose, GRP6 = female/high dose). If outliers (subjects whose response is far removed from the response of other subjects) are present, it can be difficult to find if a true difference exists. In some cases, matching as opposed to random assignment may be preferred. For example, when looking at a performance variable, the researcher may want to select subjects and assign them to groups in a way that matches them on fitness. This is another way to control for a variable that might influence results.

Defining the Independent Variable(s)

Understanding that an independent variable is the variable manipulated in a study is an important basic concept. However, how the independent variable is defined, controlled, and implemented in a study can be much more complex. First, it is necessary to distinguish between the conceptual versus operational definition of the independent variable. One can think of the conceptual variable as the "ideal" or a term that represents a broad domain. However, when deciding on the extent to which the variable can be manipulated and its effects measured, the definition must shift to that of an operational definition. Multiple operational measures could represent the domain and thus may differ from study to study. For example, if examining the effects of physical activity (PA) on blood pressure response, how is activity transformed into an operational definition (*i.e.*, total minutes of activity performed per week; weekly step counts; or just a description of the intervention frequency, duration, and intensity)? If a decision is made to use multiple levels (*e.g.*, low, moderate, and high PA), is there a standard definition based on the research literature that can be used as criteria for categorizing PA (or will the decision be arbitrary cut points)? Will the definition be influenced by the baseline characteristics of subjects that are selected?

In addition to establishing clear metrics for the operational definition of the independent variable, maintaining consistency of the treatment variable is critical. In fact, there is almost no such thing as too much control in planning the implementation of the independent variable. A lack of sufficient control reduces the chance of finding that the independent variable has a statistically significant effect (or requires more subjects to find an effect). Treatments should be administered in the same manner to all subjects. If studying the effect of heat treatment on recovery from muscle injury across several test sites, all sites should agree on the modality (*e.g.*, hot packs, ultrasound, immersion) and method (duration of heating vs. heating until reaching a set skin temperature). Inconsistencies in the treatment introduce variability, which creates issues (some unbeknownst to the researcher) that limit data analysis and interpretation.

To summarize thus far, an independent variable is intentionally "controlled" or "manipulated" in a research study in order to study an effect on the outcome or dependent variable. The dependent variable is simply what is measured or the outcome measure(s) of interest in a study that is presumably affected by the intervention (independent variable). A univariate research design uses a single independent variable, whereas multi-variable/factorial designs include more than one independent variable. It is important to control for confounding/intervening variables which could impact the results if not taken into account.

RESEARCH DESIGN DIMENSIONS: WHAT IS EXPERIMENTAL RESEARCH?

Research design can be divided into broad categories: non-experimental, quasi-experimental, and experimental. **Non-experimental** and **quasi-experimental research** can be retrospective (looking backward by collecting data or recording events which have already occurred) or prospective (looking forward by collecting new data or events that are forthcoming). Meanwhile, **experimental research** is always prospective. Non-experimental research in exercise science and sports medicine typically involves descriptive research (physiologic profiles of elite athletes or incidence of injury) or correlational studies (such as determining the association between body composition and metabolic rate). In theory, no category of research is inherently better than another. Although providing valuable information, descriptive and correlational studies lack the ability to implement true manipulation of variables (*i.e.*, control) that allows direct testing of the research hypothesis. For this reason, survey and correlational studies do not imply *causality*. Causality, by definition, implies that a change in the independent (manipulated) variable precedes and results in a change in the dependent variable.

Non-Experimental Research

Some non-experimental research appears experimental because the independent variable takes on several values within a study, or the independent variable appears to be a component of the dependent variable. For example, if examining the relationship between personal behaviors and the development of cancer, researchers could analyze medical files of patients who have been previously evaluated and look for similar characteristics in cancer patients that distinguish them from non-cancer patients. Although this retrospective research is examining differences in the dependent variable (cancer diagnosis) and the independent variables (health behaviors such as smoking, physical activity, etc.), the researcher can only use the data to form groupings based on factors that were measured to look for differences. Additionally, although the researcher may identify patterns in the data, the data itself from a retrospective study is usually collected for a different reason and may be incomplete or contain gaps that make it difficult to answer certain questions with a high level of confidence.

In order to make the same study prospective, the researcher might measure patients on baseline criteria (behaviors related to nutritional intake, exercise or physical activity level, etc.) that the researcher identifies as important to the disease and then follow the patients over time to monitor for cancer occurrence. The advantage is that the researcher is able to have more control over the data collected. In addition, they can develop inclusion/exclusion criteria to determine who is allowed in the study. Still, there is no actual intervention or manipulation of variables, and the study is descriptive in nature. Therefore, the design of the study is non-experimental.

What Makes an Experimental Design "Quasi?"

Experimental research may be subcategorized into "true" experimental and quasi-experimental design (Table 7-4). Quasi-experimental designs often closely resemble true experimental designs. If prospective, a quasi-experimental study may manipulate the independent variable

			Degree of	**Retrospective/**	**Emphasis on**
Design	**Primary Use**	**Randomized**	**Control**	**Prospective**	**Validity**
Non-Experimental	Description, examine relationships	No	Low	Can be either	
Quasi-Experimental	Causal inferences	No	Low/moderate	Can be either	External
True Experimental	Causal inferences	Yes	High	Prospective	Internal

Table 7-4 Overview of Research Design Dimensions

to determine an impact on a dependent variable; however, the quasi-experimental study is typically not as robust due to reasons such as lacking a control group or trial or failure to randomly assign subjects into intervention and control groups. In contrast, true experimental designs, often referred to as "randomized controlled trials," use random assignment to place participants into groups (*e.g.*, interventions and control) and use a control or "placebo" for comparison in order to manipulate an independent variable or variables to observe the effects on the dependent variable(s) of interest.

A quasi-experimental design is common, for example, when using a unique sample of subjects (*i.e.*, elite athletes) and reporting changes over time due to a training program or some other intervention. Unless there are sufficient numbers of subjects available to the investigator, it is difficult to randomly assign athletes to either a control or an intervention group. Thus, if simply collecting prospective data without a control group, the research would be quasi-experimental. If, however, the investigator is able to design the study so that each subject acts as its own control (*i.e.*, within-subject design) by receiving both the "experimental treatment" and the placebo or control, then the design is strengthened to experimental. Quasi-experimental designs are sometimes more appropriate for research conducted outside a laboratory in real-world settings. However, the analysis and interpretation of the results can be influenced by the setting. In these situations, random assignment may not be possible. Consider the following paraphrased abstract (13).

The purpose was to determine if girls in one school receiving counseling plus after-school physical activity intervention had greater improvement in physical activity, cardiovascular fitness, and body composition than girls assigned to an attention control condition in another school. Linear regression controlling for baseline measures showed no statistically significant group differences, but the directionality of differences was consistent with greater intervention group improvement for the dependent variables of interest.

In this example, two classes located at two different schools were studied. Because students were already assigned to a particular school and class, random assignment was not possible. One of the limitations with using intact groups is that one group may differ from the other initially on the dependent variable which could influence the study outcome. In this case, neither of the groups would serve as a good control for comparison. The authors note attempts were made to control for differences in baseline measures statistically in order to make the groups equivalent. Although this strengthens the study, as you've learned in previous chapters, random assignment would be considered the "gold standard" whenever viable. When subjects are randomly assigned to groups, statistical adjustments on pre-test measures are less likely to be needed. Any differences present in the groups are assumed to be due to random "chance" variation (model error). As sample size is increased, this variation should become more similar across groups. This idea of equal variance is an important assumption in many statistical models, and a violation of the assumption can lead to difficulties in data analysis.

Experimental Design

The key distinction between quasi-experimental and true experimental research lies in the level of control implemented to minimize variance. Sources of variance to be controlled in experimental designs primarily revolve around subject selection and their assignment as well as the manipulation of the independent variable(s) to reduce extraneous sources of influence on the results. Ideally, a large representative sample of subjects should be selected from the target population and randomly assigned to treatment/intervention and control groups (or control condition if using a within-subjects design).

Importance of a Control Group

The **control group** used in an experimental design may be a group that is measured at the same time points as the treatment group(s) but receives no treatment/intervention. In other situations, the control group may receive a "standard" condition that serves as a criterion. For example, if studying the effects of a novel drug on cancer, the control group would likely receive a treatment considered to be the standard of care. The group receiving the new drug would then be compared to the group receiving the standard treatment to determine if the newer treatment had added benefits over what is currently being used.

If using a within-subject design, all subjects receive the control or placebo condition in addition to the rest of the treatments. Placebos are also used in between-subject designs when one group of participants receives it instead of the real intervention of interest. The placebo is a dummy treatment that should not directly influence the dependent variable. A placebo is used to **blind** the participants when the researcher does not want participants to know who has been assigned to each study group or which treatment the participant is receiving. The purpose is to keep participants (single blind) and ideally both participants and study personnel (**double blind**) naïve to the study treatment so that the collection of the results and any preconceived notion participants (or researchers) have about the intervention will not influence the results.

Placebo Effect. It has been well documented that subjects receiving a placebo may perceive or show an actual benefit even though they are not receiving a treatment. This is known as the **placebo effect** and the results can be quite dramatic. In 2002, Eccles (5) reviewed eight clinical trials examining the effects of cough suppressant medication in patients with upper respiratory infections. The findings suggested that approximately 85% of the improvement related to cough suppression was due to the placebo effect, and only 15% was a result of treatment with an active ingredient. This effect has also been documented in studies involving human performance (3) for the power of a placebo for participants who were falsely informed that they were given anabolic steroids. Subjects demonstrated dramatic increases in strength compared to a baseline period of training. When using a "control" condition, it is important to carefully consider the type of placebo that might be used. In exercise science, if investigating the impact of carbohydrate drinks on exercise performance, a sugar-free, similarly flavored drink might be given (10) as the placebo. If, however, plain water is used as the control condition (9) or the participants can guess that the placebo is the fake treatment (the taste of the artificial sweetener can be easily distinguished), then the impact on performance may be questioned. This is particularly important in investigating ergogenic aids because athletes may already believe a substance will improve their performance and thus might have different motivation to give greater effort in exercise tests.

Hawthorne Effect. Another similar phenomenon that demonstrates the importance of having a control group is known as the **Hawthorne effect**. Evidence indicates that subjects may perform better simply by virtue of knowing they are being studied. This effect was coined by Henry A. Landsberger in 1950. Landsberger was examining earlier data from a study done by the Western Electric Company of Chicago, Hawthorne Works. The study examined a number of work conditions (lighting, number of hours worked, etc.) and its effects on worker productivity. One of the unexpected results was that workers seemed to improve simply by being involved in the experiment. The attention received caused the workers' productivity to increase regardless of the working conditions. After the study was completed, productivity decreased again (6).

These examples demonstrate that the control condition (placebo) or control group (group that is measured but does not receive the treatment) is an important part of experimental designs. It serves to partition out any impact on the dependent variable that might be influenced by participants' believing a condition will affect their performance or simply by being a participant in the study. By randomly assigning participants into intervention (or treatment) and control groups or using a randomized crossover design, the "true" experimental design should give a clearer picture of the effect of the intervention. These defining characteristics of an experimental design permit a better understanding of the actual treatment effect and whether the results support the use of the treatment. Like the quasi-experimental design, independent variables are manipulated to observe an effect but are designed to control for confounder variables that are not studied but can influence the study outcome. Additional discussion on controlling these extraneous variables and selection of subjects will follow.

Selection of Subjects: What to Consider

The investigator should carefully consider what the study population will look like and how the experiment might impact the specific group of participants recruited and screened for selection. Moreover, the process to obtain a representative sample from the potential pool of all possible participants deserves specific attention in order to be as free from potential sources of **bias**. For example, it is common for undergraduate and graduate student investigators to recruit other fellow college students or acquaintances based on convenience; this leads to samples that are not representative of the general population at large across a number of factors (*e.g.*, level of education, socioeconomic status, age, etc.). This may potentially influence the primary dependent variables of interest; consequently, the ability to draw large-scale conclusions would be limited. Thus, the ability to improve the retention of recruited subjects (by using a convenience sample) should be weighed against the strength of obtaining a more diverse and representative sample. The degree to which the sample represents the population of interest influences the power of the study. **Power** is defined as the ability to reject the **null hypothesis** (that no differences exist) and retain the **alternate/research hypothesis** (that differences do exist) when the research hypothesis is actually true. Because this is the key purpose of conducting research, having adequate power is critical. Power is determined by the effect or difference the researcher is trying to measure and the size of the sample chosen. Power calculations should be implemented in the research design to determine how many subjects are needed.

Inclusion and Exclusion Criteria. The researcher must determine the major criteria for a participant to qualify for selection into his or her study. These stated subject characteristics are known as **inclusion criteria**. As presented in Table 7-5 as a theoretical study aimed for the Department of Defense, inclusion criteria often specify an age range, gender, and health status. A mandatory criterion is that all participants must provide written informed consent as dictated by the institutional review board (IRB). In terms of age limits, an IRB might rely on *ACSM's Guidelines for Exercise Testing and Prescription*, 9th edition (2), to dictate the safety of including older persons to perform maximal treadmill testing without a physician present. Research studies on men only are increasingly difficult to justify for both an IRB

Table 7-5 Examples of Potential Pre-Screening Criteria for Participant Inclusion/Exclusion for a Study

Inclusion Criteria	Measure	Justification
Age: adult (age 18 years or older)	Subject self-report	Mirrors age of military population
Sex: men and women	Subject self-report	Distinguish if sex difference exists
Health status: non-obese	Percent body fat limit	Reduce between Ss variability
Fitness status: highly trained	$\dot{V}O_2$max or training history	Relevant to population
Written consent/assent	Signed consent	Required by IRB for participation

Exclusion: Specify diseases, conditions, or health behaviors which might impact dependent variables or ability of the participant to complete the study.
- Diabetes, thyroid disease, neurologic diseases, sickle cell trait/anemia, infectious diseases, cardiovascular diseases
- Pregnancy (or intention to become pregnant)
- Use of oral contraceptives, regularity of menses
- Metal or electrical implants in body or eyes (*e.g.*, pins, screws, shrapnel, plates, braces, cardiac pacemaker, hearing aid)
- History of health problems which place subjects at risk (*e.g.*, prior heat stroke or heat exhaustion that might affect exercise tolerance in the heat)
- Use of specific prescription or over-the-counter medications (*e.g.*, ephedrine/ephedra, corticosteroids, asthma inhalers, weight loss aids with amphetamines)
- Use of specific dietary supplements (*e.g.*, vitamins if urine color measured, caffeine if a performance study)
- Dietary practices (e.g., caloric restriction, hydration status, repeatability of diet)
- Recent weight loss or weight gain

Ss, subjects; IRB, institutional review board.

and funding agency. However, there are no fixed inclusion criteria. A fastidious researcher may want a homogeneous group, whereas a pragmatic researcher may want a more diverse group. Inclusion criteria should be clearly stated such that participants can easily determine if they qualify and future research can replicate findings on a similar group of subjects.

In addition to inclusion criteria, guidelines that restrict participation must also be clearly stated (*i.e.*, **exclusion criteria**). Examples might include the use of prescription medications (*e.g.*, oral contraceptives in women, corticosteroids), health behaviors (*e.g.*, smoking, excess alcohol, level of physical activity), and the presence of chronic disease (*e.g.*, diabetes, obesity). These factors are potential intervening variables that result in additional "noise" that obscures the potentially small "signal" or effect. These attributes should be carefully listed to further screen participants that meet the initial inclusion criteria (example found in Table 7-5).

Assigning Participants to Groups

After the investigator recruits the requisite number of subjects to adequately power the research design, the process of assigning participants into intervention and control groups must then be carefully developed and implemented. Ideally, this process involves either a method of randomization or subject matching on important factors that would impact the dependent variable. For example, in a weight loss study comparing different exercise regimens, it would be important to match subjects in each group according to their baseline levels of body fat at the start of the experiment so that neither group is different at the outset. Reliable and valid measures should be used for subject stratification into groups. For example, physical activity status may not necessarily be reflected solely by maximal oxygen uptake ($\dot{V}O_2$max) due to the strong genetic component in this measure. Validated survey tools or instruments should be used whenever possible to discriminate sedentary versus physically active subjects rather than a "best guess" from the investigator. If men and women were to be recruited of equivalent aerobic fitness, it is important to consider the biologic basis for $\dot{V}O_2$max by equating them based on aerobic capacity expressed relative to fat-free mass per minute (rather than liter per minute or milliliter per kilogram per minute) (14). Delimiting the physical characteristics or health behaviors that produce comparable intervention/treatment groups versus control strengthens the research design.

Controlling Additional Sources of Variability

To isolate the impact of the independent variable directly on the dependent variable, all other potential influences on the dependent variable should ideally be controlled or held constant. In reality, this is generally not possible, but it is important to account for factors that could have a primary impact on results. In the example of the mouse study (7), it is apparent that other extraneous factors might affect the dependent variable of wheel-running performance (*e.g.*, diet, prior fatigue or physical activity, exposure to day light, environmental temperature/humidity, physical or psychologic stressors, mouse genetics). These extraneous factors are considered "confounders" and might be considered **confounding or intervening variables**. If left uncontrolled, confounders may influence the effects on wheel running that are unrelated to the independent variable of interest (catechin supplementation) and result in excess noise or variability in the experiment.

The impact of confounders cannot always be teased out to understand their influences on the results of the study (*i.e.*, dependent variables). Extraneous sources of variability are considered threats to internal validity, the extent to which the observed changes in the dependent variable(s) can be attributed solely to changes in the independent variable(s). Internal validity is a critical component of experimental research that allows the determination of cause and effect; specifically, in the case of the mice population studied, catechin supplementation resulted in improved wheel running. Thus, it is imperative that known (or hypothesized) confounders are identified and a means to control or limit them implemented when possible. By the same token, it is recognized that research performed outside of the laboratory setting cannot achieve such a high degree of **internal validity** but may be more readily generalizable to real-world conditions, thus having greater external validity. **External validity** is defined as the ability to generalize a study's findings to a broader population, setting, and/or time. There is a tradeoff between internal and external validity in experimental research. Therefore, human experimental research in exercise science may sacrifice some of the internal validity inherent in animal research but gain the advantage of external validity (when properly designed).

For studies in exercise science, the importance of nutritional and other health practices along with recent physical activity should be considered in designing a study. While these might not be exclusion criteria *per se*, the adherence to "control procedures" prior to participation in the experiment is vital. Developing a simple checklist for participants to verify adherence to the pre-test procedures is a useful tool in this regard. A sample is provided in Table 7-6.

Improving the Signal Relative to Noise. The ultimate goal in an experimental research design is to dampen out extraneous noise so that the impact of the independent variable on the dependent variable can be observed and evaluated. This is known as the "signal-to-noise ratio." If the noise is minimized, then even a small signal may result in a significant effect. However, if the denominator (noise) as shown below is very large, then even a large signal may not result in a significant effect.

$$\text{Estimated Effect} = \frac{\text{Signal (impact of treatment)}}{\text{Noise (random variability)}}$$

Factors impacting both the numerator (signal) and denominator (noise) can influence the ability to estimate the sensitivity of finding an effect. An intuitively appealing measure of the signal-to-noise ratio or "sensitivity" is the mean difference between groups divided by the error of measurement. This measure is also part of the formula for the t-statistic that is used to derive the confidence limits, or P value, detecting a significant difference. Excessive variability due to subject selection, sample size, methodology, and other outside influences distort the ability to detect the signal or distinguish it from the noise. However, neither a large mean difference nor a small estimate of variation by itself dictates sensitivity, but it is the relative weight of both combined. A study by Amann, Hopkins, and Marcora (1) illustrated this concept by comparing two laboratory methods to assess endurance: a time to fatigue-cycling protocol versus a time trial protocol under conditions of either hyperoxia or hypoxia. Hyperoxia and hypoxia were the independent variables assumed to elicit a significant effect on the dependent variable (cycling performance). Despite greater variation in the time to fatigue method for assessing endurance, the sensitivity of both tests were nearly identical due to a signal that was relatively similar to

Table 7-6 Example of a Checklist to Verify Participant Adherence to Pre-Test Instructions

24-Hour History

Date: _____   Time: _____

1. How much sleep did you get last night? (Please circle one.)

| 0.5 | 1 | 1.5 | 2 | 2.5 | 3 | 3.5 | 4 | 4.5 | 5 | 5.5 | 6 | 6.5 | 7 | 7.5 | 8 | 8.5 | 9 | 10 | (hours)

2. How much sleep do you normally get? (Please circle one.)

| 0.5 | 1 | 1.5 | 2 | 2.5 | 3 | 3.5 | 4 | 4.5 | 5 | 5.5 | 6 | 6.5 | 7 | 7.5 | 8 | 8.5 | 9 | 10 | (hours)

3. How long has it been since your last meal or snack? (Please circle one.)

| 0.5 | 1 | 1.5 | 2 | 2.5 | 3 | 3.5 | 4 | 4.5 | 5 | 5.5 | 6 | 6.5 | 7 | 7.5 | 8 | 8.5 |
| 9 | 9.5 | 10 | 11 | 11.5 | 12 | 12.5 | 13 | 13.5 | 14 | 14.5 | 15 | 15.5 | (hours)

4. How long has it been since you drank a beverage? (please circle one)

| 0.5 | 1 | 1.5 | 2 | 2.5 | 3 | 3.5 | 4 | 4.5 | 5 | 5.5 | 6 | 6.5 | 7 | 7.5 | 8 | 8.5 |
| 9 | 9.5 | 10 | 11 | 11.5 | 12 | 12.5 | 13 | 13.5 | 14 | 14.5 | 15 | 15.5 | (hours)

5. When did you last have:

   - Any drugs (including aspirin), vitamins, or supplements?
   - Alcohol?
   - Caffeine?

6. What sort of exercise did you perform yesterday, and for how long?

7. What sort of physical activity have you performed today, and for how long?

8. Are you experiencing any gastrointestinal distress (*i.e.*, vomiting or diarrhea)?

9. Describe your general feelings by checking one of the following:

   __Excellent   __Very bad
   __Very, very good   __Very, very bad
   __Very good   __Terrible
   __Good
   __Neither good nor bad
   __Bad

the noise across both endurance test protocols. In summary, the louder the signal, the easier it will be to detect despite inherent variation. Conversely, weaker signals (or expected mean differences) require well-designed studies with less noise or a larger sample size to find an effect.

Other Sources of Bias. Errors in measurement may be systematic or random. Systematic error occurs when measurement error is in one direction. For example, a device to measure blood lactate might consistently read 1 mmol/L higher than the actual value. This skews the dataset by making all values higher than they should be. Random error, as the name implies, may occur in any direction and is typically expected to have a cancellation or net zero effect. Large sources of random error will result in an estimate that is imprecise but not necessarily inaccurate with respect to the mean approximation. Bias, however, occurs when unintended systematic error is introduced into the research study and leads to inaccurate results. As the risk of bias increases, the validity of the study decreases. Quality scores have been used in the past to rate a research study; however, the Cochrane Collaboration (8) favors rating studies for the risk of bias on specific design elements. Although beyond the scope of this chapter, the following experimental design elements should be evaluated in terms of risk (high, low, or unclear) for bias, subject selection bias (*e.g.*, sequence generation, group allocation concealment), performance bias (blinding of participants and personnel), detection bias (blinding of outcome assessment), attrition bias (incomplete outcome data), and reporting bias (selective outcome reporting).

Although all research studies contain bias, it is important to consider additional steps to minimize these sources. For example, if the study involves administration of a physical activity intervention, investigators should consider factors such as: Are all participants motivated in the same way during the intervention? Is the number and characteristics of participants who drop out of the intervention group different compared to the control group? Is there something inherently different about subjects who do not drop out compared to the controls? Do subjects alter other health behaviors when assigned to a physical activity intervention? Sources of bias can be reduced with an organized design plan for standardized operating procedures. Primary steps include the following: (a) Allow adequate planning in the research design stage to directly answer the research question; (b) Choose subjects that closely represent a target population at large; (c) Carefully control subject selection and administer treatments consistently to all participants/groups through detailed written instructions and methods to document participant adherence (double blinding when possible); (d) Clearly define the variables and how they are measured to ensure accuracy; and (e) Take steps to ensure data are accurate and complete (written plan for data collection, properly train personnel on procedures, pilot test, calibrate regularly, etc.).

Summary of Research Dimensions

A summary of non-experimental, quasi-experimental, and experimental designs can be found in Table 7-4. Each can make important contributions to the literature. However, as the rigor of the study design increases, so does the ability to identify causal relationships and make inferences about a treatment. Therefore, experimental designs are considered to be the most robust. With sufficiently large samples, experimental research can examine the effects of multiple independent variables on the dependent variable(s). The tradeoff is experimental designs can be more expensive and require greater time to complete, and if performed under tightly controlled conditions, they reduce the ability to generalize research findings to real-world conditions. In other words, just because an effect of an independent variable on the dependent variable is found in the laboratory, it does not mean it will translate across all populations in everyday life.

PRIMARY TYPES OF DESIGNS

Elements of experimental study design are best represented visually. Notation was developed by Campbell and Stanley (4) to describe the design. In Tables 7-7 and 7-8, this system is used:

"O" designates that a measurement observation has occurred.

"X" designates a treatment.

"R" indicates if groups were randomized (note no Rs in quasi-experimental).

Table 7-7 Common Types of Quasi-Experimental Design

Name	Campbell and Stanley (4)	Primary Advantages	Primary Disadvantages
Single Group Pre-Test/Posttest	O X O	(a) Might only be suitable for collecting pilot data	(a) Weakest research design (b) No comparison group (c) Many threats to internal validity (*e.g.*, history, maturation, practice effects, selection bias, testing, regression to mean)
Non-Equivalent Group Design	O X O O O	(a) Comparison group (b) Establishes baseline measurement for equivalency of groups and permits analysis of change scores (c) Often more suitable for conducting research in real-world settings	(a) Weak research design (b) No randomization (c) Groups may differ initially on dependent variable (d) Several threats to internal validity (*e.g.*, selection bias with one group being inherently different, history, maturation)
Time Series	O O O X O O O	(a) Multiple pre-tests and post-tests to establish pattern and reduce internal validity threats of maturation and testing (b) May be more suitable for conducting research in real-world settings	(a) No comparison group (b) Single group—no randomization (c) Greater potential for attrition over time (d) Potential threats to internal validity (*e.g.*, history, maturation)
Multiple Time Series	O O O X O O O O O O O O O	(a) Multiple pre-tests and post-tests to establish pattern and reduce internal validity threats of maturation and testing (b) Comparison group (c) Often more suitable for conducting research in real-world settings	(a) If no randomization, groups may differ initially on dependent variable. (b) Greater potential for attrition over time (c) Repeated exposure may result in improvement not related to treatment.

O, observation; X, treatment.

Table 7-8　Common Types of True Experimental Designs

Name	Campbell and Stanley (4)	Type of Design	Primary Advantages	Primary Disadvantages
Pre-Test/Posttest Control Group (also known as Randomized Controlled Trial)	R O X O R O O	Between-subjects	(a) Randomized (b) True control group (c) Baseline measure to check for equivalency of groups and changes over time not related to X (d) Design is flexible and can be expanded to include multiple Xs or X levels.	(a) May be ethical issues related to withholding treatment in therapeutic trials
Posttest Only Control Group	R X O R O	Between-subjects	(a) Simple design (b) Randomized (c) True control group (d) Useful when pretest measures are not feasible or could influence outcome	(a) Potential for non-equivalent groups if R fails (b) Potential problems with attrition due to X
Repeated Measures/ Repeated Treatment (X) Design	$OX_1OX_2OX_3O$	Within-subjects	(a) Simple design (b) Economy of subjects (subjects serve control) (c) Can counterbalance Xs to reduce threats to internal validity (d) Use of placebo/control condition for comparison (e) Reduces variability across subjects	(a) Potential changes over time unrelated to X (b) Potential carry-over effect if sufficient time is not allowed between Xs (c) Greater potential for attrition over time
Mixed Factorial Design	$R\ OX_{11}OX_{12}OX_{13}O$ $R\ OX_{21}OX_{22}OX_{23}O$	Between-subject (two levels—first subscript) and within-subject factors (three levels—second subscript)	(a) Economy of subjects (subjects serve as control) (b) Randomized (c) Can counterbalance Xs to reduce threats to internal validity (d) Use of placebo/control condition for comparison (e) Reduce variability across subjects. (f) Complex design can be expanded. (g) Can examine interaction effects	(a) Potential changes over time unrelated to X (b) Potential additive effect if sufficient time is not allowed between Xs (c) Greater potential for attrition over time (d) More complex design requiring larger sample (e) Interaction between factors can sometimes make interpretation difficult.
Completely Randomized (Full) Factorial Design	$R\ X_{11}\ O$ $R\ X_{12}\ O$ $R\ X_{21}\ O$ $R\ X_{22}\ O$	Between-subjects with multiple between factors	(a) Randomized (b) Use of true control group (c) Economy of subjects—measured only once (d) Useful when pretest measures are not feasible or could influence outcome (e) Complex design can examine interaction effects.	(a) No way to check randomization procedure (b) Posttest is only basis for making decisions about effects of X. (c) More complex design; as independent variables are added, sample size can become extremely large (d) Interaction between factors can make interpretation difficult.

R, randomization; O, observation; X, treatment; subscripts, level of factors A and B.

Each line represents a single group. Therefore, designs with two lines (*e.g.*, quasi-experimental, Table 7-7: non-equivalent group design and multiple time series; experimental, Table 7-8 all designs except repeated measures) consist of two groups, whereas other designs are single-group designs (quasi-experimental, Table 7-7: single group pre-test/posttest and times series).

Quasi-Experimental Designs

The most common types of quasi-experimental designs are outlined in Table 7-7 along with potential advantages and disadvantages. The single group pre-test/posttest only (see Table 7-7) is among the weakest of all designs and is considered quasi-experimental because there is no R of subjects or use of a control group. The non-equivalent group design (see Table 7-7) consists of two groups. Both groups are measured prior to an intervention/treatment. Then one group receives an intervention (X), whereas one does not (or sometimes receives a standard of care when unethical to withhold treatment). Both groups then are observed postintervention. This design is similar to a pre-test/posttest experimental design (see Table 7-8); however, it lacks randomization. Therefore, the comparison group may not be a true control group as described earlier (13). Notice that as a comparison group is added, threats to internal validity are reduced. A time series design simply means there are a series of observations (O) both before and after X to determine if the dependent variable differs before and after treatment. Multiple observations (O) in the time series design reduces the likelihood that extraneous factors such as maturation and testing effects may confound the results and reduce the threat to internal validity.

True Experimental Designs

Table 7-8 summarizes some commonly used experimental designs along with advantages and disadvantages. In several cases, the designs resemble quasi-experimental designs but have randomization (R) or a true control group (or control condition) which reduce threats to internal validity. Designs range from the randomized controlled trial (pre-test/posttest control group) to more complex designs that accommodate additional independent variables (mixed factorial design). However, when more factors are studied, a larger sample size is required, particularly with the completely randomized (full) factorial design which compares different groups of subjects. The advantage of a more complex design is it provides the ability to see how factors interact (*e.g.*, more similar to reality).

When considering which of these designs to select, the researcher should evaluate the potential advantage of multiple subject observations over time relative to the ability of subjects to complete the study (*i.e.*, attrition). Large amounts of missing data can create a statistical nightmare when it comes to the analysis stage. Other potential confounders such as learning effects should also be considered. Measuring subjects at baseline before the intervention can evaluate the success of randomization and allow for more powerful statistical analyses. Overall, the advantages of true experimental designs outweigh the limitations and flaws noted earlier for the quasi-experimental designs.

CONCLUSION

The design of experiments requires a balance. Independent variables (*i.e.*, treatment/ intervention) should be clearly defined, controlled, and administered using sound methods to reduce noise and enhance the likelihood that an effect can be detected. The researcher should appreciate the tradeoff with respect to the level of control for variables and the ability to translate results to real-world situations. Subject selection, allocation to groups, treatment sequence, and adequate screening for extraneous variables require planning in order to avoid potential confounders of study results. Bottom line: Investigators should carefully plan their research design (*i.e.*, implementation of independent variables and subject selection) before executing the "fun part" of doing the experiment.

GLOSSARY

Alternate/research hypothesis: hypothesis proposing that a difference exists between groups on the dependent variable; for tests of association, it is the hypothesis that there is a correlation among variables

Between-group (or between-subjects) independent variable: discrete variable (gender, age, method of training, etc.) that requires a different group of subjects to be used for each level of the variable

Bias: error introduced by the research process which potentially confounds or distorts the study's findings

Blind: study in which participants are kept unaware of information that might bias the results (such as whether they are receiving a treatment or placebo)

Confounding or intervening variables: variables which are not of primary interest in the research study but which could impact the results if not taken into account and controlled (when possible)

Constant: a characteristic that has only one value in a study

Control group: a group measured at the same time points as the treatment/intervention group(s) but receives no treatment/intervention

Counterbalancing: process of varying the sequence in which subjects receive a treatment/ intervention in an effort to prevent order effects

Dependent variable: the variable that is measured; it is the outcome measure(s) of interest in a study that is presumably affected by a treatment or intervention (independent variable)

Double blind: study in which both participants and the researchers administering the experiment are kept unaware of group assignment (such as who is receiving a treatment or placebo) to reduce bias

Exclusion criteria: conditions defined by the researcher that would disqualify potential participants from being included in the study

Experimental research: research examining causality that attempts to control or take into account all other potential confounding variables (through randomization, use of control group, etc.)

External validity: ability to generalize a study's findings to a broader population, setting, and/or time

Hawthorne effect: phenomenon in which study participants improve or change a behavior in response to being studied

Inclusion criteria: conditions defined by the researcher that participant must meet in order to participate in a study

Independent variable: the variable intentionally controlled or manipulated in a research study in order to study an effect on the outcome or dependent variable

Internal validity: the extent to which the observed changes in the dependent variable(s) can be attributed solely to changes in the independent variable(s)

Multivariate: a research design that includes more than one independent variable

Non-experimental research: descriptive or correlational research that does not imply causality

Null hypothesis: hypothesis that proposes no differences exist between groups on the dependent variable related to the independent variable; for tests of association, it is the hypothesis that there is no correlation among variables

Placebo effect: phenomenon in which study participants experience a benefit or improvement after the administration of a "sham" treatment

Power: the ability to correctly reject the null hypothesis and retain the alternate/research hypothesis; the ability to detect a difference between groups when one really exists; for tests of association, it is the ability to detect a correlation among variables when one really exists

Quasi-experimental research: research used to examine causal inferences but lacks at least one element of a true experimental design (usually randomization)

Research design: the methods and procedures an investigator uses to answer a research question

Treatment/intervention: the independent variable (*e.g.*, drug, supplement, training regimen) that is manipulated in an experiment in order to examine its effects on the dependent variable

Univariate: a research design with a single independent variable

Variable: some characteristic that can have different values and is either subject to change or can be intentionally "manipulated"

Within-group (or within-subject) independent variable: variable that is manipulated by testing each subject across all levels of the variable (repeated measures)

REFERENCES

1. Amann M, Hopkins WG, Marcora SM. Similar sensitivity of time to exhaustion and time-trial time to changes in endurance. *Med Sci Sports Exerc.* 2008;40(3):574–580.
2. American College of Sports Medicine. *ACSM's Guidelines for Exercise Testing and Prescription.* 9th ed. Philadelphia (PA): Lippincott Williams & Wilkins; 2013.
3. Ariel G, Saville W. Anabolic steroids: the physiological effects of placebos. *Med Sci Sports Med* 1972;4:124–126.
4. Campbell DT, Stanley J. *Experimental and Quasi-Experimental Designs for Research.* Chicago (IL): Rand McNally; 1963.

5. Eccles R. The powerful placebo in cough studies? *Pulm Pharmacol Ther.* 2002;15(3):303–308.
6. Franke RH, Kaul JD. The Hawthorne experiments: first statistical interpretation. *Am Sociol Rev.* 1978;43:623–643.
7. Haramizu S, Ota N, Hase T, Murase T. Catechins suppress muscle inflammation and hasten performance recovery after exercise. *Med Sci Sports Exerc.* 2013;45(9):1694–1702.
8. Higgins JPT, Altman DG, Sterne JAC. Assessing risk of bias in included studies. In: Higgins JPT, Green S, editors. *Cochrane Handbook for Systematic Reviews of Interventions.* West Sussex, United Kingdom: Wiley; 2011.
9. Millard-Stafford M, Rosskopf LB, Snow TK, Hinson BT. Water versus carbohydrate-electrolyte ingestion before and during a 15-km run in the heat. *Int J Sport Nutr.* 1997;7(1):26–38.
10. Millard-Stafford ML, Sparling PB, Rosskopf LB, DiCarlo LJ. Carbohydrate-electrolyte replacement improves distance running performance in the heat. *Med Sci Sports Exerc.* 1992;24(8):934–940.
11. Penailillo L, Blazevich A, Numazawa H, Nosaka K. Metabolic and muscle damage profiles of concentric versus repeated eccentric cycling. *Med Sci Sports Exerc.* 2013;45(9):1773–1781.
12. Reed BV, Ashikaga T, Fleming BC, Zimny NJ. Effects of ultrasound and stretch on knee ligament extensibility. *J Orthop Sports Phys Ther.* 2000;30(6):341–347.
13. Robbins LB, Pfeiffer KA, Maier KS, Lo YJ, Wesolek Ladrig SM. Pilot intervention to increase physical activity among sedentary urban middle school girls: a two-group pretest-posttest quasi-experimental design. *J Sch Nurs.* 2012;28(4):302–315.
14. Sparling PB, Cureton KJ. Biological determinants of the sex difference in 12-min run performance. *Med Sci Sports Exerc.* 1983;15(3):218–223.

Experimental Design II—Dependent Variables, Blinding, Randomization, and Matching

Andrew J. Galpin, PhD, CSCS, and Andrew C. Fry, PhD, CSCS*D, FNSCA

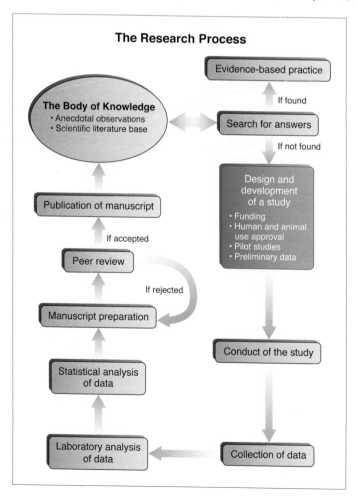

INTRODUCTION

High-quality research requires great diligence during many complex work-intensive steps (data collection, analysis, evaluation, writing, etc.) as you have learned in previous chapters. Most recognize the challenges and workload associated with these processes, as they are often tangible. For example, a study measuring changes in cellular networking pathways would likely require more time for data processing than would a similar study measuring only vertical jump performance. Yet in contrast, the time necessary for optimal experimental design is less outwardly recognizable, and as a result, inexperienced researchers often overlook it. It is common for this portion of the research process to take as long (if not longer) than every other phase combined.

Solutions to complicated problems do not arise from a single study. Thus, although the general objectives or purpose of an experiment usually develops quickly, the specifics may take exponentially longer to delineate. The research team must decide the following: Who is the subject population? What intervention should occur? What should we measure? How should we measure it? This design process often, although not always, results in a reduction in complexity or sophistication of the original idea in favor of answering a few clearly defined questions.

As a practical example, perhaps the research question is "how do warmups influence exercise performance?" The general problem is clear but certainly not "solvable" with only a single study. Only one aspect of this problem can truly be examined at once. The investigator would need to decide several factors such as what will the participant population be, what will the warmup intervention be, what will the outcome be, and how will this outcome be measured. Once this is accomplished, the researcher should explicitly state the specific purpose(s) of that individual study and not overstep it in their design or discussion. Table 8-1 lists some of the possible options when considering these study design decisions.

Scientific inquiry is often strongest when the research question is clearly identified prior to data collection. As you have learned, the order of events is traditionally as follows: (a) identify the gap in knowledge/need for research, (b) select the independent variable(s), and finally (c) select the dependent variable(s). The initial focus for the development of a solid experimental design should be identification of the independent (see Chapter 7) and dependent variables. This is undoubtedly challenging as the eternal dichotomy of science entails an inverse relationship between internal and external validity. The more control(s) used in a study (*e.g.*, dietary restrictions, hydration status, motivation, etc.), the less generalizable the results. Yet at the same time, increases in control enhance the likelihood the intervention is the actual cause of the changes in the outcome variables. This is why critical researchers select the dependent variables in a fashion that appropriately matches the level of control necessary of the study.

Numerous experimental design strategies influence the level of control. As you learned in Chapter 7, most incorporate some form of blinding into the plan so potential conscious or subconscious biases from the research team and/or participants do not influence the results. Randomization techniques also dramatically affect the study's applicability but may be complicated and confusing. All of these strategies provide unique benefits and consequences. Thus, a deep understanding of each is fundamental to truly learning appropriate scientific research design. Successful analysis and interpretation is essentially impossible

Table 8-1 Examples of Decisions to be Made When Selecting Dependent Variables for a Study on Warmup Strategies

Issue	Options	Specific Details
Population to be studied	Young/old Men/women Active/sedentary Fitness experience Athletes Rehabilitation/disabled	 Yoga, aerobics, group fitness classes Endurance, power, sprint Type of condition/disease
Intervention (warmup)	What protocol? How long will it last? How vigorous should it be? Length of time between warmup and test?	Static or dynamic Stretching Other methods/modalities
What is measured?	Strength or power Muscular endurance Oxygen uptake Performance Post-exercise soreness Injury rates	1RM, rate of force development, isokinetic, static, vertical jump, etc. Repetitive lifting task, time to fatigue task Athletic task, job site task, rehabilitation task, etc. Perception, blood marker Severity, frequency, type
How are the variables measured?	Tape measure Force plate Motion capture system Survey or questionnaire Muscle biopsy MRI Metabolic cart	 Which analysis software? Bilateral or unilateral? Countermovement or static? Markered or markerless system Video analysis

1RM, 1 repetition maximum; MRI, magnetic resonance imaging.

without this skill. Therefore, the following chapter will provide a discussion of (a) selecting dependent variables, (b) blinding, (c) randomization, and (d) matching.

SELECTING DEPENDENT VARIABLES

As explained in the previous chapter, a variable is the thing being manipulated and/or measured in an experiment. For example, these may be physical objects (*e.g.*, amount of a given protein), events (*e.g.*, frequency of smoking incidence), or time periods (*e.g.*, number of hours spent doing physical activity). The independent variable is typically the unit being intentionally manipulated by the researcher (*e.g.*, amount of carbohydrates ingested, number of reminder e-mails sent to children, type of footwear worn, etc.) but not always (*e.g.*, amount of smoking by participants when at home). The research team should have strong control over the independent variable, as it generally should not be influenced by anything else in the study. The dependent variable is the variable being measured but not specifically manipulated by the researcher. An easy trick to remembering which is the independent variable and which is the dependent variable is to switch the order. You could test how the amount of an antioxidant supplement consumed (independent variable) by a participant influenced the level of inflammation markers in the bloodstream (dependent variable), but you could not test how the level of inflammation markers in the bloodstream (dependent variable) influenced the amount of an antioxidant supplement consumed (independent variable). In another example, you could test how the temperature in a gym affected the heart rate during exercise, but you could not test how heart rate influenced the gym's temperature.

Primary and Secondary Dependent Variables

The independent variable should always at least have the potential to directly alter the dependent variable. Multiple dependent variables should be selected with admitted varying degrees of interest. If you were interested in how effective a physical activity intervention was (independent variable), measuring family income might be a poor choice as a **primary dependent variable**. This represents poor scientific practice because although an indirect correlation may exist, it is not causal and would likely not have been predicted prior to the study. Measures such as weight loss or body composition would represent more appropriate primary dependent variables. Changes in family income may be interesting and could be related to the physical activity but should be considered a **secondary dependent variable** in this scenario. Strong conclusions about this relationship would then require an additional, separately designed study.

In general, a dependent variable is the set of data the researcher analyzes. It is also the variable being predicted when using a regression equation. A primary dependent variable (sometimes referred to as a "direct marker") is the study variable most directly influenced by the independent variable. For example, if the independent variable is a particular strength training method, a primary dependent variable might be one repetition maximum strength. A secondary dependent variable (sometimes referred to as an "indirect marker") is a study variable indirectly influenced by the independent variable. For example, assuming the same independent variable (strength training method), a secondary dependent variable might be positive self-image.

Surrogate Dependent Variables

A **surrogate dependent variable** is a dependent variable that is more practical or appropriate than a primary dependent variable. In another example, the independent variable may be a particular strength training program being performed by cardiac patients and the primary dependent variable may be one repetition maximum strength indicating the efficacy of the program. The secondary dependent variables may be blood pressure and a surrogate dependent variable could be echocardiogram testing results that uses ultrasound to evaluate the heart in place of the more obvious primary dependent variable (*i.e.*, death).

The selection of the dependent variables is based on what the independent variable is most likely to influence. Let us assume a researcher wondered how strength training influences patients with Parkinson disease. The strength training would be the independent variable, but the dependent variables may be a host of direct markers (*e.g.*, force production, balance, blood flow, cognitive function, disease progression, etc.) and indirect markers (*e.g.*, spontaneous physical activity levels, mood, sleep, etc.). Admittedly, this approach is not always used or practical as resource limitations (*i.e.*, time and money) regulate dependent variable selection, which then controls research questions and independent variable selection. This order is also violated with good cause during mechanistic or exploratory research. Say a research team wanted to know if a particular gene was involved in muscle atrophy. The team may place the gene in several scenarios known to cause atrophy and measure the gene's response. In this case, the independent variable (the cellular environment) would continually change, whereas the dependent variable (activity of the gene) is fixed.

Both methods of study design are acceptable, but the former more typical manner of selecting the dependent variables previously discussed requires great care so as not to create confusion when the results seem to defy the initial logic of the hypothesis. Imagine a scenario in which a 10-week Tai Chi intervention failed to reduce resting blood pressure in a population of adults with hypertension. This does not mean Tai Chi is "ineffective"; it only means Tai Chi at this dosage, in this population, etc., is ineffective at altering this marker. However, perhaps a significant improvement in resting heart rate and stroke volume was noted. In this case, the conclusion that Tai Chi is effective or not is highly dependent on which dependent variable is selected and/or reported. This scenario highlights the importance of careful and appropriate selection of dependent variables. Several important criteria should be considered.

CRITERIA WHEN SELECTING DEPENDENT VARIABLES: RELIABILITY AND VALIDITY

The most obvious relates to the desired intention of the independent variable. If a given treatment is designed to prevent eating disorders in young athletes, the primary dependent variable should be the prevalence of eating disorders. Another critical factor is what dependent variable is most likely to respond to the treatment. A secondary dependent variable may be measurement of impairment on personal, cognitive, and social behaviors. Measuring maximal heart rate following a specific exercise training study would be a poor way of judging the effectiveness of the intervention as that marker is generally independent of training history. The dependent variable must also be both **reliable** and **valid**. That is, can the variable provide repeatable results (reliability), and does the variable measure what it is intended to (validity)? For a variable to be valid, it must be reliable. If validity and reliability for a particular measure have not been established in previous research, it should be included in the study design.

Feasibility and Subjectivity

The subjectivity or potential for bias should also be limited for the dependent variable. For example, if assessing the effectiveness of a particular drug in preventing death, the dependent variable is obviously death. Yet this measure is impractical in most situations. It is considered good scientific practice to adjust the dependent variable when it is not reasonably available, occurs too infrequently, is too expensive, is influenced by too many uncontrollable factors, or is otherwise unfeasible. Similarly, how are subjective health issues (*e.g.*, osteoarthritis or non-specific "back pain," etc.) that do not provide obvious dependent variables supposed to be treated? The best strategy in these circumstances is to pick one or more dependent variable(s) that are previously established surrogate markers. In the previous example of a drug treatment, perhaps blood cholesterol and/or the number of cardiac incidences are examined in surrogate of death. In other studies, the amount of activation of a particular inflammatory hormone and/or the response to a pain questionnaire could be measured.

Problems also arise when indirect dependent variables contradict each other. Imagine a treatment was given with the goal of improving osteoarthritis pain, and the dependent variables were an inflammatory blood marker as well as a pain questionnaire. How would it be interpreted if one but not the other improved? Both the author and any future reader would be highly encouraged to limit their conclusions about the effectiveness of the drug to its effect on that marker, not the underlying condition. It would be inappropriate to conclude that said treatment improved osteoarthritis but more accurately that it improved the sensation of pain or a particular blood marker that is related to the condition.

Dependent Variables Can Have Limitations

An indirect or surrogate dependent variable should not be considered inferior but simply needs to be recognized. Recent publications on the topic of skeletal muscle growth highlight this concept. For years, scientists have measured acute changes in signaling protein activity, gene expression, and protein synthesis as predictors of long-term skeletal muscle hypertrophy. Although a relationship between these acute markers and chronic adaptations undoubtedly exists (2,5,9), recent evidence clearly demonstrates that the relationship is not perfect (4). No one dependent variable can explain a complex phenomenon such as skeletal muscle hypertrophy and therefore, although it may not be completely responsible for the phenomenon, it does contribute to it. This by no means assuages the value of the acute dependent variables but simply reminds us of their natural limitations. In fact, without these options, a great number of studies would not be possible as they often greatly speed up and/or cheapen the cost of research. This is critical when investigating treatments with potential health implications. For example, clinical trials (*e.g.*, for a new cardiac atherosclerosis drug) normally use secondary dependent variables (*e.g.*, blood pressure testing and graded exercise test [GXT]) in the early stages of testing (*i.e.*, phase I or phase II) but typically move to more direct measures (*e.g.*, a stress echocardiography test and cardiac catheterization) during large human trials (*i.e.*, phase III).

EVIDENCE-BASED SELECTION

Regardless of the selection strategy, in most cases, dependent variables should be chosen based on scientific evidence and clearly outlined before data collection. Dependent variable selection should be supported by either previous literature or extensive pilot work. Poor scientific practice would be the selection of dependent variables postintervention, or worse, continued exploration of dependent variables until a desired outcome or conclusion is reached. This same practice is problematic when grouping or matching subjects (discussed later in this chapter) (7). Imagine a research group was interested in how safe a particular cholesterol medication was for the kidneys. Prior to data collection, they should pick variables commonly associated with kidney damage to examine. Regardless of how the treatment influenced these variables, it would be poor practice to continue exploring additional variables until a desired outcome is reached, especially if the additional measures are indirect or less established indicators of kidney dysfunction. If additional such unestablished testing is done, it exposes the participant to unneeded risks.

This is highlighted in the infamous "International Study of Infarct Survival," which trialed aspirin and streptokinase on vascular mortality in patients with acute myocardial infarction (3). This study found impressive benefits of aspirin treatment. However, when subjects were examined according to their astrological sign, the effectiveness of the treatment changed significantly. Apparently, aspirin is less effective in Geminis and Libras. Most believe this finding is a function of inappropriate post-hoc analysis, as astrological sign has no clear scientific connection to aspirin treatment. This is also an example of another unsuitable analysis technique in which excessive dependent variables are included in analysis. By simple probability, each additional dependent variable increases the likelihood of finding a significant result (see Chapter 18). The complement of dependent variables used must be carefully evaluated in order to eliminate or reduce such nonsensical outcomes.

COMPLEXITY OF DEPENDENT VARIABLES

Adding variables can also confound interpretation. Take the example of the classic human growth hormone study by Rudman and colleagues (6). In this study, the researchers took bone density measurements at nine sites (spine, hip, leg, etc.) before and after six months of hormone treatment. Significant improvements were evident for the mean bone density of the lumbar spine (L1–L4) but nowhere else. The authors then concluded that "the treatment significantly enhanced bone density." If nine sites are measured, how is one to interpret significant differences in two of the nine? How about four of the nine, or seven of the nine? Obviously, the correct answer is interpretations should be independent for each marker, but often, overall conclusions are needed. It would also be inappropriate for research to not report all variables quantified. In this example, interpretation of effectiveness of this hormone treatment would be widely skewed if all non-significant findings were not reported in the final manuscript. However, sometimes the addition of variables is warranted and/or necessary. This may happen when the purpose of the study is exploratory or mechanistic. Keep in mind, however, conclusions from this type of research should be withheld until further verification in the *a priori* manner just described.

Can Dependent Variables be Measured Reliably?

The final consideration for selection of dependent variables is the ability to measure. Each dependent variable should possess as many of the following qualities as possible: accurate;

precise; reliable; valid; and able to be collected, processed, and analyzed appropriately. If possible, identical equipment and testing procedures should be used for each participant and condition. Some testing may not require such stringent restrictions. For example, ground reaction forces from a force plate are likely similar between all laboratories, provided the instruments are correctly calibrated and analyzed. However, the magnitude of activation of a particular cellular protein could differ wildly depending on the exact analysis methods and equipment. To compare results, measurement of this protein may need to occur in the same lab, using the same preparation techniques. A blinded researcher should perform the measurement if the dependent variable is at all subjective or qualitative.

The determination of appropriate dependent variables is one of the most important steps when designing a research study. The purpose of the study can only be correctly addressed once the research question has been properly identified and the proper dependent and independent variables are established. In another example, one might want to measure blood flow in a thigh muscle with exercise, but after piloting the use of a needle probe with infrared technology inserted into the muscle, one finds a reliable value cannot be obtained. Although this technology is commonly used during brain surgery with its placement into specific vessels, its application to skeletal muscle does not work and is not worth continuing until better placement technology can be developed. Thus, measuring a more global oxygenation change in skeletal muscle may be a better variable to assess in a study of the effects of exercise cardiovascular dynamics. Thus, while you may get a measurement that is considered valid, it is not possible in this case to make it reliable enough to use as a dependent variable to evaluate the effects of exercise as the independent variable.

BLINDING

The purpose of research in some respect is to expand current knowledge. This necessitates the challenge, support, and further exploration of existing information. Hypothesizing the results of a future study is therefore innate in the research process. In other words, the investigative team will always carry some level of bias into the collection and analysis of data. Once the selection of dependent variables is complete, data collection and analysis should be carried out in a fashion which eliminates as much potential for bias as possible as you learned in Chapter 7. In some research designs, one way to remove some of the bias is by using a process, referred to as **blinding**. Both researchers and participants are susceptible to various forms of conscious and subconscious bias in favor of one treatment over another or over nothing at all. Blinding in such research designs is an effective and necessary method of mitigating research predisposition. Imagine a group of scientists were experimenting with a new treatment for hepatitis. Potential findings could help millions of people and generate substantial financial reward. These confounding factors of knowing what the treatment is must be accounted for as potential influences and blinding the treatments to both the patients and investigators alike, is the accepted approach to accomplish a solid experimental design. Therefore, the research team must be blinded to the treatment during both the experimental/drug design phase (*i.e.,* when the drug is being tested and designed in the laboratory) as well as when it is being tested on humans. The human participants in the trial may also share the desire to see a positive result and therefore must be blinded as well. Thus, using a blinded design is vital to truly test the efficacy of many interventions in which a drug, a nutritional supplement, or any treatment can be truly masked. In some cases, such blinding is not really possible; for example, studying "chewing" tobacco in which a suitable placebo with the known stimulatory effect minus the nicotine has not been engineered. In this case, a more creative design with other stimulants may be needed so as to separate out or distinguish the chewing tobacco treatment from the others including a control treatment condition where nothing is given.

The most well-known of the participant biases is the placebo effect, which you learned about in Chapter 7. This phenomenon serves to explain how an otherwise ineffective treatment somehow yields an actual or perceived improvement. For example, if a subject was given a nutritional supplement that he or she believed improved maximal strength, this person's strength may actually improve when tested, regardless of the physiologic effectiveness of the supplement. The inverse may also occur when a subject believes a particular intervention is not effective. This may cause the subject to intentionally or unintentionally perform worse when tested. Other psychologic factors such as motivation, competitiveness, self-efficacy, etc., significantly influence performance, further highlighting the need for blinding.

Bias is inherently limited when the participant cannot consciously influence the dependent variable and its measure is objective (*e.g.*, bone mineral density via a DEXA analysis, blood cholesterol levels, etc.). However, it is a major concern when the dependent variable is either partially or completely subjective (*e.g.*, circumference of a muscle tracing, score on a rate of perceived exertion scale, etc.), can be consciously manipulated (*e.g.*, maximal exercise performance), or both. Although basic research ethics hopefully eliminates direct alterations caused by the scientists, it may happen inadvertently. For example, more verbal motivation may be given unintentionally during the treatment condition, causing the participant to perform better. Thus, standardizing the audience effect is one example of experimental control as to how subjects will be motivated during each experimental session. For all of these reasons, the general solution is to keep as many people blinded to as much information as plausible as allowed by an institutional review committee or ethics board. Many times, this can also be done at the level of analysis where ultrasound scans, biochemical assays, and other readings are performed by laboratory personnel who are blinded to the treatment condition of what they are assessing. Circumstances do exist in which blinding the participants, researchers, or both are difficult, impossible, or even unnecessary. Proceeding without blinding may be acceptable in these situations.

Non-Blinded Experiments

Non-blinded experiments are those in which neither the researcher nor the participant are blinded. These tend to be simpler in design, execution, and cost. Some argue that they possess the most external validity and represent the most realistic and real-life scenarios because humans do not typically engage in self-blinded treatment. Although non-blinded studies are the most susceptible to bias, sometimes they are the only option. It would be unethical to deny a cancer patient treatment with a new drug, which is believed to help their condition, in lieu of a placebo or less effective treatment. Likewise, it would be almost impossible to blind participants or researchers if the effectiveness of a diet and nutrition plan were being compared to a surgical weight loss procedure. Non-blinding is commonplace in human performance laboratories, as participants and researchers can often quickly identify the testing condition, treatment, or exercise.

The drawback to the non-blinding approach is that definitive conclusions of effectiveness are difficult to make. Statistical considerations may also arise as people frequently withdraw from studies when they are randomized into a treatment group that they perceive as less effective. For example, say a participant liked the idea of being in a resistance training group but then with randomization is put into an endurance training group and therefore drops out as he or she really did not have his or her heart or mind into this type of exercise. This leaves disproportionate participant numbers between the groups and necessitates special statistical or study design considerations. Another concern is the protection of results from both the study team and the participants. This must be maintained until data collection is complete. If breached, communication between participants may alter expectations and outcomes. Non-blinded members of the research team are just as susceptible to this form of expectation bias.

Single-Blind Experiments

Single-blinded experiments are those in which only the participants are blinded. These share some of the conveniences of the non-blinded approach in that they are typically faster, easier, and cheaper than a double-blind study. They also increase the confidence in determining the effectiveness of the independent variable compared to non-blinded experiments. Instances other than convenience also occur that make a single-blind design more appropriate than a double-blind. This is particularly true when one group is at more risk than the other is. The research team has the responsibility of identifying adverse events and ending the experiment as quickly as possible if one condition increases the risk of harm beyond a reasonable level. Psychologic studies that intentionally manipulate outcomes or provide false feedback also require a single-blind study design. By nature, single-blind studies dramatically reduce (if not eliminate) the probability of subject bias; however, they do not address researcher bias. This can only be accomplished by double blinding. Sometimes, as will be discussed later, it may be appropriate to single blind the treatment but double blind the analyses.

Double-Blind Experiments

Double-blinded experiments are those in which both the researcher and the participant are blinded. This provides the greatest control but also requires the highest level of organization. Regardless of the blinding style (single or double), it is important that the blinding is not broken at any point. As stipulated by institutional review or ethics boards, the code must be broken if an injury or adverse reaction to a treatment occurs; the medical monitor will then break the code to determine whether there is linkage to the treatment or not. The research team should pay particular attention to securing results, as discussed earlier, as well as ensuring participants cannot reasonably "break" the blinding code. For example, if a study necessitates providing a consumable product (*e.g.*, food, beverage, supplement, etc.), all groups or conditions should receive a product with a similar size, feel, smell, taste, texture, and consistency (*i.e.*, placebo treatment). This increases the likelihood of maintaining blinding. Indeed this may be challenging. Early research on fish oil supplements were routinely unintentionally non-blinded because a common side effect of the supplements were "fishy" burps and/or breathe. One way to account for how well the blinding was maintained is to include some marker of perception following data collection. This can be done by simply administering a questionnaire to all volunteers asking if they knew which condition was which. Admittedly, this form of quality control is not typical but can be quite important.

Often, single-blinded or non-blinded studies can be performed in a double-blind fashion. Some investigators choose to blind a portion of the research team but not the others. Likewise, often new members will be brought on as part of the research group to specifically serve as blinded members. This is perhaps the best approach as it provides the control of the double-blind method while allowing the flexibility of the non-blinded approaches. The blinded members may be used during the data collection or analysis (or both), depending on the nuances of the study. Nutritional supplement studies frequently use this idea. One team member may be responsible for allocating and coding all supplements and placebos into storage containers labeled as only Treatment A or Treatment B. The team members for delivering the supplements, performing the testing, and analyzing the results would not know which treatment was the actual supplement and which was the placebo until after the processing was complete and the code was broken. Likewise, the participant would also be blinded.

If the study design requires researcher manipulation or otherwise does not allow for blinding to occur during data collection, a blinded member of the team may hold the sole responsibility of data processing. Data are collected in an open fashion but delivered to the analyzing member without participant information. Anonymity would only be broken after completion of analysis (*i.e.*, blinded analysis). Similarly, a blinded researcher could be used only during the data collection process. This is particularly useful (and probably always needed) when the dependent variables are partially or completely subjective.

RANDOMIZATION

Introduction

Several levels of control must be acquired in order to confidently establish that an independent variable influenced a dependent variable. Of most importance is to ensure that no portion of the testing procedure itself accounted for any change or variation in performance. This is typically done by subjecting participants to the testing procedure multiple times under several conditions ("crossover design") or by simply assigning all participants into different groups. This process of assigning individuals to a particular treatment group is known as **randomization** and functions to minimize both selection and accidental bias. Grace, Muench, and Chalmers (1) brilliantly illustrated the importance on randomization in a classic 1966 study. This review found that approximately 72% (or 34/47) of studies which did not randomize treatment groups reported conclusions which endorsed a particular surgical procedure (portacaval shunt) for the treatment of patients with portal hypertension. Shockingly, this same conclusion was drawn in only 25% of the trials in which volunteers were randomized.

Random selection is not the same as **random assignment**. Random selection means the pool of subjects was selected from the entire population of potential subjects in a completely random manner. On the other hand, random assignment occurs after an available pool of subjects has been identified; they are then randomly placed into different groups or conditions based on the independent variables being used. Although both processes are random in nature, they are not identical.

Although it is typically preferred, sometimes randomization is unnecessary, practically unrealistic, and/or may produce ethical dilemmas. One example would be the comparison of leg strength between professional rugby versus hockey players. Assigning hockey players to the rugby group or vice versa would defeat the purpose of the study. In this example, subjects are specifically assigned to their group based on the inclusion criteria of the study, not a randomization process. Ethical considerations arise when a given treatment is thought to have a major influence on health, lifespan, and/or living quality. The researchers could not ethically place individuals into a treatment group legitimately thought to be inferior or less effective. However, when randomization is appropriate, it should be done in a highly organized fashion for a number of reasons (Fig. 8-1).

Avoid Accidental Bias

Avoiding accidental bias is an important consideration needed in the removal of investigator/subject selection and/or accidental bias. Imagine a study that asks participants to perform an agility test before and after eight weeks of exercise training. The study would likely require

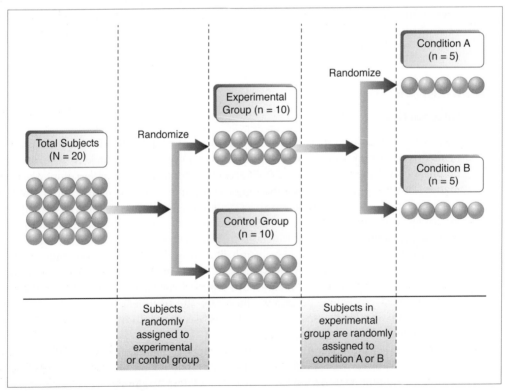

FIGURE 8-1:   Randomization of subjects in two different conditions.

some number of participants to perform the agility testing and exercise intervention. Meanwhile, a separate group would also perform the agility testing before and after eight weeks but would not engage in the exercise training. The former group would be considered the **experimental group**, with the latter being the **control group**. Participants must be assigned to both groups based on a specific and organized allocation process. Assigning group distribution based on the volunteer's personal preference (or personal selection) produces massive bias. Those most interested will inevitably give the most effort during the agility testing, and they will also be the most likely to choose to be a part of the training group. Uninterested volunteers will do the opposite. This results in an automatic bias of motivation and interest in success toward the training group, which would likely result in false positive findings regarding the effectiveness of the training program. Randomizing group allocations will limit uneven distributions of motivation or any other factor influencing the findings.

Another important reason arises with overall volunteer enrollment. Interested parties may decide to participate because the potential treatment is of value or significance to them (*e.g.*, 12 weeks of a free personalized exercise program, etc.). This is problematic if the treatment cannot be reasonably blinded, especially if the dependent variables are personally subjective (*e.g.*, level of happiness, quality of sleep, self-worth, etc.). Enrollment in the study and assignment to condition are therefore best when randomized. Keep in mind that the process itself should remain unknown and unpredictable to any participant. If not, potential volunteers may consciously select their enrollment date/circumstances to ensure allocation into their desired group. Randomization methods such as, "The first X amount of subjects get the experimental condition, and the second X amount get the control condition," or "every other" are easily breakable and ineffective. In fact, these methods are not random by definition.

Accidental Bias

Selection biases are less of an issue in double-blind studies but are highly problematic in single- or non-blinded designs. Accidental bias, on the other hand, can influence all three study designs. Again, as previously discussed, another reason randomization must be highly organized to regulate accidental bias. This refers to situations in which random or unforeseeable covariates (*e.g.*, gender, race, dietary habits, weather, world events, etc.) significantly influence the outcome. Random assignment of groups is a researcher's only method of accounting for such instances. This is particularly important if the study occurs over an extended timeline.

Avoiding Unequal Group Representation

Uneven group distribution and small sample sizes are the primary cause of accidental bias. Thus, another reason to strategically plan your randomization scheme is to ensure adequate statistical support. This results in less complex statistical analyses because the confidence covariates are equally balanced between the groups. Investigators who typically use smaller sample sizes are highly encouraged to employ this practice, regardless of participant awareness and/or selection bias. Randomization can be simple or complex (*e.g.*, block, stratified, crossover, etc.) and can occur at the individual or group (*e.g.*, an entire school district, a hospital, a section of time, etc.) level. The following section will discuss multiple methods of randomization.

Simple Randomization

Depending on how many groups and/or the study design, **simple randomization** techniques such as pulling from a hat, using tables, or even flipping a coin may be perfectly acceptable. More sophisticated designs or large-scale studies may require the use of specialized randomization software, lists of random numbers, websites, or other programs. The advantages of these methods are ease, convenience, and cost. The major disadvantage of simple randomization is group distribution can be unequal at any given point. For example, consider a study requiring 20 subjects in which the researchers choose to randomize using the coin flip technique. Because it is actually more likely than not that the distribution of that coin flip will be something besides 10 heads and 10 tails, randomization would end in some number other than 10 being allocated to either the control or the experimental group (*i.e.*, uneven distribution). Uneven group sizes reduce the statistical likelihood of identifying an effect and may also weaken the quality of the research in the eyes of reviewers or readers. In order to minimize this problem, the researchers must either dramatically increase the sample pool (as the distribution of heads and tails will eventually even out) or end the randomization process after one group reaches its enrollment requirements. In other words, after one of the groups is filled, all remaining enrollments will be directly assigned to the other group. This is by definition not random and causes a problem if the trial is stopped early because of funding, time, subject availability, or any other reason.

Block Randomization

A different scheme called **block randomization** (Fig. 8-2), which groups participants together in blocks prior to the start of the study, can help reduce imbalances in the number of participants per group. The order in which the intervention is assigned to each block is still randomized and continued until all participants are randomized. For example, imagine a scientist wishes to have both experimental (A) and control (B) groups equal by every fourth person enrolled in the study (*i.e.*, they never want the group enrollments to differ by more than four). In this case, the block size is four. The possible combinations of randomized entry into the block would be AABB, ABAB, BAAB, BABA, BBAA, or ABBA. The order of each block (AABB, ABAB, etc.) would be randomly selected, and each would not be used again until all six have been used at least once. Let us assume sequence 1 (AABB) is randomly selected as the first block. This means the first and second participants enrolled in the study would be randomized to condition A. The third and fourth participants would be assigned to B. Another block would be randomly chosen (*e.g.*, BABA), and participants 5–8 would then be assigned to conditions B, A, B, and A, respectively. This means conditions A and B are guaranteed to be equal (two in each) after every four total volunteer enrollments. In fact, the number of participants in each group (A and B) will never differ by more than the block size divided by two (in this case, $4/2 = 2$). This process would continue until the desired total enrollment is reached. Randomization of the block order is important when subject selection bias is a concern, as simple patterns are easily identifiable and broken. Obviously, the larger the block size, the more difficult this becomes.

Block randomization allows termination of enrollment at virtually any time, a consideration particularly important when the participant number is large. It is also logistically

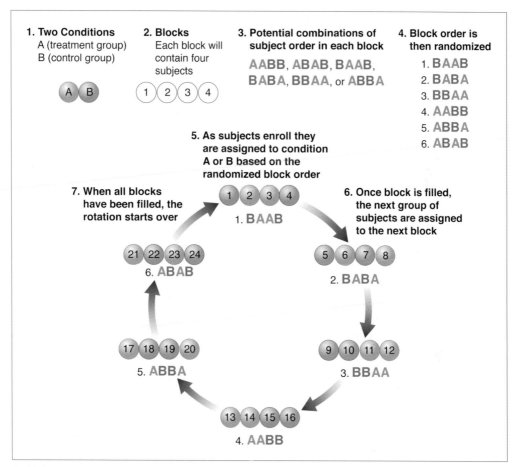

FIGURE 8-2:   Block randomization.

a simple process when groups are limited to two and block sizes are small (*e.g.*, two, four, or six). However, studies that necessitate three or more groups and/or block sizes of more than six become exceedingly complex, quickly. Another possible issue with block randomization is the condition of the final subject in each block is easy to identify. Most handle this concern by randomizing the length of each consecutive block (*e.g.*, block 1 = ABAB, block 2 = ABBBAA, block 3 = BABA, block 4 = BA, etc.).

Stratified Randomization

Stratification helps improve comparability between groups for factors the research team feels may influence the findings. In this model, subjects are divided into various subgroups or "strata." For example, perhaps the research question revolves around the amount of physical activity a population engages in following a given intervention. If the researchers knew from previous research a specific relationship exists between previous physical fitness and the effectiveness of the intervention, it would be critically important to group the subjects (before the study) based on their overall fitness level (*e.g.*, those least physically fit, those in the middle third of fitness levels, and those most fit). The high intergroup variation would statistically hide the effectiveness of the intervention had the subjects not been prestratified. Another major advantage of stratification is it allows collapsing/grouping of data from large groups. If the level of fitness in our example earlier did not influence the effectiveness of the intervention, all three strata could be combined and analyzed collectively. This saves time, increases statistical power, and can make data easier to interpret.

Stratification must be determined prior to randomization. In this case, volunteers should be specifically assigned into a stratum but still randomized into the condition (*e.g.*, treatment or control) by either simple or block strategies. One could think of this process almost like performing several small studies within a single larger one. This may increase enrollment requirements, commanding more resources, but may be a necessity.

Stratification can be done following the collection of data if two criteria are met. First, enough participants are available to sufficiently represent each group. Second, the need for stratification is clearly articulated, logical, and supported by previous research. A "failure to find significance with normal randomization" is not a reason that falls under any of these categories. This is perhaps the biggest criticism of stratification as it allows the potential for unnecessary grouping of participants for convenient analytic purposes. Some refer to this technique as "data mining." Post-hoc stratification is also acceptable in circumstances in which novel findings are unexpectedly identified. This is common in mechanistic or exploratory science but is not entirely unheard of in other forms of research as well. In reality, post-hoc stratification is likely responsible for numerous discoveries.

Crossover Randomization

Crossover randomization reduces sample size requirements because individual participants are exposed to all testing conditions. Unlike stratification, participants receive each treatment, thus serving as their own control. Randomization into separate treatment groups is therefore unnecessary. For example, a crossover study on the influence of listening to music during exercise would ask participants to perform the exercise testing once while listening to music and once while not listening to music (*i.e.*, control). This cuts the amount of participants in half compared to recruiting a separate pool of subjects for the testing (*i.e.*, listening to music) and the control conditions (*i.e.*, not listening to music). This becomes particularly important when studying a specialized population, as sample sizes might be intrinsically restricted. A crossover design also enables personalized responses to be directly compared between conditions because each subject serves as their own control.

A crossover design, however, is not always possible because it assumes exposure to the independent variable, or the testing battery will not have a lasting effect. Picture a study that examines the effectiveness of two different motivational strategies on smoking cessation. Crossover would be inappropriate considering participants must receive both motivational strategies in addition to the no-motivation (or "control") condition. This is obviously problematic as one treatment would invariably carry over to the next. A similar example taken to an extreme would be if a treatment was actually so successful it eliminated or cured the disease or disorder. Bringing participants back to receive the control/placebo condition would be unnecessary. The best way to handle this concern is to use a washout period between conditions. Depending on the details of this study, this period may be as short as 24 hours or as long as several months. This approach is often used during nutritional supplement trials. Volunteers will usually ingest the supplement/placebo for a matter of weeks, enter a washout period of several weeks or months, and then return for the next round of supplement/placebo. A crossover design can be either random or non-random.

Sometimes, the testing battery itself denotes the same carryover concern. Novel tasks are particularly susceptible because basic learning of the test or skill may produce improvements beyond the potential of the intervention. In other words, a treatment, which genuinely improves performance by 8%, may be concluded as ineffective if practicing the dependent task alone improves performance by 35%. To account for this, researchers typically provide extensive familiarization before the start of actual data collection. For all of these reasons, a study such as a biomechanical analysis of gait pattern while wearing different footwear would be a much better candidate for crossover randomization. However, this still requires some form of randomization (usually simple) for the order of intervention for each volunteer (*i.e.*, which shoe condition they use first). This ensures (or at least increases the chances) any influence of order (*e.g.*, learning, training, maturation, etc.) is minimized.

MATCHING

Sometimes, every form of randomization is unwarranted. Study designs and questions frequently exist, which require the purposeful placement of participants into specific groups (**matching**). This strategy was used in a recent analysis of the cardiovascular and muscular function of champion cross-country skiers older than 80 years old compared to age-matched non-athletes (8). Because a particular trait (*i.e.*, age and exercise training history) was key to the study, volunteers were intentionally grouped into either the athlete or the non-athlete group. This matching approach is particularly useful when cross-sectionally studying humans. Groups should be reasonably matched in number (*i.e.*, sample size) and for as many traits as possible (*e.g.*, age, lean body mass, activity, diet, health, etc.), except those of interest. The important aspect of matching is that it attempts to eliminate the variance in the study. For example, if you were to do a training study, you would want to match on activity/training status so as not to impact the various dependent variables monitoring its effects. A participant already running each week will not respond as great to an endurance training program as one who has never trained. The same can be said for strength training. So you want each group to have the same opportunity for gains in the relevant dependent variables (*e.g.*, maximum oxygen consumption, one repetition maximum strength, etc.).

SUMMARY

The ability to delineate the necessary dependent variables is undoubtedly one of the most important parts of creating a well-designed research study. As is clear from the rest of this text, there are numerous other decisions that need to be made as well. Knowing which variables are most valid for the purposes of a study can help increase the legitimacy of the project. Additionally, proper assignment of subjects to the various conditions and treatments will also help ensure a successfully completed study.

ACKNOWLEDGMENTS

The authors would like to thank Justin Nicoll for his assistance with the figures.

GLOSSARY

Blinding: experimental approach in which information that may lead to intended or unintended bias is concealed from the participant, researcher, or both

Block randomization: design approach that groups experimental units together, usually by a source of variability that is not of primary interest to the researcher

Control group: participant group in which the independent variable is delivered in such a fashion that it minimally influences the dependent variable

Crossover randomization: experimental design strategy that requires all participants be exposed to all testing conditions, allowing each participant to serve as his or her own control

Double-blinded experiment: experimental approach that requires the independent variable given to the participant be hidden from both the researcher and the participant

Experimental group: participant group in which the independent variable is delivered in such a fashion that its influences on the dependent variable can be measured

Matching: purposeful placement of research participants with similar characteristics into opposing experimental or control groups

Non-blinded experiment: study in which both the researcher and the participant are aware of the participant's treatment condition

Primary dependent variable: the study variable most directly influenced by the independent variable

Randomization: process of assigning individuals to a particular treatment group

Random assignment: method used to indiscriminately place participants into different experimental or control groups

Random selection: the arbitrary process of selecting research participants from a given larger pool or population

Reliability: ability of a measure to remain consistent

Secondary dependent variable: a study variable indirectly influenced by the independent variable

Simple randomization: using techniques such as flipping a coin or drawing from a hat to arbitrarily assign research participants to experimental or control groups

Single-blinded experiment: experimental approach that requires the independent variable given to the participant be hidden from the research or the participant

Stratification: dividing research participants into various subgroups based on previously known characteristics to arbitrarily assign them to experimental or control groups

Surrogate dependent variable: a study variable that is more practical or appropriate than a primary dependent variable

Validity: ability to accurately quantify the intended measure

REFERENCES

1. Grace ND, Muench H, Chalmers TC. The present status of shunts for portal hypertension in cirrhosis. *Gastroenterology.* 1966;50(5):684–691.
2. Hartman JW, Tang JE, Wilkinson SB, et al. Consumption of fat-free fluid milk after resistance exercise promotes greater lean mass accretion than does consumption of soy or carbohydrate in young, novice, male weightlifters. *Am J Clin Nutr.* 2007;86(2):373–381.
3. ISIS-2 (Second International Study of Infarct Survival) Collaborative Group. Randomised trial of intravenous streptokinase, oral aspirin, both, or neither among 17,187 cases of suspected acute myocardial infarction: ISIS-2. *Lancet.* 1988;332(8607): 349–360.
4. Mitchell CJ, Churchward-Venne TA, Parise G, et al. Acute post-exercise myofibrillar protein synthesis is not correlated with resistance training-induced muscle hypertrophy in young men. *PLoS ONE.* 2014;9(2):e89431. doi:10.1371/journal.pone.0089431.
5. Mitchell CJ, Churchward-Venne TA, West DW, et al. Resistance exercise load does not determine training-mediated hypertrophic gains in young men. *J Appl Physiol.* 2012;113(1):71–77.
6. Rudman D, Feller AG, Nagraj HS, et al. Effects of human growth hormone in men over 60 years old. *N Engl J Med.* 1990;323:1–6.
7. Sleight P. Debate: subgroup analyses in clinical trials: fun to look at—but don't believe them! *Curr Control Trials Cardiovasc Med.* 2000;1(1):25–27.
8. Trappe S, Hayes E, Galpin A, et al. New records in aerobic power among octogenarian lifelong endurance athletes. *J Appl Physiology.* 2013;114(1):3–10.
9. Wilkinson SB, Tarnopolsky MS, Macdonald MJ, Macdonald JR, Armstrong D, Phillips SM. Consumption of fluid skim milk promotes greater muscle protein accretion after resistance exercise than does consumption of an isonitrogenous soy-protein beverage. *Am J Clin Nutr.* 2007;85(4):1031–1040.

The Unique Challenges of Field Research

Douglas Casa, PhD, ATC, FACSM, FNATA, Rebecca L. Stearns, PhD, ATC, Jason P. Mihalik, PhD, CAT(C), ATC, and Matthew S. Ganio, PhD

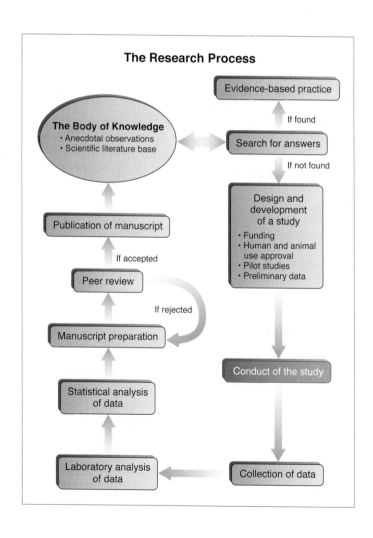

The Research Process

- Evidence-based practice
- If found
- The Body of Knowledge
  - Anecdotal observations
  - Scientific literature base
- Search for answers
- If not found
- Design and development of a study
  - Funding
  - Human and animal use approval
  - Pilot studies
  - Preliminary data
- Publication of manuscript
- If accepted
- Peer review
- If rejected
- Manuscript preparation
- Conduct of the study
- Statistical analysis of data
- Laboratory analysis of data
- Collection of data

INTRODUCTION

This chapter discusses the role and logistics of field research studies within the scientific research landscape. Such studies are done outside of a controlled laboratory setting and can vary considerably (*e.g.*, collecting blood from runners immediately after a marathon, testing of soldiers during a sustained operations field exercise, examining heart rate responses during a soccer game). Understandably, field research studies have their own benefits as well as limitations when compared to the traditional laboratory model. This chapter provides an overview of these benefits and challenges with specific insight into the logistics of planning, designing, analyzing, interpreting, and building future field research studies.

THE NEED FOR FIELD RESEARCH

Many scientists have long critiqued the lack of external validity of controlled laboratory studies. Many of the claims are justified. The lack of naturally occurring environmental influences, competitiveness, and extreme physiologic responses are all valid claims which make us consider the reality that laboratory studies, although offering great value, have limitations. The field study offers us a chance to examine the real-life responses that have the most meaning to us. Field research studies also have great limitations that must be recognized so that we do not overstep our conclusions and hinder the progress of scientific discovery. The use of field- and lab-based research studies may offer the best opportunity to allow a variety of valuable research questions to be addressed surrounding a particular topic. The importance of field research to address a question is related to the topic under investigation (*e.g.*, a field study would be more appropriate to answer the question of heart rate responses to a game or match than a laboratory study in which the active domain could not be simulated, whereas a controlled laboratory study in an environmental chamber would be better to examine the impact of equipment on heart rate under different environmental conditions). Thus, the need for field-based or laboratory studies is highly related to the question and topic being investigated.

RESEARCH DESIGN IN FIELD RESEARCH STUDIES

The strength of field research studies can be measured by their impact on clinical practice. How is this measured? Ideally, double-blind randomized clinical trials would be performed. Unfortunately, ethical restrictions prevent many athletic injuries to be studied in this capacity. For example, how could one ethically randomize the injury mechanism by which an athlete was to sustain a concussion and then ensure they were injured in such a fashion? As an additional example, what are the ethical implications of randomizing athletes to heat stroke interventions known to be less effective than cold water submersion? The answers to many of these questions are outcomes of comparative effectiveness research studies. These studies are designed to inform healthcare decision-making in a timely and effective manner, partly due to its ability to include clinicians, patients, policymakers, and health plans as primary study stakeholders. The seven steps identified by the Agency for Healthcare

CONCEPT BOX 9-1 The Importance of Basic Research Methods

Field studies can be valuable, but basic research methods cannot be forgotten. For example, in the area of heat and hydration research, many field research studies that were published in the early and mid-2000s made the finding that percent dehydration is not related to core body temperature during intense endurance exercise (11,15,24). This was in complete disagreement to the numerous laboratory findings that had found an approximate 0.4°F increase in body temperature for every additional 1% body mass loss (3,21,23). But the authors of these studies (11,15,24) failed to recognize that in a field study where intensity is variable, an increase in dehydration could often mean a decrease in intensity (because the subject did not feel well or was less physiologically able). Because intensity is the key determinant of core body temperature, a decrease in intensity would mean a decrease in body temperature. Paradoxically, the exact opposite response was found in field research studies as compared to lab studies. Intensity in laboratory studies could be controlled and monitored, and the progressive dehydration (and maintained intensity) meant a gradual increase in body temperature, which was exacerbated with more dehydration. This relationship was found to be most consistent during intense exercise in the heat.

When this paradigm was examined in a controlled field study, the exact same relationship that had been consistently reported in the lab studies (4,17,26) was observed. The controlled field study offered an opportunity to maintain intensity while manipulating hydration levels. The result was reflective of the best aspects about field research studies (competitiveness, natural sport setting, environmental reality) and laboratory studies (control, research question isolation, crossover design). It also highlighted how investigators must understand the limitations and benefits of both types of studies. In the closing statement of the paper by Casa and colleagues (4) an insightful summary of the process is provided:

> In conclusion, it seems likely that the physiologic and performance decrements associated with dehydration that have been consistently shown in a laboratory setting exist when athletes perform athletic activities in a natural sport setting. The differences that have been noted between laboratory and field settings are linked to the methodologic challenges in a field setting, which make it harder to isolate the effects and are not due to the absence of the physiologic effects themselves. (4)

Research and Quality (1) illustrate how one should build on previous findings to develop a clinically sound and meaningful research agenda (Fig. 9-1).

A field study is one that is conducted outside a controlled laboratory setting. This does not imply that a field study is inherently less controlled or less meaningful than any other study. However, it does mean that there may be unique situations and limitations that have to be considered. Field research studies follow the same scientific methods as any other study using well designed and implementing controls that are possible for the field context being studied. However, the planning, execution, and interpretation of the findings may differ in field research studies versus what we think of as the "traditional" (*i.e.*, laboratory building with testing capabilities in a multifaceted investigator controlled environment) laboratory-based studies.

When embarking on a field study, it is important that the investigator considers the type of research design. Each research design has advantages and disadvantages (*e.g.*, one needs to examine a game to get actual heart rate responses but one cannot control the conditions of the game) that should be considered, but more often than not, the research question drives the research design. For the purposes of this discussion, we will only describe

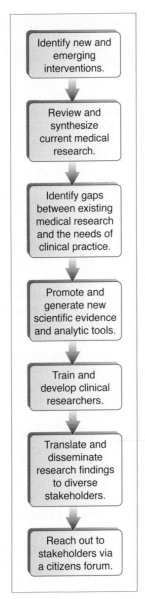

FIGURE 9-1:   The seven steps for developing a meaningful research agenda as identified by the Agency for Healthcare Research and Quality (1).

quantitative prospective studies. It is important that the researcher understands the advantages and disadvantages of common prospective field-based study designs. Some common study designs taking place in field settings are (a) observational/correlational (also referred to as **natural field study**) design, (b) **between-subjects design**, and (c) **within-subjects** (*i.e.*, repeated measures) **design** (also referred to as a **controlled field study** design).

Observational field research studies are ones in which the subjects are already planning on executing a task and the researchers are simply observing various outcome variables.

The outcome variable can be as simple as finish times in a marathon or more involved like assessing body temperature after the marathon. It is important that the measurements taking place do not influence the subjects as in the naturally occurring field study mentioned previously. For example, although subjects may already be drinking fluid during the marathon, if they are part of a research study in which they know their fluid consumption is being measured, they may subconsciously drink more than usual. This is known as the "Hawthorne effect" (14), which you learned about in Chapter 7. Observational studies have the advantage of making and/or collecting data on subjects in their "natural" settings. Observational research can help better define a problem that laboratory research can address or other field studies help expand on. They often lend themselves to large datasets. However, given the nature of the design, the interpretation of the findings are often correlational in nature. Without a scientific intervention, it is difficult to conclude that relationships observed are causal (13).

On the opposite end of the spectrum, there are within-subjects (repeated measures) field research studies. These types of studies can look very similar to a laboratory-based study but just occur in a field setting. Sometimes they are used when findings from a laboratory-based study are being "confirmed" (and validated) in a field setting. They are also useful when certain research questions cannot be answered in a laboratory-based setting. For example, examining the pacing strategy of the cycling peloton cannot be effectively done in a laboratory. In a repeated-measures field study, subjects arrive at a site and follow the explicit instructions of the researcher, just like they would in a laboratory-based study. Given that most lab-based studies have an intervention and/or repeated trials, there are several considerations that are unique to this type of field study design. With repeated trials, all factors need to be held constant (*i.e.*, there should be no design differences from the prior trial) day to day except for the intervention. However, unlike in a laboratory setting, in a field setting, it is very difficult to control extraneous factors on different testing days (*e.g.*, the weather). A potential way to account for this is to counterbalance the number of subjects with the intervention on each testing day. Repeated measures field studies allow the investigators to examine a research question in a setting that may be a little more applicable than a laboratory-based study. This is also an example of the controlled field study design mentioned earlier. However, unavoidable differences on various testing days may increase variability of the data that should be accounted for (see the section called "Statistical Issues to Consider in Field Research Studies" later in this chapter). In some cases, if the confounding variables are measured or anticipated, one can use them as a "covariate" in the subsequent statistical analyses.

A blend between a repeated measures field study and observational field study is a between-subjects field study. Similar to an observational study, the subjects may already be going to execute a certain task (*e.g.*, a marathon). The investigator decides that they want to invoke an intervention and compare the outcome to other subjects that do not have the intervention. However, due to the nature of the setting and the design, only a select number of the subjects will receive the "treatment" and the others will be control subjects (*i.e.*, no treatment). Following from the example earlier, a research question may be, "Does a prescribed fluid volume ingested during a marathon influence finish time?" The investigator would still observe individuals that were already going to run a marathon, but prior to the race, half of the subjects would be assigned a prescribed fluid intake volume. The other half would not have any intervention at all (*i.e.*, the control group). Race times would be examined after the race to see if the prescribed fluid intake influenced the outcome. There are inherent advantages and disadvantages to this type of field study design. Between-subjects designs allow the researcher to see if changes occur when the subject has some type of intervention. However, it is difficult in this type of design to associate a causal effect between the intervention and outcome variable (13). Part of the reason for this is a lack of control of many confounding variables and the inability to manipulate the outcome variable systematically. In other words, this research is often restricted to making correlational relationships and inferences. One potential way to overcome this barrier, if the situation allows for it, is to have a repeated measures design, as previously discussed.

BENEFITS, DRAWBACKS, UNIQUENESS, AND LIMITATIONS/ASSUMPTIONS OF FIELD RESEARCH

Naturally occurring field research studies (observational) are studies that take place within the natural confines of the practice, game, or race. Nothing is contrived in order to address the research question. The athletes participate in regularly scheduled workouts and practices. Studies with elite football players (8), youth hydration studies (7), high school football players (29,30), endurance road cycling (2), and triathletes (12) are examples of naturally occurring (observational) field research studies. In all of these studies, data was collected within the confines of the athlete's exercise or competition. Therefore, the exercise session was not altered, but data was collected during opportunities such as natural rest periods and transitions before or after exercise.

Examples of between-subjects design studies include those in which an intervention group of youth athletes were educated regarding their hydration habits (20), or another in which triathletes were split into control and intervention groups immediately following an Ironman Triathlon race to examine the effect of a recovery aid (25), and lastly, a comparison of cooling rates between cold water immersion at two different road races (19).

Examples of within-subjects (*i.e.*, repeated measures or a controlled field study design) include those in which trail runners competed multiple races on different days while receiving different treatments for each race or trial (4,26,31) or another that examined prerace hydration beverages when mountain bike racing (28), and lastly, a study that examined different rehydration beverages following exercise (10). All of these studies had subjects repeat the same trial in the field but provided different interventions with each trial.

As briefly discussed earlier, some of the main benefits of field research studies include the following: (a) they are in a real sport setting (actual competition or training or close approximation); (b) naturally occurring competition and competitive drives as well as associated psychophysiologic states; (c) potential for extreme physiologic demands and responses; and (d) an abundance of potential subjects in the same place at same time. The potential for extreme physiologic responses is a particularly unique benefit. Field studies observe aspects of real-life situations which could not be created in the laboratory.

The institutional review boards (IRBs) have in many cases rightfully tightened regulations on the physiologic monitoring process during lab studies, thus making any insights into the competitive field environmental extremes not possible to study. For example, in the realm of thermal physiology studies, the core body temperature cutoff is often 103–105°F depending on the university. When body temperature is measured in a field setting, an athlete may be competing at 104.6°F (and be completely fine without symptoms of heat stress), but participants reaching these pre-determined imposed temperature thresholds in the laboratory setting would not be permitted to continue activity. It is important that the local IRB is aware of this possibility so that the investigators do not have to prematurely stop exercise. Considering extreme physiologic responses represent a major area of interest, the field setting creates a laboratory that is limited only by the desire, abilities, and physiological capacity of the individual being studied. This is extremely exciting for the researcher who works in this area. Obviously in a practice or competition situation, where investigators possess information that could benefit the medical staff, they should be quick to share this information in order to maximize the health and safety of subjects. Even when presented with these advantages, field research studies also create several disadvantages researchers should recognize. In any investigation, the protection of the participants is of primary importance. One must balance ethics, safety, and value of the realtime observations in any field study.

The first disadvantage is the lack of true experimental control. Environmental conditions, level of competition, conditions of the exercise area (field, trail, road, etc.), time of day, and exercise intensity are often dictated by team administrators and self-pace of the athletes themselves. Many steps can be made to counteract the influence of limited control including, for example, setting well-defined parameters for testing. However, this is only possible in the controlled field study. Because control is out of the investigator's capability to manipulate, there is much more of a gamble in the naturally occurring field study. For example in one summer, when conducting a football research study examining heat and hydration issues, the high ambient temperature did not break 60°F on one of the research days. This is an example of the inherent challenge associated with these types of field studies (*i.e.*, one cannot control the weather).

Another disadvantage of field research studies is that it is often difficult to have a crossover design. For example, research studies examining the Ironman Triathlon World Championships did not allow for a crossover design. Subjects could not return two weeks later and compete again to participate in the other experimental condition. In these circumstances, you need to work diligently to counterbalance your trial groups and also pursue larger sample sizes than those of laboratory studies due to the inherent increase in variability associated with subjects that are not serving as their own controls. This is much easier to manage in a controlled field study but still difficult if you are asking for an extreme task to be performed. Field research studies also make it difficult to isolate the specific effect being studied due to the many intervening variables that may disguise the effect. Also, extremely large research teams are often needed to study a large number of people at the same time. This can directly impact the research budget making some field studies cost-prohibitive. This is very different than interacting with one individual at a time in a lab study. For many field research studies, one can have routinely more than 20 research assistants onsite during data collection. Although the experiment often can be completed quite quickly in a field study, much help is needed during the data collection.

LOGISTICS OF MOVING A LAB AND PERSONNEL, AND BUDGET CONSIDERATIONS IN FIELD RESEARCH STUDIES

A well-designed field study is the basis for success; however, a deep understanding and realistic expectations of how data within a specific field study can be collected will strengthen the study design, even in the face of unexpected events (*i.e.*, a subject does not finish, poor weather, equipment failure, etc.). For field research studies, it is just as important to consider the potential pitfalls that are common to field research studies and use this information to inform a strong research design capable of overcoming these limitations. There are three main considerations that can guide researchers to successful research studies:

1. Logistics of moving a laboratory
2. Person power requirements
3. Budget and cost considerations

Logistics of Moving a Laboratory

When moving a laboratory, researchers should take into account three large factors:

1. Onsite resources and transporting necessary equipment
2. Weather considerations
3. Communication ability

Onsite Resources and Equipment

Because equipment can be very expensive, transporting a laboratory requires careful packing, handling, shipping, and planning. Therefore, before departing for an offsite location, researchers should consider if there are any collaborators near the study research that could loan equipment for the onsite analysis needs of the research study. Depending on the needs of the study, many resources may also be available within the research study location, and analysis by another party may present a more cost-effective alternative considering the costs of moving a lab and shipping samples. This will largely depend on the distance that is being traveled and the analysis being performed, but nonetheless, it is an option. Careful consideration should also be given to your institution's policy on transporting equipment off campus and any liability that may be associated with this.

If equipment is shipped or driven to the site, it is important to verify the accurate functionality of the equipment prior to departure and also upon arrival. Be sure to check manufacturer instructions regarding threats to the equipment's accuracy. For research studies that are done at a site farther than a driving distance from the laboratory, any equipment that is transported should be sent with enough time to safely ensure its arrival and functionality prior to data collection. This also requires careful planning and coordination in respect to the person who can receive this shipment depending on how much time you will have onsite prior to the start of data collection. Depending on the number of items being transported, it may be prudent to transport via a wood pallet, but this method can be costly (a 4-ft × 4-ft 500-lb pallet can cost a lot of money when shipped from the East Coast to West Coast) and best used when large pieces of equipment are being transported.

It is also important to ensure that the resources needed for the study equipment will be readily available. A preliminary site visit and careful examination is vital in this phase of study preparation ending with a needs analysis and action plan for solving the deficiencies identified. Power outlets, extension cords, water sources, lighting, tables, data sheets, biohazard containment, removal, etc., all need to be secured for onsite use. It is best to coordinate with the entity either managing the event or the institution hosting it. Approval and assistance by these individuals will provide much easier access to the event, greater availability of resources, and better ability for the subjects to be able to find and reach you. However, all of this planning can take a large amount of time for which you should budget. Some field research studies can take a year or longer to secure these arrangements. In addition, it is highly recommended that the research team bring a printer. Although data sheets and questionnaires can be printed ahead of time, it is always best to be able to freely print new items or print off a few more copies of necessary documents. It may also be important to locate the closest copy center in the event it is needed.

Weather Considerations

Changing or unexpected weather can cause changes not only in the ability of the research team to collect data but also in the accuracy of instruments being used. Lab equipment that is sensitive to external environments needs to be used indoors, likely in a hotel room or rented space. Rain, snow, heat, cold, lightning, and security threats are all possible. Not unlike an emergency action plan to prepare for medical emergencies, research teams should have plans onsite to help protect expensive equipment and valuable personnel should inclement weather or other uncontrollable factors alter the research team's ability to collect data. If these extremes can cause changes to the event itself, researchers must be prepared to consequently alter the study design. If the field research study is being done within a controlled field study, this is an important element to consider in the design of the study. Many tools, such as weather history for the projected data collection days, can be helpful to minimize the chance for weather-related complications.

Communication

Communication in a field location can be a vital component of success for a field research study. Researchers must be able to quickly and effectively communicate with other members of the team, and subjects need to be able to contact the research team both prior to onsite arrival and also while onsite. These challenges have been lessened with great improvements in technology such as smartphones and tablets, but it is still suggested that researchers provide clear and complete instructions, maps, and contact information to subjects prior to their arrival onsite. Therefore, in the event that the subject is not able to contact you prior to or upon his or her arrival, he or she will still have all the necessary information. Securing subjects prior to onsite arrival by the research team and minimizing recruitment that is done onsite greatly improves the likely number of subjects recruited, reduces the possibility for subject attrition, and provides subjects more time to understand the study requirements and expectations. In the least, it is recommended that one researcher can serve as a point of contact for subjects who will be accessible via phone or e-mail at all times (given the consideration that wireless internet may not always be available). A master list of cell phone numbers is recommended for the research team members, which should be programmed into each researcher's phone. If cell phone service is limited, handheld radios are recommended, especially when the research team may be distances apart throughout data collection.

Personnel

Field research studies demand a much greater amount of personnel than do traditional laboratory studies. This is mainly because field research studies are usually centered around races or athletic events when the research team is collecting data on all the study participants at one time or does not have control over timing of when subjects arrive and when data collection occurs. Depending on the event and time point of the data being collected, researchers' formation for data collection may differ. Field researchers have found that pods (mobile groups of two to four researchers that can collect a variety of variables; Fig. 9-2), stations (subjects move from various variable-specific stations for data collection; Fig. 9-3), and one-on-ones (when a researcher works directly with one subject for all the data collected; Fig. 9-4) all have their advantages and disadvantages. Table 9-1 provides a summary of the features of these various setups and examples. As one example of pod use, researchers worked with high school football players during their preseason practices to collect various variables during short five-minute practice breaks (30). As an example of station use, researchers examined body cooling strategies in athletes and used various stations following exercise bouts to implement cooling and also collect paper-based variables (9).

The authors have found it advantageous to have study-specific T-shirts, hats, and clothing (usually brightly colored) so subjects can quickly identify researchers. Having a large banner with the study or university name is also helpful for subjects to identify the

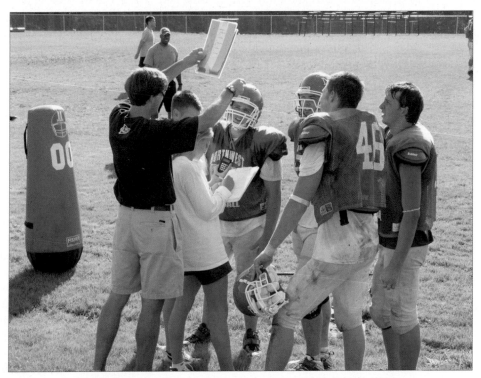

FIGURE 9-2:   An example of a pod-based data collection formation.

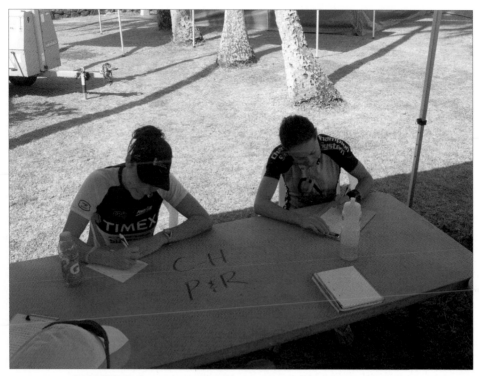

FIGURE 9-3:   An example of a station-based data collection formation.

research team. Likewise, to identify subjects, the authors have used brightly colored rubber bracelets, stickers on helmets, or bib and jersey numbers.

Budget and Costs

Field research studies provide some budget benefits, largely because researchers' time and overhead costs are greatly compacted or reduced. However, during data collection, it usually means a few long sequential days of work. Unique budgeting items for a field study include considerations for shipping costs (for supplies and samples), researcher transportation (car or air), car rentals, gas costs, lodging, food costs, onsite costs for lab location (hotel or rented space), and sometimes costs for items such as dry ice to properly store and/or ship samples.

With the large number of researchers required for field research, when traveling to an event, it can be beneficial to rent a vacation rental or similar property to save money on hotel costs and also food (which can be cooked and prepared by the staff instead of going out to eat for every meal). Also remember to factor in extra room for any car rentals, as you will likely be bringing extra bags with you for equipment in addition to personal bags. If you take a flight, try to use an airline that does not charge you for baggage; this way, each researcher can bring his or her personal bag as well as one with non-fragile research items.

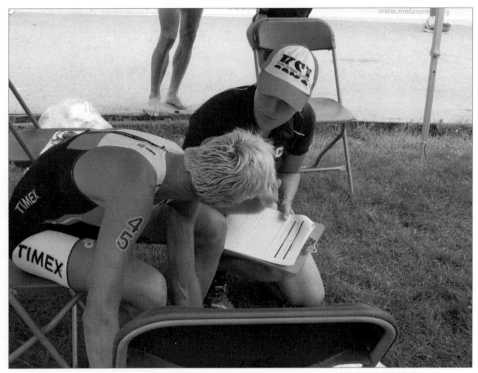

FIGURE 9-4:   An example of a one-on-one–based data collection formation.

Overall, although the logistics of a field study can be large and complicated, careful, precise, and complete planning can help to manage a lot of the stress that can occur with field research study data collection. It is highly recommended that researchers practice their planned data collection methods as best as possible (and even budgeting time onsite prior to the start of official data collection) to identify any weaknesses and implement strategies to address these weaknesses prior to data collection.

INSTITUTIONAL REVIEW BOARD SUBMISSION AND PLANNING LOGISTICS

The process of managing a field study offers some unique considerations, particularly as it relates to IRB submissions. Given that field research studies will often happen off of the campus where the IRB is housed and may require additional independent IRBs to be involved, your study may require some special—and advanced—planning. Before you submit items to your own IRB, you need to consider the following:

1. Other universities that will need IRB approval (either of fellow researchers who will be assisting you or you will be at the site of the university for the data collections)
2. Permissions that need to be ascertained in order to have the approval of the necessary entities
3. Logistical planning regarding setup, data collection, access to the subjects and areas

Table 9-1 Advantages and Disadvantages of Various Field Data Collection Techniques		
	Pods	**Stations**	**One-on-One**
Number of Researchers Required	Two to four per pod	Varies, usually one to three per station	One per subject
Advantages	1. Researchers are mobile and can move to subjects. 2. Researchers can collect information from a number of subjects at one time.	1. Allows researchers to be specialized in data collection that may be technically difficult 2. Large subject and data variable capacity 3. Variables requiring more subject time can be completed	1. Ensures all data is collected for each subject 2. Improved subject satisfaction with participation 3. High flexibility of researcher's responsibility
Disadvantages	1. Restricted in data volume capacity (due to mobility of researchers and how much they can carry) 2. Best designed for data that is collected within minutes (body temperature, perceptual scales) 3. Technical or specialized variables may not be possible (*i.e.*, blood draws).	1. Subjects may accidentally skip a station. 2. If stations are specialized, researchers are restricted to their specialty (less researcher flexibility).	1. Requires researchers to be highly competent in all procedures and variables collected 2. Time-intensive for researchers 3. Low subject capacity

4. Ancillary support staff that should be in the loop
5. Specific IRB issues related to monitoring and reporting

Before submitting your materials to your IRB, you will need permissions from the relevant entities. This can include athletic directors, head coaches, race medical directors, race directors, team physicians, head athletic trainers, head strength and conditioning coaches, hospital chief executive officers (CEOs), league commissioners, owners of facilities, superintendents, principals, etc. A full explanation of the purposes and procedures of the study will need to be explained to these individuals so they can make an informed decision as to whether to participate in the project. Their approval letter will be needed for the IRB submission process.

The process of having multiple sites approving a single IRB protocol can be cumbersome. Our experience has found that it is best to provide ample time (make the first submission to the home IRB six months before start of data collection) to allow for the multiple review procedures that take place. The optimal situation is to gain approval from your home IRB then have the other IRBs offer reciprocity without the need for a full approval process. With recent changes to the regulations that IRBs must respect, "rely-on" procedures are becoming more commonplace and easier to obtain. In the unlikely event that the secondary site requires full IRB approval, it can create a difficult situation with multiple versions of the same document, which can create an awkward and cumbersome process. Any researcher who is assisting with the data collection needs to obtain permission from his or her home IRB to assist with the study. This protects all parties involved and is an important legal and ethical consideration.

You will need to have plan in place in order to properly write up your IRB materials. It is important to directly involve the event planners with the research coordination needed to address the project directly. Some of these include coordination regarding field access, finish line access, medical tent access, details regarding where your lab will be set up, when you will have access to subjects, e-mails and contact with athletes and/or participants, and contingencies for when problems (weather, cancellations, delays, etc.) arise. Efforts should be made to reach out to field maintenance staff, police/safety staff, fire staff, assistant coaches, etc., regarding details of setup and logistics to gather additional insights and be as well-prepared as possible.

Given that the investigative team may be responsible for medical care (controlled field study) or potentially not in charge (naturally occurring field study), the team needs to make specific arrangements with the IRB regarding what type of care will be provided and the chain of command that will take place. Additionally, if you are not in charge of care, a policy must be developed to outline the process of informing appropriate people (medical staff, coaches, parents, etc.) regarding relevant medical data that is acquired that may be important to enhance safety and care. For example, if you are recording body temperature, you may stop a participant in a controlled field study when he or she reaches 104.5°F, but in a naturally occurring field study, you may need to inform the head athletic trainer so he or she has the information and opportunity to act as he or she wishes to optimize the care for which he or she is responsible. In controlled field research studies in which the researchers are creating risk, they are responsible for providing appropriate care if a problem arises. We highly encourage the researchers to be sure an athletic trainer or other appropriate medical care is always onsite during these circumstances. This person would coordinate the care in these cases.

STATISTICAL ISSUES TO CONSIDER IN FIELD RESEARCH STUDIES

The statistical tests used for field study data are no different than data from other types of studies. However, there are considerations and potential issues that should be acknowledged before conducting a field-based study. The biggest factor dictating the statistics performed is study design. The statistics used for an observational study are much different than a repeated measures design. It is important to consider this at the onset of the study because it will likely have an impact on the number of subjects needed to answer the research question with adequate statistical power (16,22).

A well-organized and well-executed field study will have the same degree of internal and external variability as any other study. However, some of the logistical hurdles and settings in which a field study may take place provide a real threat to controlling variability and missing data. For example, a mass event like the Ironman Triathlon provides a unique study population in a unique setting, but careful planning considering every scenario must be done prior to the event. *A priori* decisions and related questions to consider could be: What if multiple subjects finish at the same time and post-race data is needed on all of them immediately? What if some of the subjects do not finish the race? These and similar questions should be asked ahead of time because the answers have implications for how the data will be handled, the statistics performed, and even the number of subjects needed to answer the research question.

Proper statistical power for the number of subjects needed is a vital calculation in order to recruit enough subjects if attrition is expected in a field study, For example, if the research question can only be answered with complete datasets of individuals that finish the race, more subjects will be needed if it is expected that some individuals may not finish the race. This is the equivalent of attrition that occurs in any other study. However, depending on the field setting, the **attrition rate** may be higher than it is in other types of studies. The degree of attrition is also dependent on the type of field study employed. A lower attrition rate may be expected in a field-based study that is a repeated measures design. If subjects are conducting multiple trials similar to a laboratory-based study, there may be flexibility in subjects repeating a trial. This is a viable option if the protocol allows for it and all of the other extraneous factors are controlled as much as possible (*e.g.*, choosing a date with similar weather conditions). However, the attrition rate may be higher in an observational field study in which subjects are performing an arduous task that has a high rate of failure (*e.g.*, Ironman Triathlon). Regardless of the study design, it is difficult to predict attrition, so researchers often try to have more subjects than needed (within ethical boundaries) to have statistical power even after attempting to take attrition into account.

Similar to attrition, how to handle missing data should be considered before embarking on a field study. If the logistics of data collection are carefully planned, missing data may not be an issue, but the nature of field research studies lends themselves to unforeseen barriers. When data collection requires a large number of researchers, it is important that each researcher is well-trained on how to collect the data. If circumstances present themselves in which some missing data is inevitable, the priority must be given to data that is most salient to the research question. There are many different ways to handle missing data, but the most important aspect is to minimize bias by handling it objectively (27). Just like other studies, though, large amounts of missing data compromise the integrity of the study by way of influencing variability and statistical power. Similar to dealing with attrition in planning a field study, missing data can be "planned for" by recognizing it is a real possibility. Increasing subject size helps maintain statistical power when enough missing data forces the researcher to eliminate a subject from the analysis.

INTERPRETING RESULTS, FORMING CONCLUSIONS, AND BUILDING UPON PREVIOUS FINDINGS

At this point, we hope that we have impressed upon you the unique challenges of field research. Field research presents a rare opportunity to explore clinical phenomena directly in the environments in which they naturally occur. Studying head trauma directly on the football field, exploring heat tolerance at major marathon events, and applying injury prevention programs on the soccer pitch are all examples of field research that have considerably advanced our understanding beyond that which could have been discovered in a laboratory setting. It is no surprise that funding agencies are becoming increasingly interested in field research studies because they permit the translation of laboratory discoveries to field application.

A strength of field research studies, particularly in those addressing injury management (*e.g.*, concussion management, heat illness interventions, etc.), is the opportunity to apply clinical interventions in real-life unaltered settings. This is illustrated through the following example: A team of clinical researchers is interested in determining the best way to treat serious heat illness. In a laboratory setting, they establish that cold water submersion appears most effective at lowering core body temperatures in study participants who are subject to a treadmill fatigue protocol. Bound by their institutional ethics board, the researchers are required to stop the study participants when core body temperature reaches 103°F, even though they recognize that serious heat illness typically occurs at core body temperatures exceeding well above this threshold. Although cold water submersion works for these study participants, how well will this intervention work in athletes who compete—needlessly and recklessly—to the brink of heat exhaustion, or worse, heat stroke? In field research studies, particularly observational field studies (*e.g.*, marathons in which researchers may only interact with competitors once the race has been completed), it is thus possible to translate laboratory findings to clinically meaningful environments. What is not permitted in laboratory settings is often an observable event in field research studies. Much of our understanding of human tolerance and the required medical interventions when these tolerances are exceeded have been the result of well-designed field research studies.

A key determinant to a well-thought out research agenda is the investigator's ability to build on previous findings. This is no truer than in field research studies. Injury events—particularly for rare events—make widespread studies difficult to carry out. Thus, researchers must maximize their access to patient populations and apply study interventions when the opportunities present themselves. Follow-up studies must build on these findings because limited access to patient populations may continue. Duplicating one's own findings, although sometimes valuable, is a commodity that often cannot be met with the financial and patient-access restrictions of important field research.

Interpreting Results

A key strength of field researchers is the ability to analyze data in an objective and structured manner. This textbook provides the reader with the necessary statistical methods to make meaningful statistical comparisons. However, statistical significance does not equate to clinical significance. For a pairwise comparison, a statistically significant finding is one in which the null hypothesis that two groups are equal is rejected. The differences in the group means are largely attributed to the independent variable (*i.e.*, grouping variable) and not likely due to random chance. But what is the magnitude of the difference? How does this relate to the reliability and precision of the test measures? More important, how clinically meaningful are these results? We will present the following methods to address the clinical meaningfulness of clinical data: (a) effect size, (b) reliability change index, (c) sensitivity and specificity, and (d) predictive value.

Effect Size

An **effect size** is a measure of the strength of a phenomenon. Effect sizes are not intended to be used in isolation but rather in combination with inferential statistics and their associated statistical significance findings. Because the computation of effect sizes rely on data obtained from samples, researchers should recognize that they are estimated with error (as are inferential statistics). Many methods exist for computing effect sizes, and they are largely dependent on the study design and the nature of the statistical analyses employed. The most recognized method to determine the effect size between two group means is the **Cohen's *d***, and it is computed by subtracting the means of two groups and dividing by a standard deviation for the data:

$$d = \frac{\overline{x_1} - \overline{x_2}}{s}$$

where $\overline{x_1}$ represents the mean of group 1, $\overline{x_2}$ represents the mean of group 2, and *s* represents the standard deviation for the data. Cohen (6) originally qualified the magnitude of these effects sizes as "small" (0.2–0.3), "medium" (0.5), and "large" (greater than 0.8).

Reliable Change Index

Reliable change index (RCI) methodology determines a test result representing a clinically meaningful change as opposed to normal variability in test performance. Reliable change methodology has been revised over the years to encompass both the reliability and the practice effects of an instrument (5). Reliable change incorporates the reliability and variance of a measure to produce a value that can be defined as change that occurred beyond the scope of measurement error or variability. Consider the following example: Researchers are exploring a novel test metric they believe will help with concussion diagnosis. They apply the test to a group of healthy athletes at baseline and repeat the testing in those following a suspected concussion. They perform a paired-samples t test (comparing the pre- and post-injury means) and make the conclusion that because the analysis yielded a significant difference, their new test metric is an effective tool for diagnosing concussion. The analyses identify that the post-injury 5-point drop in performance was statistically significant. There is no mention of the test's reliability or expected learning effects with repeat testing. Your enthusiasm for this new test metric would likely be tempered if you learned that test-retest performance variability observed in healthy participants might exceed as many as 9 points.

Context is critical in interpreting results for clinical application. The RCI combines Pearson correlation coefficients (*r*) across test sessions in addition to the means; standard deviations (SD); the standard error of the measurements from test sessions 1 (SEM_1) and 2 (SEM_2); the standard error of the difference (SE_{diff}); and the z-score associated with the 95% (z = 1.96), 90% (z = 1.684), and 80% (z = 1.282) confidence intervals, respectively, to compute the predictive RCI values for each outcome measure (formulas below). This methodology allows researchers to provide clinicians with values by which observed departures from baseline are 80%, 90%, or 95% likely attributable to the condition of interest and not what one might expect from typical test-retest performance variability.

$$SEM_1 = SD_1 \sqrt{1 - r}$$

$$SEM_2 = SD_2 \sqrt{1 - r}$$

$$SE_{diff} = \sqrt{SEM_1^2 + SEM_2^2}$$

$$RCI = SE_{diff} \times \text{z-score}$$

Sensitivity and Specificity

The validity of a diagnostic test is often evaluated in terms of its ability to accurately assess the presence (**sensitivity**) or absence (**specificity**) of the medical condition. The sensitivity of a device is its ability to identify a patient as having the condition when he or she does, in fact, have the condition (*i.e.*, ability to identify a true positive). The specificity of a device is the ability of identifying a patient as *not* having a condition when he or she does *not* have the condition (*i.e.*, identifying true negatives). These values are very simple to compute and provide a straightforward presentation of clinically meaningful data related to novel diagnostic metrics studied in the field (Table 9-2).

$$Sensitivity = \frac{A}{A + C}$$

$$Specificity = \frac{D}{B + D}$$

Predictive Value

Clinical tests must also be *useful* adjuncts to clinical expertise, and we determine this use by assessing a screening tool's **predictive value**. An instrument must be an efficient use of time and resources if it is to be applied to clinical practice. We evaluate clinical usefulness through positive predictive value (PV+) and negative predictive value (PV−). The PV+ is the likelihood that someone who tests positive on the novel device actually has the condition. Alternately, PV− is the likelihood that someone who tests negative on a novel device actually does not have the condition. Although seemingly similar to sensitivity and specificity, these definitions are uniquely distinct. Sensitivity and specificity relate the performance of the novel device to an existing gold standard. However, PV+ accounts for false positives, and PV− accounts for false negatives. The PV+ and PV− are often neglected in clinical studies. Although a novel device that is 75% sensitive to identifying a condition seems a great tool for clinicians, that would be tempered if the PV+ is a mere 10%. This would mean that of all people who test positive for a condition on the novel device, only 10% would have the condition.

$$PV+ = \frac{A}{A + B}$$

$$PV- = \frac{D}{C + D}$$

Table 9-2 Novel Device Results

		Gold Standard Diagnostic		Total
		Positive	Negative	
Novel Device Results	Positive	A (true+)	B (false+)	A + B
	Negative	C (false−)	D (true−)	C + D
	Total	A + C	B + D	A + B + C + D

Concept Box 9-2   **Example from the Field**

Commercially available helmet- and chin strap–based head impact indicators purportedly measure the forces associated with head impacts and alert coaches and athletes when these impacts exceed pre-determined tolerance thresholds during sports participation. These thresholds vary among currently available head impact indicators and are widely unsupported by the research literature. One device in particular employs a low threshold (approximately 75 g) so that its device can capture as many injury events as possible, increasing its apparent sensitivity and enhancing its market presence in the field. A field study of head impact biomechanics is conducted and observes over 280,000 head impacts and identifies 24 head injuries in the process (18). The observations can be summarized as follows:

The sensitivity (18/24 = 75%) and specificity (274,763/283,324 = 97.0%) of the head impact indicator may suggest clinical use. However, the PV+ (18/8,579 = 0.2%) is clinically meaningless. Would you rely on a device to identify 8,579 athlete incidents requiring a comprehensive sideline concussion evaluation only to identify 18 injuries? The cost, time, and clinical usefulness of this product are not supported in the field given this important clinically interpretable outcome (PV+).

		Diagnosed Injury Resulting from Head Impact		Total
		Yes	No	
Head impact indicator threshold (75 g) exceeded	Yes	18	8,561	8,579
	No	6	274,763	274,769
	Total	24	283,324	283,348

CONCLUSIONS

Field research can be a fulfilling challenge for clinical and exercise science investigators. More importantly, it is a necessary and logical extension of applying laboratory discoveries to advance the evidence base for our clinical practice. Armed with the right perspectives and an understanding of clinical interpretation of one's findings, the impact of field research on advancing the field can be considerable. A number of statistical methods exist to analyze field data in a robust manner, but the field investigator must consider the additional steps required to interpret these data and translate them into clinically meaningful outcomes that will elicit changes in patient care. Beyond patient care and injury aspects of clinical medicine, it should now be obvious that the wide array of field studies also involve other topics as well. A wide variety of field studies have been done in sports from studying small-sided games in soccer to stress of tennis matches, to techniques in weight lifting meets, to the stress of wrestling matches, etc. Other areas of military research use field studies to evaluate basic training or operational demands. So in conclusion, field studies represent an important investigative approach in a host of different topics in exercise and sport science, military research, and sports medicine and demand the same insightful rigor for study design and conduct as traditional laboratory-based experiments.

GLOSSARY

Attrition rate: natural or expected reduction in total subjects that are able to complete all research procedures (either due to illness, injury, fitness ability, etc.); important to account for when anticipating the number of subjects needed to recruit and therefore obtain enough statistical power

Between-subjects design: a blend between a repeated measures controlled field study and observational field study; this occurs when subjects are already going to execute a certain task, but some are assigned to a treatment or intervention, whereas others will serve as controls or no treatment; allows researchers to see if changes occur with some type of intervention but is often restricted to making correlational relationships and inferences

Cohen's *d*: a method used to determine the effect size between two group means

Controlled field study: also see within-subjects design; when similar controls from a laboratory-based study are placed within a field setting; in a repeated trials controlled field study, subjects are asked to return multiple times to serve as their own control for numerous trials

Effect size: a measure of strength for an examined phenomenon based on differences in group means and standard deviation of the data

Natural field study: also see observational field research; studies in which the subjects are already planning on executing a task and the researchers are simply observing various outcome variables; have the advantage of making and/or collecting data on subjects in their natural settings but without scientific intervention, it is difficult to conclude that relationships are causal

Observational field research: also see natural field study; studies in which the subjects are already planning on executing a task and the researchers are simply observing various outcome variables; have the advantage of making and/or collecting data on subjects in their natural settings but without scientific intervention, it is difficult to conclude that relationships are causal

Predictive value: either the likelihood that someone who tests positive on a novel device actually has the condition (positive predictive value) or the likelihood that someone who tests negative on a novel device actually does not have the condition (negative predictive value)

Reliable change index: a methodology to determine if a test result represents a clinically meaningful change as opposed to normal variability in test performance; combines Pearson correlation coefficients in addition to the means; standard deviations; the standard error of the measures; the standard error of the difference; and the z-score associated with 95%, 90%, and 80% confidence intervals

Sensitivity: the validity of a diagnostic test in terms of its ability to accurately assess the presence of a medical condition (the ability to identify a true positive) when compared to a gold standard; usually used in conjunction with specificity

Specificity: the validity of a diagnostic test in terms of its ability to accurately assess the absence of a medical condition (the ability to identify a true negative) when compared to a gold standard; usually used in conjunction with sensitivity

Within-subjects design: also see controlled field study; when similar controls from a laboratory-based study are placed within a field setting; subjects are asked to return multiple times to serve as their own comparison for numerous trials

R E F E R E N C E S

1. Agency for Healthcare Research and Quality Web site [Internet]. What is comparative effectiveness research? Rockville (MD): Agency for Healthcare Research and Quality; [cited 2013 November 17]. Available from: http://effectivehealthcare.ahrq.gov/index.cfm/what-is-comparative-effectiveness-research1/
2. Armstrong LE, Casa DJ, Emmanuel H, et al. Nutritional, physiological, and perceptual responses during a summer ultra-endurance cycling event. *J Strength Cond Res.* 2012;26(2):307–318.
3. Armstrong LE, Whittlesey MJ, Casa DJ, et al. No effect of 5% hypohydration on running economy of competitive runners at 23 degrees C. *Med Sci Sports Exerc.* 2006;38(10):1762–1769.
4. Casa DJ, Stearns RL, Lopez RM, et al. Influence of hydration on physiological function and performance during trail running in the heat. *J Athl Train.* 2010;45(2):147–156.
5. Chelune GJ, Naugle RI, Lüders H, Sedlak J, Awad IA. Individual change after epilepsy surgery: practice effects and base rate information. *Neuropsychology.* 1993;7:41–52.
6. Cohen J. *Statistical Power Analysis for the Behavioral Sciences.* 2nd ed. Hillsdale (NJ): Lawrence Erlbaum Associates; 1988.
7. Decher NR, Casa DJ, Yeargin SW, et al. Hydration status, knowledge, and behavior in youths at summer sports camps. *Int J Sports Physiol Perform.* 2008;3(3):262–278.
8. DeMartini JK, Martschinske JL, Casa DJ, et al. Physical demands of National Collegiate Athletic Association Division I football players during preseason training in the heat. *J Strength Cond Res.* 2011;25(11):2935–2943.
9. DeMartini JK, Ranalli GF, Casa DJ, et al. Comparison of body cooling methods on physiological and perceptual measures of mildly hyperthermic athletes. *J Strength Cond Res.* 2011;25(8):2065–2074.
10. Fiala KA, Casa DJ, Roti MW. Rehydration with a caffeinated beverage during the nonexercise periods of 3 consecutive days of 2-a-day practices. *Int J Sport Nutr Exerc Metab.* 2004;14(4):419–429.
11. Godek SF, Bartolozzi AR, Burkholder R, Sugarman E, Dorshimer G. Core temperature and percentage of dehydration in professional football linemen and backs during preseason practices. *J Athl Train.* 2006;41(1):8–14; discussion 14–17.
12. Johnson EC, Pryor JL, Casa DJ, et al. Bike and run pacing on downhill segments predict Ironman triathlon relative success. *J Sci Med Sport.* 2015;18(1):82–87.
13. Kuhn JE, Greenfield ML, Wojtys EM. A statistics primer. Types of studies in the medical literature. *Am J Sports Med.* 1997;25(2):272–274.
14. Landsberger H. *Hawthorne Revisited: A Plea for an Open City.* Ithaca (NY): Cornell University; 1957.
15. Laursen PB, Suriano R, Quod MJ, et al. Core temperature and hydration status during an Ironman triathlon. *Br J Sports Med.* 2006;40(4):320–325; discussion 325.
16. Lipsey MW. How to estimate statistical power. In: *Design Sensitivity: Statistical Power for Experimental Research.* Newbury Park (CA): SAGE Publications; 1990. p. 69–91.
17. Lopez RM, Casa DJ, Jensen KA, et al. Examining the influence of hydration status on physiological responses and running speed during trail running in the heat with controlled exercise intensity. *J Strength Cond Res.* 2011;25(11):2944–2954.
18. Lynall RC, Laudner KG, Mihalik JP, Stanek JM. Concussion-assessment and -management techniques used by athletic trainers. *J Athl Train.* 2013;48(6):844–850.
19. McDermott BP, Casa DJ, O'Connor FG, et al. Cold-water dousing with ice massage to treat exertional heat stroke: a case series. *Aviat Space Environ Med.* 2009;80(8):720–722.
20. McDermott BP, Casa DJ, Yeargin SW, Ganio MS, Lopez RM, Mooradian EA. Hydration status, sweat rates, and rehydration education of youth football campers. *J Sport Rehabil.* 2009;18(4):535–552.
21. Montain SJ, Coyle EF. Influence of graded dehydration on hyperthermia and cardiovascular drift during exercise. *J Appl Physiol.* 1992;73(4):1340–1350.
22. Park L, Schutz RW. "Quick and easy" formulae for approximating statistical power in repeated measures ANOVA. *Meas Phys Educ Exerc Sci.* 1999;3(4):249–270.
23. Sawka MN, Latzka WA, Mattot RP, Montain SJ. Hydration effects on temperature regulation. *Int J of Sport Med.* 1998;19:S108–S110.
24. Sharwood K, Collins M, Goedecke J, Wilson G, Noakes T. Weight changes, sodium levels, and performance in the South African Ironman Triathlon. *Clin J Sport Med.* 2002;12(6):391–399.
25. Stearns RL, Casa DJ, DeMartini JK, et al. Examination of performance and hydration responses in elite triathletes during the Ironman World Championship Triathlon. *J Athl Train.* 2012;47(3):S26.
26. Stearns RL, Casa DJ, Lopez RM, et al. Influence of hydration status on pacing during trail running in the heat. *J Strength Cond Res.* 2009;23(9):2533–2541.
27. Tabachnick BG, Fidell LS. Cleaning up your act: screening data prior to analysis. In: *Using Multivariate Statistics.* New York: HarperCollins; 1989. p. 59–89.
28. Wingo JE, Casa DJ, Berger EM, Dellis WO, Knight JC, McClung JM. Influence of a pre-exercise glycerol hydration beverage on performance and physiologic function during mountain-bike races in the heat. *J Athl Train.* 2004;39(2):169–175.
29. Yeargin SW, Casa DJ, Armstrong LE, et al. Heat acclimatization and hydration status of American football players during initial summer workouts. *J Strength Cond Res.* 2006;20(3):463–470.
30. Yeargin SW, Casa DJ, Judelson DA, et al. Thermoregulatory responses and hydration practices in heat-acclimatized adolescents during preseason high school football. *J Athl Train.* 2010;45(2):136–146.
31. Yeargin SW, Casa DJ, McClung JM, et al. Body cooling between two bouts of exercise in the heat enhances subsequent performance. *J Strength Cond Res.* 2006;20(2):383–389.

Veracity of Data: Understanding Validity and Reliability

Lori L. Ploutz-Snyder, PhD, and Jessica M. Scott, PhD

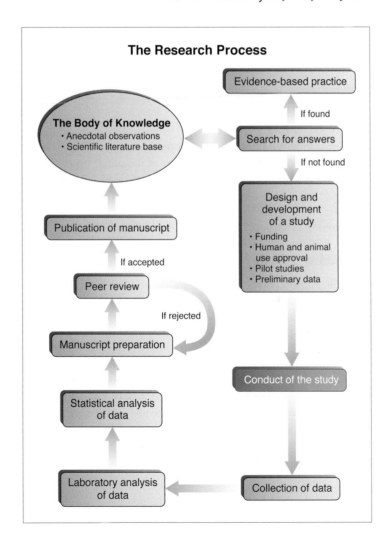

INTRODUCTION

To ensure that research findings are trusted and believed, scientists must be extremely thorough in examining the merit of the data they use. In conference presentations, journal articles, and thesis defenses, researchers routinely make complex choices regarding the trustworthiness of data. If asked "how do you know that you are indeed measuring what you want to measure?" and/or "can you be sure that if you repeat the measurement you will get the same results?" researchers must be able to provide clear answers. As we will see later in the chapter, an integral part of **validity** is **reliability**, which is related to the consistency, or repeatability, of a measure. These principles are fundamental to the scientific method.

VALIDITY

An often cited definition of "validity" is that of Hammersley (2): "An account is valid or true if it represents accurately those features of the phenomena, that it is intended to describe, explain, or theorise." Although this would seem to be an all-inclusive description, many other definitions also exist:

- "An agreement between two efforts to measure the same thing with different methods" (2)
- "The measure that an instrument measures what it is supposed to" (3)
- "Are we measuring what we think we are?" (3)

Validity is simply the extent to which a test measures what it is supposed to measure. The question of validity is raised in the context of the three points: (a) the form of the test, (b) the purpose of the test, and (c) the population for whom it is intended. Therefore, important questions to ask are "will this test provide the information I need for the decision I need to make?" and "is this the best test for what I am researching?" The types of validity can be divided into three basic types: content, criterion, and construct.

Content Validity

Content validity often pertains to learning in an educational setting. For example, if a professor wants to test knowledge on lower body muscle anatomy, a test that focuses on muscle origin and insertion points in the arm would be considered to have low content validity, whereas a test requiring students to draw and label muscles of the leg would have high content validity.

Content validity also involves using logic or common sense to determine if it's reasonable to assume a test is valid. To use an elementary example, consider a football coach who wants to compare the speed of his players. He decides to measure the time it takes each player to sprint 40 yards and then ranks his players from fastest to slowest using the data he acquires. In this case, lower sprint times indicate higher speeds, clearly a measure of what the coach intended.

Criterion-Oriented Validity

Measurements used in investigations are frequently validated against a well-established criterion, or "gold standard." Before getting into the two types of **criterion validity** (concurrent and predictive validity), it is important to consider how criterion validity is assessed.

Regression

Typically, a statistical technique known as "product-moment correlation" or **regression** is used to establish criterion-related validity. It may involve two variables, such as the relationship between height and weight. It may also involve three or more variables (multiple regression), such as the relationship between cardiovascular fitness and body weight, percentage fat, and muscular endurance. The coefficient of correlation, or **interclass correlation**, is a quantitative value of the relationship between variables and can range from 0.00 to 1.00 in either a positive or negative direction. A **positive correlation** exists when a large value for one variable is associated with a large value for another variable. For example, the correlation between height and weight is positive; to some extent, height is a valid indicator of weight; taller individuals tend to be heavier than shorter ones (Fig. 10-1). A **negative correlation** exists when a small value for one variable is associated with a large value for another variable or vice versa. Figure 10-2 depicts a negative correlation between bodyweight and pull-ups; heavier individuals can typically complete fewer pull-ups than can lighter individuals.

The number associated with the correlation indicates the strength of the correlation. A perfect correlation between variables is 1.00 and no relationship at all is 0.00. A high correlation between a test and a criterion suggests evidence of criterion validity and indicates that the test can predict the criterion with good precision. It is important to pause here and remember that correlation only describes the

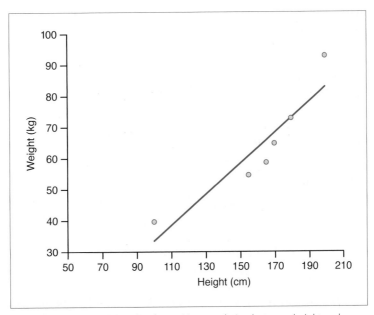

FIGURE 10-1: Example of a positive correlation between height and weight; taller individuals tend to be heavier than shorter ones.

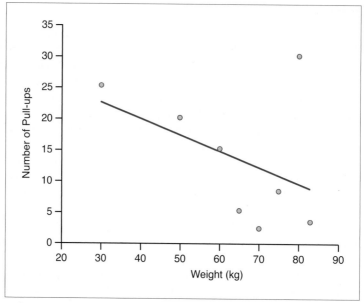

FIGURE 10-2:   Example of a negative correlation between bodyweight and pull-ups; heavier individuals can typically complete fewer pull-ups than lighter individuals.

mathematical relationship between two variables. *It does not imply any cause or effect or directionality of relationship.* Using the example earlier, being heavier does not cause someone to perform fewer pull-ups. Although the relationships may be true for a group of subjects, there are almost always other contributing factors; in this case, factors such as arm strength, body composition, and prior training will influence pull-up performance. For example, in Figure 10-2, the scores do not fall on a straight line. One heavy individual can perform many pull-ups, likely due to strength and prior training. Correlation is an excellent tool for evaluating criterion validity; however, it should not be overinterpreted.

Bland-Altman

One problem with regression is that the two variables might be highly correlated, yet there could be substantial differences in the two measures across their range of values. For instance, two devices can measure $\dot{V}O_2max$: a metabolic cart, recognized and accepted as a gold standard for assessing aerobic capacity, and a new portable machine. The two devices are highly correlated (a high value from one device corresponds to a high value from the other device) yet produce different outputs. Therefore, another method often used to assess criterion validity is with a **Bland-Altman plot** (Fig. 10-3) (1). Bland-Altman plots create a visual representation of how well two methods agree. Rather than a statistical test, it is intended to demonstrate both typical differences

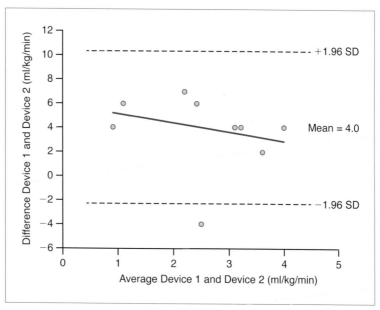

FIGURE 10-3: Example of a Bland-Altman plot, which creates a visual representation of how well two methods agree. The basic concept of Bland-Altman's approach is the visualization of the difference of the measurements made by the two methods, then plotting the differences (y-axis) versus the mean of the two readings (x-axis). Additional reference lines, 95% upper (0 + 1.96 standard deviation) and 95% lower (0 − 1.96 standard deviation) are also overlaid on the same scatter plot.

between the measures and any patterns such differences may take. The use of the plot is that it is not affected by the range, whereas a linear regression shows the strength of the linear association but not how closely the two measures agree. The Bland-Altman plot allows the user to focus on differences between the measures and understand the clinical relevance of these differences. The basic concept of Bland-Altman's approach is the visualization of the difference of the measurements made by the two methods, then plotting the differences (y-axis) versus the mean of the two readings (x-axis) (see Fig. 10-3). Additional reference lines, 95% upper (0 +1.96 standard deviation) and 95% lower (0 −1.96 standard deviation) are also overlaid on the same scatter plot. When there is no systematic bias, it is easy to see the differences are symmetrical around zero.

In the example of comparing two devices that measure metabolic gases (see Fig. 10-3), the limits are very wide, indicating the new device is not valid. Additionally, with a mean difference between devices of 4 mL/kg/min, the Bland-Altman plot illustrates that the new device (device 2) typically underestimates aerobic capacity. Bland-Altman plots have become an essential requirement in validity or method comparison studies. Indeed, Bland and Altman's original paper has been cited on more than 26,800 occasions—compelling evidence of its importance in medical research.

Concurrent Validity

Concurrent validity often involves examining an instrument with some criterion administered at the same time (*i.e.*, concurrently). Sometimes, a researcher wishes to substitute a shorter, more easily administered test for another that is more difficult to implement. For example, magnetic resonance imaging (MRI) is the gold standard used to measure muscle size. However, it is expensive and uses specialized equipment typically available only in a medical setting. Ultrasound is an inexpensive and portable alternative to using MRI. To determine whether ultrasound is a valid measure of muscle size, both an MRI and ultrasound measurement of muscle size should be administered in a group of participants. If a satisfactory relationship exists, researchers can conclude that ultrasound is a valid measure of muscle size. There is a particularly important but often overlooked concept in this statement related to a "satisfactory relationship." It is essential that the researcher understand the topic area and the measurement techniques completely enough to make a subjective judgment regarding the suitability of different measurement techniques.

For example, using the earlier example, assume that MRI is the gold standard measurement of muscle size and can reliably measure vastus lateralis size within 1%. But a single MRI scan is too expensive, and the researcher would need to travel 50 mi to the nearest scanner. This might make implementing MRI scanning impractical. The researcher then considers ultrasound because it is readily available for a low price in a good location. The next question becomes, "How good is ultrasound for measuring muscle size?" Is it valid compared to MRI? In other words, does it give the same answer as MRI? How reliable is it? Essentially, do you get the same number with every ultrasound scan, or does it vary from measurement to measurement? The answers to these questions must be evaluated in the context of the particular research study. Consider two different situations. In one study, previously sedentary subjects will perform 10 weeks of high-intensity weight lifting that is expected to increase leg muscle size by 30%. It is necessary to have a measurement tool that can detect large (30%) changes in muscle size. It is not necessary to precisely measure very small changes. In this case, it would be quite easy to accept ultrasound as a surrogate measurement technique because its validity compared to MRI is well within the 30% range. On the opposite extreme, if the goal were to take highly trained weight lifters and make a small change to their training program in an attempt to increase their leg muscle size by 2%, the measurement technique would need to be far more precise, valid, and reliable, and ultrasound would not be a good choice as it may not be able to detect such a small increase.

Thus, it is critically important to understand the magnitude of change that is expected and select a measurement tool that is "good enough" for that particular application. In some cases, a less reliable test might be good enough, such as when large effects are expected. However, a less reliable tool will add to the variance in the measure but ultimately needs to be a valid measure of the dependent variable.

Predictive Validity

When the criterion is looking at some later behavior, for example, when entrance examinations are used to predict later success, **predictive validity** is the major concern. Because several predictors are likely to have greater validity than the correlation between any one test and the criterion, multiple regressions are often used. For example, the most accurate method to measure percentage of body fat is with hydrostatic weighing; however, the most commonly used field test of percent body fat is skinfolds. The thickness of skinfolds at various points on the body are entered into equations to predict body density, which is then converted to percent body fat. These easily administered field tests have proven concurrent validity and have accordingly become an acceptable measure for many applications. As discussed in the previous paragraph, it is important to know how precisely or accurately you need to measure body fat before selecting a technique. For evaluation of large changes such as those associated with a diet and exercise program, it is likely acceptable. With skinfolds having about a 4% error factor, one would want to know that interpretation of a 10% outcome could be 6% or 14% in actuality, and if this is acceptable range, then the measurement tool of skinfolds may work. How accurate your measurement needs to be to interpret success or proper placement in a range will also determine what measurement tool you want to use. Understanding your dependent variables and its meaning and interpretation is also important for choices made for a measurement tool. For detecting very small changes, it is probably not acceptable. It is critical to know what type of measurement accuracy is needed for a particular study.

One limitation of such tests is that the validity tends to decrease when the prediction is used in a new sample. Using a skinfold equation derived from young males to predict body fat of young females would likely have a low validity coefficient. A technique to help estimate the accuracy of a prediction formula is called **cross-validation**. With this technique, the same tests are given to a new sample from the same population to check if the formula is accurate or not. For instance, a researcher could administer skinfold and dual energy x-ray absorptiometry (DEXA) tests to a sample of 200 people and then use multiple regression on the results from 100 of them to develop a prediction formula. This developed formula could then be applied to the other 100 subjects to see how accurately it predicts percent body fat for them. This cross-validation of your regression formula which has its own inherent measurement error in it is vital to using a formula population wide. Also, larger n sizes may be needed to reduce any error even more.

Construct Validity

Construct validity is the degree to which a test measures an intended hypothetical construct, that is, a test that measures abstract characteristics rather than concrete characteristics. Anxiety, self-efficacy, and creativity are examples of hypothetical constructs. Compared to body weight, which is directly observable, these traits cannot be seen or directly measured. Therefore, the variable being measured is also known as a "construct" because it is constructed of measures that indicate the relative or absolute quantity of the relevant characteristics. For example, a researcher wants to validate a measure of creativity. She has a hypothesis that creativity increases when subjects are outdoors; therefore, being outdoors is correlated to the creativity scores and in this way has some construct validity. Whether this association is valid also depends on the degree to which the creativity test actually measures creativity. So validity has a few different perspectives in context with other tests. Ultimately, validity is related to how close the measure is to the actual direct measurement of a variable. So typically, one measures a gold standard and then uses another measure to see how closely the second measure is correlated to the gold standard one so it can show good construct validity and be used as well.

The known group difference method is also sometimes used to establish construct validity. Assume that you develop a test of basketball skills, and your construct is dribbling ability. To determine the construct validity of your test, you administer it to three groups of students: individuals who completed an introductory basketball course, individuals who completed an advanced basketball course, and members of the varsity basketball team. If the group mean scores accurately discriminated between skills levels, the test has construct validity. However, if the means were not consistent with the performance-defined groups, this is evidence that the test lacked construct validity.

Factors Affecting Validity
Choice of Criterion

A good criterion has high reliability, high objectivity, and high correlation with the construct of interest. A gold standard criterion is one that is generally accepted as the best measure at the time of the respective construct. For example, $\dot{V}O_2max$ (the maximum amount of oxygen a person can use) is considered the gold standard measure for aerobic fitness. Underwater weighing used to be the gold standard for body composition until DEXA was put forth and now it is considered the new gold standard. Thus, other measures of aerobic fitness such as distance walked in six minutes should be evaluated against $\dot{V}O_2max$ to determine validity.

Population

When a population contains subgroups that differ in age, gender, experience, body size, etc., these aspects also produce variance in test scores. Variance caused by such characteristics in the population is not measurement error because it is not random; rather, this variance is bias, meaning that subjects who are alike on certain characteristics tend to be consistently different from other subjects.

Objectivity

Low objectivity introduces measurement error, thus decreasing validity. To avoid variety in subjective interpretations such as "hot" or "large," standardized measurement tools are crucial. This eliminates much of the perceptive variability of individual observers.

RELIABILITY

An integral part of validity is reliability, which is related to the consistency, or repeatability, of a measure. A test cannot be considered valid if it is not reliable, so if a test cannot consistently yield the same results in successive trials, the test cannot be trusted. A test can be reliable but not valid; a researcher can consistently and reliably measure weight on a broken scale, but the results will not be true or valid. Furthermore, any results must be repeatable;

other researchers must be able to perform the same experiment under the same conditions and generate the same results.

MEASUREMENT ERROR

A first step in establishing reliability is to ensure measurement error is reduced as much as possible and then understand what error should be expected given the circumstances. There are several possible sources of measurement error:

1. The participant. Numerous individual factors may influence measurements such as mood, motivation, fatigue, and specific knowledge. These errors can be minimized by putting constraints on the subjects before testing. For example, before a $\dot{V}O_2$max test, subjects could be asked to have a small meal; ensure they are well-hydrated; not perform intense exercise in the prior 24 hours; abstain from alcohol, caffeine, and nicotine during the prior eight hours; and have had a good night's sleep the night before. Such subject constraints can be helpful in reducing variability in personal performance.

2. The testing. Errors in testing could be due to lack of clarity or completeness in direction, or poor test conditions such as noise or a slippery surface when conducting a running test. Different test operators may not be consistent in exactly how they conduct the test. Taking the previous example of conducting a $\dot{V}O_2$max test, it is important to have standardized instructions for subjects and conduct compelling coaching and encouragement during the test to give an exhaustive effort. One distracted operator checking his phone and providing minimal encouragement will likely produce very different results from an engaged operator providing formidable cheering.

3. The scoring. Exercise science applications sometimes use scoring to evaluate physical performance such as in judging gymnastics or figure skating or evaluating older adults' ability to perform tasks of everyday living. Error in scoring is related to the experience of the scorers (how familiar the scorer is with the behavior being tested) or attentiveness of the scorer (inattention to detail could produce measurement error). For instance, when assessing a child on throwing and catching skills, he or she can be rated on a scale of 1–5 on how often he or she steps with the opposite foot to throw, if his or her arm is straight or not, and if he or she looks at the target. An inexperienced scorer may rate a child who stepped once with the wrong foot with a 3, whereas an experienced scorer recognizes the majority of the trials were conducted correctly and rates the child with a 4.

4. The equipment. Measurement error due to instrumentation includes obvious causes such as inaccuracy and lack of calibration of gas analyzers when measuring $\dot{V}O_2$max. To reduce measurement error due to equipment, it is crucial to calibrate or "zero" equipment before each test. Weighing an athlete on an uncalibrated scale causing a 5-lb error will make a large difference on his or her aerobic capacity relative to body weight!

Interpreting Test Reliability

In addition to limiting measurement error, it is important to consider how reliability is assessed. Two commonly used methods for sport scientists to assess reliability are correlation coefficient and standard error of measurement.

Intraclass Correlation

The correlation technique used for computing the reliability coefficient differs from that used for establishing validity. As previously described, to establish validity, interclass correlation is often used to examine the relationship between two different variables. In contrast, to provide estimates of reliability for a repeated measure, intraclass correlation (ICC) should be used. **Intraclass correlation** provides estimates of systematic variance (the procedure for calculating ICC is the same as that of a simple analysis of variance [ANOVA] with repeated measures and will be discussed in Chapter 18). As an example, previous studies have shown that there is a learning effect on peak aerobic tests in heart failure patients with reduced ejection fraction. A group of researchers want to determine whether there is a learning effect in heart failure patients with preserved ejection fraction, and therefore conduct two peak tests. An ICC of 0.92 was found between tests. Because reliability is defined as good (greater than 0.75), moderate (0.5–0.75), and poor (less than 0.5) (4), researchers concluded that there is no learning effect in heart failure patients with preserved ejection fraction, and only one peak test is necessary in this population—an important finding saving much time and resources for future investigations.

Standard Error of Measurement

Reliability can also be expressed in terms of the **standard error of measurement** (SEM). It is an estimate of how often you can expect errors of a given size. SEM is the "standard deviation" of measurement error. SEM provides a measure of how much an individual's score can be expected to vary because of measurement error. The formula for SEM is

$$SEM = (s\sqrt{(1 - r)})$$

where s is the standard deviation of scores, and r is the reliability coefficient for the test. For example, in the measurement of cardiac output from impedance cardiography, assume the standard deviation is 6.6 and the test-retest correlation is .90. The SEM would be

$$SEM = (6.6\sqrt{(1 - 0.90)}) = 2.1\%$$

Note that the SEM is governed by the variability of test scores and the reliability of the test. If there was a higher reliability coefficient, the SEM would obviously decrease.

Methods of Establishing Reliability

It is significantly easier to establish reliability than validity, and three commonly used methods are outlined here.

Test-Retest Reliability

Test-retest reliability is the degree to which scores are consistent over time. It indicates score variation that occurs from testing session to testing session as a result of errors of measurement. There are two types of test-retest reliability. **Intrarater reliability** assesses the stability of an individual scorer. For example, if a student wants to determine if she can reliably acquire skinfolds, she could acquire skinfolds on several occasions. **Interrater reliability** evaluates the reliability of several scorers. For example, two technicians could acquire ultrasound images on the same subject on the same day. If similar results (*i.e.*, a high ICC and low SEM) are obtained between the two technicians, they would be considered reliable.

Another form of test-rest reliability is reproducibility, which is a benchmark on which the reliability of an experiment can be tested. Reproducibility is tested by a replication study, which is independent and ideally generates identical findings or extends its generalizability. It is important to understand that replicating results is not essential for validity, although it certainly helps. Often, due to sheer feasibility, replication studies are not possible. Yet one can reproduce many different types of studies, many times not understanding the importance because reviewers too often say "we already know this" or "this study has already been done." However, without multiple studies validating the same concept, theories, principles, and even laws cannot be produced. So it all starts with the individual investigator being able to reproduce his or her own measures, day to day or year to year. Then, studies from the literature can be reproduced. Does a short-term progressive heavy resistance training program result in the same percentage improvements in untrained men or women each time it is performed with similar training and testing equipment? Ultimately, when many studies testing a similar hypothesis show similar results, solid theories and principles can be developed. Obviously, attempting to replicate a large study such as the Framingham Heart Study, an experiment that has been going on for over 60 years, would be very impractical over the short term. However, other studies like it can be initiated and one day researchers can see if the results are similar or not as history moves on and new independent variables exist in the population (*e.g.*, improved exercise habits due to "exercise is medicine," etc.).

Equivalent-Forms or Alternate-Forms Reliability

This form of reliability involves two tests that are identical in every way except for the actual items included. It is often used when it is likely that test takers will recall responses made during the first session *and* when alternate forms are available.

Internal Consistency Reliability

This type of test involves acquiring multiple measures within a day, usually at a single testing session. For example, an isometric strength test can be administered several times within a day. The test requires the subject to exert maximum effort for six seconds. The recommended test procedure is to administer a warmup trial at 50% effort and then two trials at maximum effort. The average of the two maximum trials is the individual's score. If there is high internal consistency, and the results from the two trials are similar, then the test is likely reliable.

SUGGESTIONS FOR RESEARCH DESIGN

To delineate several tips on how to improve validity and reliability throughout the scientific method, below is an example of a student who wants to determine whether short high-intensity or prolonged low-intensity aerobic exercise lowers blood glucose more in her classmates. She hypothesizes that high-intensity exercise will lower blood glucose more than low-intensity exercise.

1. Designing the experiment: Make sure goals and objectives are clearly defined and operationalized. Several factors must first be outlined. For example, how will blood glucose be measured? When will blood glucose be measured? How will exercise intensity be determined and measured? What exercise equipment will subjects use? Will subjects be given a standard meal before the exercise tests? A poorly designed study could encompass several of these areas resulting in an experimental design with low reliability and validity. For example, the student might not control pre-exercise diet, obtain blood glucose samples at different times post-exercise in all subjects, or use ratings of perceived exertion (clearly a subjective index) as a measure of exercise intensity. Instead, the student decides to give her subjects a standardized meal, obtain blood pre- and post-exercise at set times with a finger prick, and measure blood glucose with an automated glucose analyzer available in her laboratory. She wants to base her high- and low-intensity exercise sessions on maximal aerobic capacity, but she does not have access to a metabolic cart. What are her options? She could use age-predicted maximal heart rate to prescribe exercise intensities; however, this method has limitations. She decides to conduct a peak cycle test to measure peak heart rate to prescribe exercise intensities. To ensure further quality control, she makes sure the two exercise sessions are equivalent in work output.

2. Gathering the data: Piloting or pre-testing can help increase validity and reliability. The student testing blood glucose must ensure methods of obtaining and analyzing blood samples are reliable and valid; otherwise, any observed change after exercise could be considered false. Instead of assuming blood collection and analysis are reliable and valid, she conducts pre-testing. She recruits her lab mates and obtains blood samples at different times and calculates her reliability with ICC or SEM. Because she is using an automated glucose analyzer, she compares the results of the automated analyzer against a clinical dry chemical analyzer with a Bland-Altman plot to ensure there is good agreement between the automated analyzer and the gold standard (clinical dry chemical analysis). These pre-test findings can then be included in the final report as evidence of sound scientific methods.

3. Analyzing and interpreting results: Cause and effect can only be established by well-designed experiments. The student completed the experiment and found that high-intensity exercise did indeed lower blood glucose more than low-intensity exercise. When reporting results, all steps contributing to the validity of the experiment must be clearly outlined. We can assume the student identified inclusion and exclusion criteria for subjects (*e.g.*, individuals with Type 2 diabetes were excluded), completed all testing in a timely manner (*e.g.*, the high-intensity and low-intensity exercise sessions were completed on different days), calibrated all equipment (*e.g.*, once validity is established for the automated analyzer it was calibrated daily), and conducted appropriate statistical analyses. If these actions are taken, the student can be confident in her results.

SUMMARY

Numerous measurement issues apply when conducting research, and in this chapter, two key concepts—validity and reliability—were discussed. Criterion validity (including concurrent and predictive validity) and construct validity are two of the most commonly used methods of validating measures in research studies. The topic of test reliability has generated thousands of studies and discussions among researchers but it is important for each lab and each individual investigator to establish the reliability of a measure before using it in a study. A measure that does not yield consistent results cannot be valid. The rationale for using an intraclass coefficient instead of an interclass coefficient when determining reliability was presented, as was the concept of standard error of measurement. Additionally, various methods of estimating reliability including stability, alternate forms, and internal consistency were outlined. Understanding validity and reliability is extremely important for any scientist and is a crucial foundation of any research design. A well-designed experiment containing validity and reliability is the best way to ensure results stand up to rigorous questioning.

GLOSSARY

Bland-Altman plot: creates a visual representation of how well two methods agree

Concurrent validity: relates one measure to another criteria obtained at the same time (*i.e.*, concurrently)

Construct validity: the degree to which a test measures an intended hypothetical construct (*i.e.*, a test that measures abstract characteristics rather than concrete characteristics)

Content validity: often addressed in academic and vocational testing and involves using logic or common sense to determine if it is reasonable to assume a test is valid

Criterion validity: a measure of how well a variable predicts an outcome

Cross-validation: a technique used to help estimate the accuracy of a prediction formula

Interclass correlation: a quantitative value of the relationship between variables and can range from 0.00 to 1.00 in either a positive or negative direction. Values closer to 1 indicate a stronger correlation

Interrater reliability: evaluates the reliability of several scorers

Intraclass correlation: provides estimates of systematic variance

Intrarater reliability: assesses the stability of an individual scorer

Negative correlation: when a large value for one variable is associated with a small value for another variable

Positive correlation: when a large value for one variable is associated with a large value for another variable

Predictive validity: refers to the degree to which any measure can predict independent future or past events

Regression: estimates the relationship among variables and is used to establish criterion-related validity

Reliability: related to the consistency, or repeatability, of a measure. A test cannot be considered valid if it is not reliable

Standard error of measurement: an estimate of how often you can expect errors of a given size (*i.e.*, the standard deviation of measurement error)

Test-retest reliability: degree to which scores are consistent over time; indicates score variation that occurs from testing session to testing session as a result of errors of measurement

Validity: the extent to which a test measures what it is supposed to measure

REFERENCES

1. Bland JM, Altman DG. Statistical methods for assessing agreement between two methods of clinical measurement. *Lancet.* 1986;1(8476):307–310.
2. Hammersley M. Some notes on the terms "validity" and "reliability." *Br Educ Res J.* 1987;13(1):73–81.
3. Kerlinger F. *Foundation of Behavioral Research.* New York (NY): CBS Publishing; 1986.
4. Shrout PE, Fleiss JL. Intraclass correlations: uses in assessing rater reliability. *Psychol Bull.* 1979;86(2):420–428.

Unique Features in Animal Research

Michael R. Deschenes, PhD

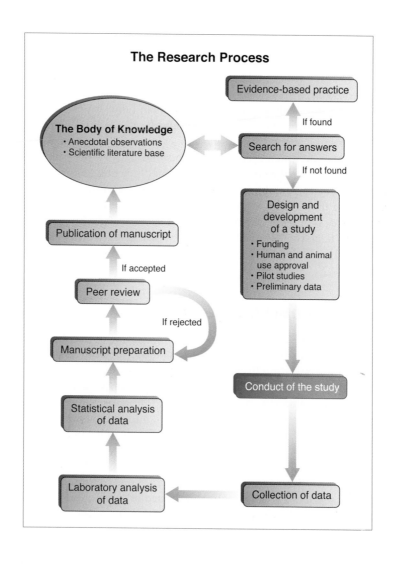

INTRODUCTION

In the field of exercise science, much of the research reported in the literature is generated by investigators working in the Human Performance Laboratory of various research universities and institutions. In the United States, this focus on human performance can be traced back to the Harvard Fatigue Laboratory operated by David Bruce Dill, a pioneering and prolific exercise physiologist, from 1927 to 1946. Many of the young scientists who studied under Dr. Dill at that facility went on to establish their own laboratories investigating human performance and physiologic responses to exercise and/or environmental stress. Even today, much if not most of the research conducted in the field of exercise science uses human subjects. This is reasonable because our primary interest in the field lies in expanding our knowledge of how humans respond to an acute exercise session or adapt to a prolonged (*i.e.*, weeks or months) program of exercise training and how these adaptations may improve the health and functional capacity of the human organism.

However, in many circumstances, it is necessary to use animal subjects to conduct scientific research. This could be because it is not realistic to logistically use human subjects when large volumes of tissue are needed to examine the effects of exercise or if the tissue is not easily accessible in the human body. It may also be that the experimental intervention to be investigated might be dangerous or even lethal—such as a new drug or surgical procedure—and as such must first be tested for safety on animals. Finally, animals are often used as research subjects when the principal goal of the experiment is to better the circumstances or health of these animals rather than for the benefit of humans. Examples of this may include examining fish from polluted waters to determine their health issues or perfecting vaccines to protect animals from contagious diseases. In truth, the use of animal subjects has a long and fruitful history in research, particularly that of a biomedical nature and has resulted in many of the most fundamental and useful experimental findings of how the body and its physiologic systems work.

USE OF ANIMALS IN BIOMEDICAL RESEARCH

Although the use of animal subjects in the discipline of exercise science is relatively new, particularly in the United States, their use in biomedical research has much earlier beginnings, dating back even centuries into the past. Indeed, the ancient and noted Greek physician Galen was known to perform surgeries on animals to reveal basic facts on mammalian anatomy and function in the 2nd century A.D. And Claude Bernard, the 19th century French scientist commonly referred to as the "father of modern physiology," routinely used animal subjects in his experiments to unravel the workings of various physiologic systems. In the very late 19th century, Ivan Pavlov famously used dogs to demonstrate the concept of conditioning by measuring how dogs learned to salivate at the ring of a bell after associating that sound with the presentation of food. In the 20th century, a myriad of seminal biomedical breakthroughs were made possible by the use of animal subjects, including the isolation of the hormone insulin in 1922 and the production of an effective vaccine against polio in the

1950s. Today, animals play a vital role in perfecting organ transplantation techniques as well as in engineering specific tissue replacement procedures. Some of the most important biomedical advances made possible by the use of animal models are presented in Table 11-1.

In fact, it was also in the 20th century that the use of animal models in biomedical research in the United States actually became mandatory with the establishment of the **Food and Drug Administration** (FDA) by the federal government in 1938. This organization stipulates that any newly developed food additives, cosmetics, and drugs be tested first on animals to confirm that they are benign and produce no harmful effects before they can then be tested on human volunteers. The FDA was instituted after a number of women

Table 11-1 Chronology of Important Biomedical Advances Since 1900 Made Possible by the Use of Animal Models	
Year	**Medical Breakthroughs**
1900	• Treatment of rickets and other vitamin deficiencies • Passive immunization against tetanus and diphtheria • First tissue transplantation
1920	• Discovery of thyroid hormones • Discovery of insulin
1930	• Vaccination against tetanus • Development of modern anesthetics • Development of neuromuscular inhibitors
1940	• Therapy for rheumatoid arthritis • Identification of antibiotics (penicillin, streptomycin) • Treatment of leprosy
1950	• Oral vaccination against polio • Development of chemotherapies for cancer treatment • Open heart surgery
1960	• Vaccination against German measles • Bypass surgery on heart • Discovery of antihypertensive drugs
1970	• Extinction of smallpox • Heart transplantation • Discovery of non-addictive analgesics
1980	• Implantation of artificial hearts • Vaccines against hepatitis B • Treatment for AIDS • Development of cholesterol-lowering drugs • Treatment of leukemia • Use of ultrasound to destroy kidney stones
1990	• Development of minimally invasive surgical techniques • New diagnostic and therapeutic techniques for cancer
2000	• Decoding the genome in fruit fly, mouse, rat, and man

were left blind by the effects of a newly formulated but untested eye makeup and more than 100 people died as a result of consuming a new cough syrup that contained an additive that proved toxic in humans. As a result of the efforts of the FDA, food and drug product safety is much more effectively assured than at any other time in our history.

Concerns for Animal Well-Being

Largely as a result of these major biomedical breakthroughs of the 20th century, concerns were raised about the safety and well-being of the animals that participate as subjects in the experiments that benefit humans. In fact, this concern for experimental animal welfare had its beginnings even before the 20th century. In 1876, Britain passed the Cruelty to Animals Act to assure that measures would be taken to do what was possible to limit the pain and suffering of animals included in experimentation. Not all experiments result in pain. Many are quite harmless and directly benefit animals. Due to similar concerns, in 1866, the first American Society for the Prevention of Cruelty to Animals was established in New York City, and the American Anti-Vivisection Society was formed in 1883. More directly related to biomedical research, the federal **Animal Welfare Act** was passed in the United States in 1966 to guarantee acceptable standards for the treatment and safety of research animals. Although mice and rats—which comprise more than 90% of the animals used in research—are not covered by the Animal Welfare Act, they are protected by the Public Health Service's *Guide for the Care and Use of Laboratory Animals*.

As a result of these organizations and their oversight efforts along with a general concern for the well-being of animals, the number of animals used in research sharply declined in the second half of the 20th century. At the turn of the 21st century, however, there was an increase in the number of animals used in biomedical research, with the species of choice being mice and zebra fish. This uptick in animal use can be attributed to the **Human Genome Project**, which sought to identify and sequence all the genes in human DNA. It was successfully completed in 2003, thus opening up vast potential for research on the genetic causes of diseases and illnesses. Mice have been used in these efforts not only because 90% of their genetic pattern overlaps that of humans but also because laboratory methods have been refined to develop strains of transgenic mice in which specific genes can either be deleted or added to the DNA of the mouse. This in turn enables researchers to determine what role specific genes and their proteins may have in the onset or cure of the diseases that all too often shorten lives or compromise the quality of life of those afflicted. Due to technical difficulties, scientists have had little success in generating transgenic rats, so mice have become the species of choice for transgenic investigation.

Although the genetic profile of the **zebra fish** features less similarity with that of humans (there is only about an 80% overlap), it displays other biologic features that make it particularly useful in biomedical research. Its embryonic development, although similar to the process observed in humans, actually occurs outside the maternal fish in a transparent pouch and occurs at a strikingly three-day pace of completion. These features, combined with the fact that scientists can create specific and precise genetic mutations in the embryo, enable the visualization—recall that the pouch containing the embryo is transparent—of how such mutations impact the development of specific organs during embryogenesis.

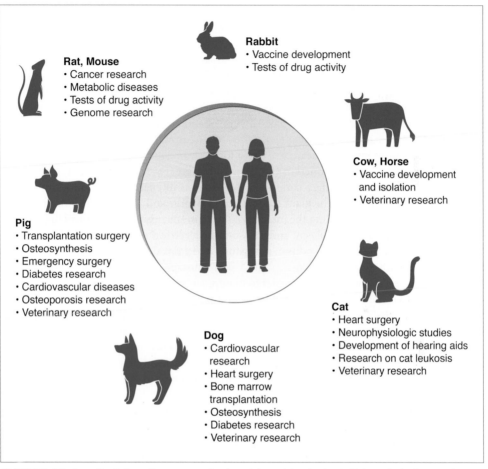

FIGURE 11-1: Depiction of important animal models participating in vital biomedical advances that have improved the health of mankind.

Some of the different species of animals used in biomedical research throughout history and advances made possible by them are depicted in Figure 11-1.

Selection of Animal Species

Obviously, a crucial issue in performing research with an animal model is the proper selection of the most appropriate animal species. Generally, it is best to select a species in a phylum that is close to that of humans so that the structure and function of given cells, organs, and even organ systems closely resemble those found in humans. As such, mammals are most commonly used for the conduct of biomedical research as the major organ systems (*e.g.*, cardiovascular, neuromuscular, immune) of mammals are similar in form and function to those same systems in the human organism. Accordingly, researchers may enjoy high levels of confidence that findings gleaned from animal subjects will effectively transfer to humans. Proper research design in studying the efficacy of various treatment procedures calls for subsequent testing on human volunteers before those procedures are deemed acceptable for use in a larger human sample.

Periodically, non-mammalian animal models can be used to optimize our insight into the workings of fundamental physiologic processes which may or may not be directly useful in the prevention or treatment of disease conditions or injury. Two outstanding examples of the invaluable contributions made by non-mammalian animal models are the squid and the fruit fly. The squid (*Loligo opalescens*) has neuronal axons that are particularly large and are unmyelinated. Researchers (3–6) took advantage of these facts to reveal the essential elements of neural function (*i.e.*, how action potentials are generated) and how those electrical impulses are then conducted down axons to enable communication with postsynaptic cells. Because the **giant squid axon** is so large and accessible, neuroscientists were able to place electrodes into the interior of the axon (*i.e.*, axoplasm), control the flow of ions into and out of the axoplasm, and measure the electrical charge generated by the flow of various ions, particularly sodium, potassium, and chloride. The fact that such a large axon remains without myelination—a lipid-based substance that is normally found wrapped around larger axons—made it easier to manipulate and place electrodes in the axoplasm as well as to estimate the speed at which action potentials migrate down axons toward postsynaptic cells. The lack of myelination dramatically slows down the rate of the conduction of electrical impulses down the axon, thus enabling an accurate assessment of the speed of neuronal conduction. It is not an overstatement to say that the giant squid axon made possible our earliest understanding of neurophysiology and that even today the knowledge gained by those early experiments forms the foundation of treatments used to counter a host of neuronal diseases.

Similarly, the **fruit fly** (*Drosophila melanogaster*) is an invertebrate and comes from a biologic phylum that is quite distant from that of humans (*Homo sapiens*). Still, the ordinary fruit fly is responsible for much of our early and still relevant, knowledge of genetics. The main reason for this is the short lifespan of the fruit fly (approximately 30 days) and the fact that it lays many eggs in a single brood. Accordingly, it is possible to study many generations of the fruit fly over a relatively short experimental period. This in turn has allowed scientists from as early as 1910 to directly observe how genetic variations—either occurring spontaneously or through breeding efforts—alter phenotype in subsequent generations and even how such genetic manipulations may impact survivability and lifespan. Because of the characteristics of the fruit fly, much was learned about the effects of genetic variation and manipulation long before transgenic technology was developed with mice. Even today, the common fruit fly provides important information about genetics and heritability.

USE OF ANIMALS IN EXERCISE SCIENCE RESEARCH

Although many of the research projects of interest in the discipline of exercise science can be answered with the use of human subjects, some research questions can only be answered with the use of an animal model. Animals may be necessary when certain interventions will be performed that may cause too much inconvenience and physical discomfort, when intact but isolated physiologic systems are required, or when the experiment must result in euthanasia.

When animals must be used as experimental subjects, all procedures must be approved beforehand by proper oversight committees. The rigor of these committees overseeing animal research often exceeds those standards protecting the safety and well-being of human subjects. The principal justification of this is that unlike humans, animals do not have the ability to decline to participate in the research project. In short, informed consent cannot be obtained from animal subjects. Before approval to do a research project is granted by an **Institutional Animal Care and Use Committee** (IACUC), it must be demonstrated that the knowledge to be gained by the project will be useful and helpful enough to humans or other animals that it will outweigh the intervention imposed on the animals, their discomfort, or even their loss of life. It must be emphasized that this is a decision that is not taken lightly by IACUCs. In considering the cost-to-benefit ratio of the proposed research, the investigator must demonstrate his or her assessment of the **three Rs** which inform decisions on animal research. The three Rs stand for *reduction, refinement,* and *replacement.*

To address *reduction,* investigators seek to limit the number of animals used during experimentation to the bare minimum necessary to provide statistical power and appropriate levels of confidence in the results produced by the experiments. In fact, this is one of the areas in which the use of an animal model can have a distinct advantage. That is, compared to humans, there is less inter-individual genetic variability among rats and mice of the same strain, and accordingly, experimental results are more consistent with less inter-individual variability. This fact enables the use of a small number of animals per treatment condition to provide the desired statistical power. An additional advantage to using animals in experimental research is that the animal model permits more control over extraneous and potentially confounding variables such as the amount and type of food made available, environmental conditions such as temperature and humidity, and even the number of light hours the animal is exposed to on a daily basis. (Bear in mind that rats and mice are nocturnal creatures, and they display more activity in the dark than in the light.) Tight control over these variables and others act to reduce the degree of variability evident in the data produced by the experimental procedures and again strengthens the investigator's confidence in the experiment accuracy.

The second R to be considered when using animals in research is *refinement.* In application to animal experimentation, this refers to the elimination of pain and stress imposed on animals, and if severe enough, such as surgical procedures, the use of analgesia and anesthesia to do so. Analgesic drugs work by relieving the sense of pain while recovering from a painful procedure such as surgery. Examples of analgesics include aspirin, ibuprofen, and acetaminophen; note that these are normally taken after the procedure to alleviate the resulting pain. In contrast, anesthetic drugs act to mask the sensation of pain, as opposed to relieving it, and these are administered prior to the pain-inducing procedure so the pain is not felt during that procedure. Examples include procaine, lidocaine, isoflurane, and even ether, and like all anesthetics, their effects are reversible. Some anesthetic drugs induce general anesthesia affecting the entire body and even resulting in loss of consciousness (isoflurane), whereas others result in local, confined areas of loss of sensation and typically are injected into the area. Today, researchers are obligated to use pain-relieving/numbing drugs when at all possible if their experimentation will likely cause pain in their animal subjects.

Finally, the third R refers to *replacement.* Here, the researcher must defend his or her use of an animal model as opposed to other experimental models such as computer simulation, or cell cultures. In fact, a number of excellent computer simulation programs have been developed to demonstrate basic physiologic processes; these make effective teaching tools. However, when trying to determine how an organism or physiologic system will respond to a new intervention (*i.e.*, drug, surgical procedure, environmental intervention), these computer simulations are not nearly as effective simply because the basic biologic or mechanistic knowledge pertaining to the intervention has yet to be gained, making predictions difficult and risky. Similarly, although cell culture studies can provide much valuable insight as to how certain cells respond to various interventions, the fact that those cells are isolated complicates the scientist's ability to ascertain how a disruption in one specific cell type will affect other types of cells comprising an organ system, especially within the whole organism. Obviously, such interactions among cells and/or physiologic systems can be observed and recorded only by testing in whole animals. That said, cell culture research is an outstanding way of gaining an initial or preliminary understanding of the effects of an intervention such as a newly developed drug. One way of appreciating the value of the three Rs is to view survey data which show that when people are made aware of considerations of reduction, refinement, and replacement by oversight committees, they are far more likely to support the use of an animal model in conducting research (2).

Models of Increased and Decreased Physical Activity

Investigators in the field of exercise science are interested in documenting responses and adaptations to both increased activity and decreased activity. In both cases, animal models have been effectively used. Even though cats, dogs, mice, and even birds have been used in performing exercise science research, rats in particular lend themselves to research in exercise science. More so than mice, rats are docile, easy to handle and physically manipulate, and they demonstrate less natural, spontaneous locomotor activity, making it easier to accurately quantify the work performed during exercise training sessions and the sessions' effects on various physiologic systems.

Certain strains of rats (*Rattus norvegicus*) show specific characteristics that have proven to be of special value to exercise scientists over the years. For example, for those interested in the role that physical activity might play in managing bodyweight, the Zucker rat is often used, as it naturally becomes obese shortly after birth. In addition to excess bodyweight, the Zucker also naturally exhibits difficulty in managing blood sugar levels much in the same way that obese humans do. Thus, this strain of rat has been important in the investigation of how exercise works to not only counter excess bodyweight but also how exercise may manage the associated resistance to insulin observed among the obese (7,9).

Other strains of the common laboratory rat have played instrumental roles in our comprehension of how aging impacts various physiologic systems and whether exercise training can effectively attenuate those natural biologic declines. The Fischer 344 rat has been used in innumerable aging studies, including those that seek to assess the effects of exercise in aged organisms. The Fischer 344 is useful because it grows at a much slower rate than most other strains. For example, a 10-week-old male Fischer 344 male rat weighs about 230 g, whereas a 10-week-old Sprague-Dawley male rat weighs about 400 g, a body mass making exercise training less feasible and the animal more lethargic. Moreover, the Fischer 344 stays remarkably healthy through old age compared to other strains. More recently, the Brown Norway strain of the lab rat has been developed to assist in the study of aging. These rats have a longer average lifespan (approximately 30 months) than other strains of rats including the Fischer 344, which on average lives 24–26 months (11). But like the Fischer 344, the Brown Norway remains healthy during old age, perhaps even more so than the Fischer 344.

Laboratory rats typically live for just over two years, and in estimating corresponding age in "human years," a simple rule of thumb that is often used is that one month in the lifetime of a rat is roughly equivalent to three years of a human's life. For example, a 20-month-old rat is the chronologic equivalent to a 60-year-old human. A caveat is in order here when comparing durations between rats and humans. When conducting an exercise training investigation using rats, this same proportionality does not apply. That is, a one-month training protocol completed by a rat is not the same as having a human complete a three-year training regimen. Indeed, the physiologic adaptations demonstrated by trained rats proceeds along the same timeline as those made by a human participating in exercise training. Rat adaptations following 10 weeks of training can be expected to be quite similar both in nature and extent to those observed in a human as a result of the same 10-week training protocol. The effects of disuse follow a similar pattern. It should also be noted that the soleus muscle, which is often targeted in exercise training or disuse studies, shows similarity in myofiber-type composition between humans and rats (*i.e.*, 80%–90% slow-twitch, or type I, fibers), but in contrast, this same muscle is dominated by fast-twitch, or type II, myofibers in mice.

Running is the preferred exercise mode when determining the impact of increased activity (exercise) with the murine model. This can be performed on specially built motorized treadmills that accommodate rodents, on treadmills built for human use that have been customized to be used with small animals, or even with running wheels placed in animal housing units that are suited to the spontaneous running activity of mice. Compared to mice, rats demonstrate less spontaneous running activity and are generally better suited to running on motorized treadmills where, initially at least, motivation can be provided in the form of light electric shocks or a blast of air. It should be noted, however, that running styles used by rats can vary substantially both from each other and from humans. Whereas humans and many, but not all rats run at a steady, consistent pace, some rats use a "stop-and-go" approach to treadmill running. More specifically, rats will allow the moving treadmill belt to carry them to the back of the running compartment and then sprint to the front of the compartment, stop, and allow themselves to be carried to the back once again to simply repeat this pattern the entire time they are running. Some of these rats eventually will choose to run in a steady pattern maintaining an even pace, but most do not and instead continue to show the stop-and-go running pattern throughout the training regimen.

Another popular form of endurance exercise that can be performed by small animals is swimming in tepid water (hypothermia can occur quickly in small animals). A major drawback in the use of swimming exercise is that it is not as easy to quantify the amount and intensity of work done as it is with treadmill running, or even with running on a wheel. Although it is simple to merely record the amount of time in the water a rat might spend, it is more difficult to determine how much of that time the rat spends actually swimming as opposed to floating. The researcher must also be sure to use a barrel or a can of proper dimensions to facilitate swim training among rats. A shallow wading pool designed for use by small children will not suffice, as rats will easily leap up onto the edge of the pool and avoid swimming altogether. A deeper barrel must be used so that adequate water depth can be used without allowing the surface of the water to get too close (*i.e.*, 2–3 ft) to the edge of the barrel or can, thus preventing rats from climbing onto the edge to avoid swimming. One must also consider that if more than a single rat is placed in a swimming chamber at a time, they will often seek each other out in attempts to crawl on each other trying to use the other as a flotation device, avoiding the need to swim.

Finally, proper safety issues must be taken into account. Because they are in water, it is possible that due to excessive fatigue from swimming, the animal(s) might drown. Accordingly, it is essential to have a researcher nearby at all times while rats are swimming. Likewise, it is necessary to observe rats or mice running on treadmills. This is to be sure that if some sort of accident occurs (*e.g.*, a foot or tail becomes ensnared in the moving treadmill belt), corrections can be made to prevent serious injury and to ensure that animals are actually running while the treadmill is in operation. If it appears that an injury to the animal has occurred, do *not* immediately reach in with an uncovered hand to help the animal. This is almost sure to result in a painful bite to unprotected skin. First, stop the treadmill belt, allow a brief time for the animal to calm down a bit, and place a thick glove over the hand to be used to assist the distressed animal. Even under safe conditions, anecdotal evidence suggests that approximately 20% of rats are non-compliant to treadmill running, and those rats often devise techniques (often ingenious ones) to avoid running, even while the treadmill belt is working. It is best to begin an exercise project by identifying these exercise avoiders and assigning them to the control group, or simply using them for another experiment that does not involve exercise.

Although efforts to find an animal model to perform endurance exercise have proven quite successful, finding an effective model to emulate resistance exercise (*i.e.*, weight lifting) as performed by humans has proven to be more elusive. Several models have been used including a ladder climbing protocol with additional weight added to the animal—usually a rat—either by attachments to the tail or by dressing the animal with a weighted vest. To motivate the rat to climb the ladder, either a quick blast of cold water or air to the tail end of the animal has been found to be effective. Another resistance training model that has been used is to have the animal push against a weighted bar with the inducement of a food reward. Even birds, specifically the quail, have been used as a model for resistance training by attaching a weight to a single wing, which instinctively compensates by lifting to counteract the pull of the weight with a continuous isometric muscle contraction. If used properly, including a progressive increase of the weight/resistance applied, all of these models result in significant increments of muscle strength and size. However, they often are not viewed as accurately mimicking the high intensity, keenly motivated efforts demonstrated by humans during their own resistance training sessions.

Exercise scientists are also interested in how the body responds to periods of reduced physical activity or even the total absence of activity (*i.e.*, disuse). In particular, the neuromuscular and musculoskeletal systems are of interest due to the many and varied interventions that may result in unloading (an alternate term is "unweighting") of those systems. For example, following surgeries such as knee or hip replacement, or even surgery to correct damage to ligaments and tendons, researchers are curious to assess the decline of muscle function and mass, or even of bone density, as a result of post-operative bed rest and subsequent crutch-assisted ambulation. Animals can be fine models used to study basic and applied research questions concerning biologic adaptations to unloading. In part, this is because rat muscle has striking similarities in form and function to human skeletal muscle—with the exception that rats and mice, but not humans, express type IIB myofibers (10)—and because a number of models of unloading have been developed for those animals. **Hind limb suspension**, in which the animal is lifted by its tail to eliminate weight-bearing activity of the hindquarters, has become popular as a model of reduced activity because no surgery or drug administration is necessary. Generally, rats adjust rather quickly—usually within hours—to the suspended condition. Still, there are concerns to be considered. Such concerns include the fact that rats often become seemingly depressed in the 24-hour unloaded state, and as a result of this, along with the physical challenges of eating standard rat chow in the suspended position, affected rats tend to eat less and lose significant body mass. This can be remedied, at least in part, by not isolating rats while they are unloaded so that they can see and smell other rats (they must not be allowed to come in physical contact, however) to avoid depression and by crushing the food pellets they are fed in order to make it easier for them to eat using only their front paws.

Other methods of eliciting decreased activity of limb musculature include **immobilization** whereby movement of the limb in question is prevented either by way of casting or splinting. Applying a hard casting material around the leg may require general anesthesia or methods to restrain the animal so that the material can be applied and allowed to harden without interference from the animal. In turn, splinting requires the placement of wooden or plastic sticks on either side of the leg which are then secured in place with a strong adhesive tape maintaining the leg at a fixed angle. Both casting and splinting bring about negative modifications in muscle function and mass that are similar to the procedure of hind limb suspension, but there can be problems with rats trying to chew and bite off the cast or splinting material.

To observe total disuse of limb musculature, surgical denervation procedures have been used to eliminate neural activation of limb muscles, and neurotoxins have been administered to paralyze muscles. Although denervation and toxin administration are excellent models to allow researchers to examine what a total absence of activity does to the neuromuscular and musculoskeletal systems, those models are inappropriate for researchers who are trying to understand effects of and recovery from more prevalent conditions such as post-surgical repair or from injury such as sprains and strains. Overall, it is fair to say that there is much popularity of hind limb unloading and immobilization among the research community, including those interested in the effects of microgravity encountered during space travel. Indeed, NASA researchers almost exclusively use the hind limb suspension model in attempts to reveal microgravity-induced modifications of neuromuscular and musculoskeletal function. Still, in determining the effects of both increased and decreased physical activity, scientists cannot always be certain that what they observe among animal subjects as a result of experimental interventions will necessarily be noted among humans. Indeed, there are both advantages and disadvantages to using animal models when performing biomedical and exercise science research; a number of these are presented in Table 11-2.

Table 11-2 Advantages and Disadvantages to Using Animal Models in Biomedical and Exercise Science Research

Advantages	Disadvantages
• Similarity of design and function of physiologic systems with those of humans	• Physiologic systems do not always closely mimic those in humans
• Faster rate of aging enabling more efficient study of effects of senescence	• Experimental results cannot be assumed to be transferable to humans
• Larger number of experimental subjects can be studied	• Can be non-compliant to many exercise regimens
• More control of important external variables such as diet, temperature, exercise, etc.	• Can be costly to maintain (*i.e.*, food, shelter, medical care) animals
• Transgenic technology facilitates understanding of the role of genes	• Ethical concerns with use of other sentient beings as subjects for experimentation
• Testing of newly developed drugs and medical procedures before trials are performed on humans	• Absence of informed consent for participation in research
• Less inter-individual variability (due to less genetic variability) provides greater statistical power	• No adequate model for advanced workings of human brain
• Short lifespans enable genetic studies (generational carry-over)	• Can generate controversy among the general public
• If necessary to successful completion of experiment, animals can be euthanized	• Can be dangerous (bites, etc.) to those handling animals
• Some, especially mammals, have similar genetic profiles to those of humans	
• Experimental results many times directly benefit other animals	

Use of Large Animals in Biomedical and Exercise Science Research

Although rats and mice are by far the most frequently used mammals in the conduct of scientific investigation (see Fig. 11-2), large animals have also been valuable contributors. For example, studying the cardiopulmonary systems of the horse while galloping—this must be done with the assistance of specially designed treadmills—provides insight into their highly developed oxidative metabolic systems for exercise scientists to allow comparison with the oxidative metabolic system of the human body. In addition, biomedical scientists use the model of the immediately post-exercise horse to improve our understanding of some lung diseases in humans. The severely taxed equine cardiopulmonary system suffers rupture of pulmonary capillaries resulting in leakage of blood into the lungs' alveolar spaces, which is a condition experienced by humans with some forms of lung disease.

Another large animal model often used in biomedical research is the pig. In fact, much of the critical work done to enable sophisticated cardiac surgery in humans was first performed on swine because of the great similarity in their hearts (*i.e.,* valves and vessels) to the size, structure, and function of valves and vessels found in the human heart. Even today,

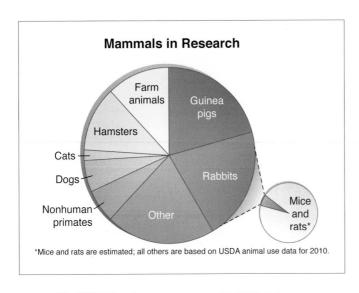

Mammals in Research

Farm animals

Guinea pigs

Hamsters

Cats

Dogs

Rabbits

Nonhuman primates

Other

Mice and rats*

*Mice and rats are estimated; all others are based on USDA animal use data for 2010.

FIGURE 11-2:   An illustration displaying the proportion of rats and mice used in biomedical research relative to other mammalian species.

the lives of many humans are spared every year by surgically replacing a damaged human heart valve with a healthy one obtained from a pig.

The domestic dog, although representing less than 1% of all the animals used in research, has a long history of serving scientists in their pursuit of understanding how the body works. In the modern era, the first known example of using the dog model in scientific research can be traced back to the 1600s when William Harvey was performing his landmark investigations revealing how the circulatory system functions. But even today, dogs play a vital role in disease research as they spontaneously develop many of the same illnesses that afflict humans including cancer, arthritis, chronic obstructive pulmonary disease (COPD), and even heart disease. A distinct advantage to using the dog model is the ease in the handling and training that these animals offer. Man and dog have cohabited through centuries of evolution becoming familiar to and trusting of each other. Additionally, dogs are generally anxious to please their human caretakers, making them easier to train than any other species. Moreover, with the many breeds available, it is fairly easy to select a breed or mix of breeds—mongrels are often used in research—that exhibits characteristics and behavioral tendencies that the investigator may desire.

Another large animal with a long history as serving as an animal model for scientific researchers is the standard domestic cat. In the 1800s, Claude Bernard regularly used cats in the performance of his many investigations designed to gain insight into the workings of various physiologic systems. In particular, cats are featured in investigations of the nervous system and reflex responses, illustrating the connectedness of the sensory and motor branches of that system. In an oft-cited study, V. Reggie Edgerton of the University of California at Los Angeles used the spinalized cat model to demonstrate that the spinal cord alone, without input from the higher motor cortex area of the brain, is capable of generating coordinated movements of the four legs to generate locomotor activity, although cats without brain function are awkward relative to what is seen in normal cats (8).

In another classic and highly referenced study investigating the functional characteristics of the neuromuscular system, Robert E. Burke (1) in the 1970s used a cat model to determine how that system is capable of performing such a wide array of tasks. These included everything from involving slight force exerted for extended periods of time to those requiring much force produced rapidly but of brief duration (1). By directly stimulating hundreds of motor neurons in the hindquarters of anesthetized cats, Burke and his colleagues (1) were able to identify three categories of **motor units** (*i.e.*, a single motor neuron and all the myofibers it innervates). These categories are (a) slow (S), which very gradually develop only meager amounts of peak force but exhibit endurance characteristics; (b) fast fatigue-resistant (FR), which reach peak force levels that are greater than those of slow motor units and display moderate resistance to fatigue; and (c) fast fatigable (FF) which even more rapidly achieve an even higher peak force output but have limited ability to maintain such force. It is due to the existence of these three different types of motor units that we now understand how it is that a single whole muscle can display such a wide range of contractile properties.

Perhaps the most controversial animal used in the conduct of research is the nonhuman primate (*i.e.*, monkeys and apes). These animals bear the closest resemblance to human beings genetically, physiologically, and, importantly, in terms of brain structure and function. As a result, they in some ways make outstanding animal models for research while at the same time and for the same reasons, they generate the most ardent resistance to their use as biomedical research subjects, although less resistance is expressed to the work of anthropologists who study interactions among them in the wild.

In the United States, most nonhuman primates that are used to perform laboratory-based research are domestically bred specifically for use in research (*i.e.*, purpose-bred), although some are still imported from other countries such as China, Peru, Philippines, and Mauritius. In terms of biomedical research, most of the work with these highly intelligent animals is to better understand functioning of the brain and also to increase our understanding of vision because the process of sight in monkeys is similar to that in humans. Nonhuman primates have also played essential roles in research related to HIV, stroke, cognition, hepatitis, and in the development of immunizations. Because primates, much like humans, are naturally social beings who opt to live together in small groups or colonies, behaviorists routinely observe their interpersonal behavior to promote an appreciation of the behavior of humans when placed in social settings.

CONCLUSIONS

It is clear that animal models have historically played a vital role in our understanding of human physiology, pathology, and behavior. Animals continue to participate in biomedical and exercise science research in various roles and for disparate purposes, and it is virtually certain that animals will continue to be invaluable in mankind's research pursuits. Despite bold technical advances made over the past decade, computer simulations and even cell culture studies—the two most promising replacement models for animal research—simply cannot replace direct investigation into the dynamics and interactions of various physiologic systems and the organism as a whole living unit. Examining the effects of perturbations to those systems in living organisms whether by new surgical procedures, administration of newly developed drugs, dietary alterations, exercise training, or neuromuscular disuse will continue to require the use of animal research models, at least for the foreseeable future.

Assuming this to be true, the question becomes one of proper care and treatment of animals used to conduct scientific investigation. This is to be ensured by animal research oversight and ethics committees along with the determination that the potential good to be derived by performing research with animal subjects outweighs the potential pain, discomfort, and in some cases, even the deaths of these animals. The historical records show that with few exceptions, the benefits have markedly outweighed the risks, resulting in better, healthier lives for both humans and animals. As humans, we owe a great debt of gratitude to the animals that have and continue to make possible the many and magnificent breakthrough discoveries achieved by biomedical and exercise scientists.

GLOSSARY

Animal Welfare Act: U.S. federal statute designed to guarantee human treatment of laboratory animals; does not apply to rats and mice

Food and Drug Administration: U.S. federal agency charged with assuring the safety of food and drugs

Fruit fly: small invertebrate animal used to study genetics mainly due to its short lifespan

Giant squid axon: large, unmyelinated axon found in the squid used to study neurophysiologic properties

Guide for the Care and Use of Laboratory Animals: document produced by the U.S. Public Health Service providing guidelines for proper use of animals in research, including rats and mice

Hind limb suspension: technique use to impart muscle unloading on rats

Human Genome Project: massive collaborative scientific project revealing the entire genetic code of humans

Immobilization: technique used to decrease limb muscle activity

Institutional Animal Care and Use Committee: research oversight committee of a university or research institution that must approve any investigation using animal subjects before the project begins

Motor unit: single motor neuron and all the muscle fibers that it innervates

Three Rs: consideration of reduction, refinement, and replacement in the use of animal models for research

Zebra fish: small fish commonly used to study embryonic development

REFERENCES

1. Burke RE, Levine DN, Zajac FE III. Mammalian motor units: physiological-histochemical correlation in three types in cat gastrocnemius. *Science.* 1971;174(4010):709–712.
2. Festing S, Wilkinson R. The ethics of animal research. Talking point on the use of animals in scientific research. *EMBO Rep.* 2007;8(6):526–530.
3. Hodgkin AL, Huxley AF. Propagation of electrical signals along giant nerve fibers. *Proc R Soc Lond B Biol Sci.* 1952;140(899):177–183.

4. Hodgkin AL, Huxley AF. A quantitative description of membrane current and its application to conduction and excitation in nerve. *J Physiol.* 1952;117(4):500–544.

5. Hodgkin AL, Katz B. The effect of sodium ions on the electrical activity of giant axon of the squid. *J Physiol.* 1949;108(1):37–77.

6. Hodgkin AL, Katz B. The effect of temperature on the electrical activity of the giant axon of the squid. *J Physiol.* 1949; 109(1-2):240–249.

7. King PA, Horton ED, Hirshman MF, Horton ES. Insulin resistance in obese Zucker rat (fa/fa) skeletal muscle is associated with a failure of glucose transporter translocation. *J Clin Invest.* 1992;90(4):1568–1575.

8. Lovely RG, Gregor RJ, Roy RR, Edgerton VR. Weight-bearing hindlimb stepping in treadmill-exercised adult spinal cats. *Brain Res.* 1990;514(2):206–218.

9. Moral-Sanz J, Menendez C, Moreno L, Moreno E, Cogolludo A, Perez-Vizcaino F. Pulmonary arterial dysfunction in insulin resistant obese Zucker rats. *Respir Res.* 2011;12:51. doi:10.1186/1465-9921-12-51.

10. Smerdu V, Karsch-Mizrachi I, Campione M, Leinwand L, Schiaffino S. Type IIx myosin heavy chain transcripts are expressed in type IIb fibers of human skeletal muscle. *Am J Physiol.* 1994;267(6, pt 1):C1723–C1728.

11. Turturro A, Witt WW, Lewis S, Hass BS, Lipman RD, Hart RW. Growth curves and survival characteristics of the animals used in the biomarkers of aging program. *J Gerontol A Biol Sci Med Sci.* 1999;54(11):B492–B501.

CHAPTER 12

Ethical Principles in Human and Animal Research

Matthew D. Barberio, PhD, Margaret K. Bradbury, MS, CGC, MSHS, and Monica J. Hubal, PhD

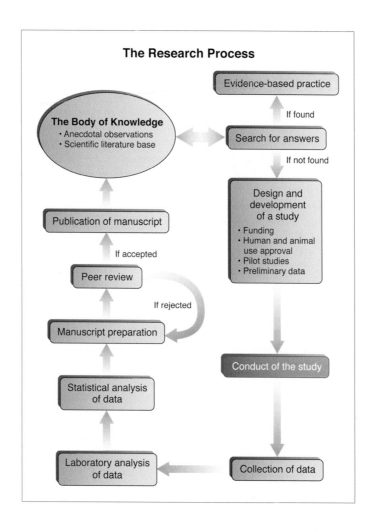

INTRODUCTION

Research is an exciting process with the ultimate goal of enhancing the body of knowledge within a given field. As you begin your introduction to research in the fields of exercise science, human performance, and health sciences, it is important to understand the proper conduct expected of scientists. As an individual involved in research, you may encounter situations in which you will ask the question, "Is this the right way to conduct my research?" The answer to such a seemingly simple question requires you to understand the moral guidelines and protective regulations to which the scientific community must adhere. As students, you serve an important role not only in conducting research but also in protecting yourself, your mentor, your colleagues, your institution, and (most importantly) your research participants from scientific misconduct. Scientific research serves a vital role in society, and protecting the integrity of the entire process is important in maintaining the public's trust. In this chapter, you will find a short history of how current guidelines were developed, a brief summary of current rules and regulations, and an exploration of how these guidelines must adapt to changing landscapes within the world of research.

ETHICAL THEORIES RESEARCH

Derived from the Greek word "ethos" (meaning habitual way of behaving), **ethics** can be defined as the establishment of a set of guidelines for morally acceptable conduct within a theoretical framework. These guidelines are a roadmap for how we should act in all facets of everyday life, including our work as researchers. However, not all individuals, groups, or cultures follow the same ethical guidelines, and ethical theories continue to be debated as time passes. For example, within normative ethics (the study of ethical actions), there are multiple competing theories on how one should answer moral questions. A follower of deontology ("duty" or "obligation" ethics) believes that it is the act and the motive of the act itself, not the consequences of the act that determines "good." The tenets of consequentialism, which state that to act morally "right," one must consider the consequences of his or her action. Another major approach of normative ethics is virtue ethics, in which the virtue of a person's character determines ethical behavior.

These differing theoretical frameworks are examples of the complexity of ethics as a field of study, which is also made more complex by the needs of the field to adapt to changes in society over time. So how does a student make sense of all these rules? As a researcher, to whom does your primary obligation or duty belong? What makes one's character virtuous? Is it OK to do harm if the consequences promote good?

Although these are questions that cannot be expected to be answered simply, the ethical system of principlism contains a solid general framework within which you can work. Principlism's foundation is rooted in four moral principles:

1. Autonomy: The right to govern oneself.
2. Beneficence: One should act to do good.
3. Non-maleficence: One should not do harm.
4. Justice: Benefits and burdens should be equitably distributed.

Principlism has formed the general basis for moral judgments in research involving human subjects in the United States. We will discuss these principles in more detail later in this chapter. First, we will briefly discuss historical events and cases that have highlighted the need to develop guidelines to protect research subjects.

UNETHICAL EXPERIMENTATION IN HUMAN AND ANIMAL RESEARCH

History is littered with examples of unethical research practices in the name of science and medicine. For centuries, naturalists and others have ventured into unethical practices in pursuit of medical advancement in some of the earliest medical research on record. Unfortunately, modern times are no stranger to unethical conduct in scientific experimentation either, and the following examples represent only a couple of the most egregious cases that eventually led to the establishment of more concrete guidelines for ethical conduct.

Nazi Medical Experiments

Without consent or permission, medical doctors from Nazi Germany conducted numerous studies on unwilling participants, including Jewish prisoners, disabled individuals, and others. In some experiments, individuals were exposed to freezing water and cold air temperatures for long durations to study hypothermia and rewarming (4). In other studies, sections of muscles, bones, tendons, and nerves were removed from unanesthetized individuals to study regeneration of these tissues. Although the result of the experiments themselves often resulted in death, those who survived, purposefully or not, were frequently killed at the conclusion of the observations. Those unfortunate enough to survive such cruelty were often left mutilated, dismembered, and psychologically devastated. Other experiments included exposure of subjects to chemical weapons (such as mustard gas), high altitudes (66,000 ft), radiation, and biologic diseases (such as malaria) (4). In the aftermath of these atrocities, these doctors defended their actions by arguing that no law—international or national—regarding medical experiments in humans prevented these experiments. At the end of the trials that would follow, during which many of the doctors were convicted, the Nuremberg Code was published and accepted as the first international standards for ethical scientific conduct for use of humans in research. More information regarding Nazi medical experimentation can be found in the Holocaust Encyclopedia on the U.S. Holocaust Memorial Museum website at http://www.ushmm.org/learn/holocaust-encyclopedia (16).

Tuskegee Syphilis Study

Although some examples of unethical practices come from extraordinary circumstances such as crimes during war, other examples come from more unexpected circumstances. In 1932, the U.S. Public Health Service (PHS) began a study to analyze the long-term effects of untreated syphilis (at the time a disease for which there was no known cure) in a population. With compliance of the Tuskegee Institute (now Tuskegee University), 600 impoverished African American men from rural Macon, Alabama, were selected to receive free medical care, burial insurance (so autopsies could be performed), transportation, and meals for participation in the study. Among the participants, 301 had previously contracted syphilis, whereas 299 had not. No participants were informed of the actual intentions of the study and were told they were being studied for "bad blood," which in local dialect covered multiple maladies.

For 40 years, this population was routinely monitored for occurrence of syphilis. Remarkably, despite the fact that penicillin had been discovered to cure syphilis and was in routine medical use in the early 1940s, the natural history study did not adopt its use. Not only were participants not being treated for a now fully treatable disease, they were being enticed to continue in the study by receiving written offers for "last chance for special free treatments." The study continued until 1972, when PHS venereal disease researcher Pete Buxtun and John Heller broke the story in the July 25 edition of the *Washington Star* (now part of the *Washington Post*). Buxton had written of his concerns in a letter to the PHS as early as 1966 and leaked the information to the press early in the 1970s. Following congressional hearings and ad hoc advisory committees, $9 million was allotted when a monetary settlement with surviving participants (about $38,000 each) and families of deceased participants (about $15,000 each) was reached. Not only did the actions of this study fracture the public trust of research but it also left the African American community understandably reluctant to participate in research or seek preventative medical care. The public outcry and condemnation from the medical community following this study would leave a lasting legacy on human research in the United States (18).

Experimental Animal Surgeries

Breaches of ethical misconduct are not isolated to human research, and in 1965, the magazine *Sports Illustrated* published an article chronicling the story about a stolen dog—Pepper the dalmatian. Pepper had been taken from the yard of her owners in Pennsylvania and sold to a hospital in New York City, where she died during an experimental animal procedure. The following year, *Life* magazine published an article detailing the horrific living conditions that dogs and cats were subjected to at animal dealer facilities. It is suspected that these actions (dog-napping) and the conditions of animal facilities were prevalent around the country at that time. Much public outcry was heard following these articles, and the Animal Welfare Act (Laboratory Animal Welfare Act of 1966, Public Law 89–544) was signed into law by President Lyndon B. Johnson.

REGULATION AND OVERSIGHT OF HUMAN AND ANIMAL EXPERIMENTATION

Following the atrocities committed by the Nazi regime during World War II, 23 Nazis (20 medical doctors) were charged with war crimes, crimes against humanity, performing medical experiments on prisoners of war and civilians of occupied countries, and membership in a criminal organization. The most common defense used by the doctors regarding unethical experimentation is that no law existed that delineated legal experimentation from illegal. As a result of the **Nuremberg Trials**, as they are collectively called, the **Nuremberg Code** was published in 1947 as codified ethical principles for human experimentation (15,17). Lacking legal force for actual implementation in any country, the Nuremberg Code served as the basis for the U.S. Department of Health and Human Services (DHHS) Code of Federal Regulations. The Nuremberg Code can be read in its entirety on the DHHS website (17), provided in Table 12-1.

Table 12-1 Useful Websites on Research Ethics	
Document	**Web Address**
The Nuremberg Code (17)	http://www.hhs.gov/ohrp/archive/nurcode.html
Declaration of Helsinki (21)	http://www.wma.net/en/30publications/10policies/b3/
The Belmont Report (18)	http://www.hhs.gov/ohrp/humansubjects/guidance/belmont.html
ACSM Code of Ethics (1)	http://www.acsm.org/join-acsm/membership-resources/code-of-ethics
American Physiological Society Guiding Principles for Research Involving Animal and Human Beings (2)	http://www.the-aps.org/mm/Publications/Info-For-Authors/Animal-and-Human-Research

In June of 1964, The World Medical Association (WMA) published its ethical guidelines in the **Declaration of Helsinki**—*Ethical Principles for Medical Research Involving Human Subjects* (21). Since its inception, the Helsinki Declaration (as its commonly referred to) has been reaffirmed, revisited, and clarified by the WMA in 1975, 1983, 1989, 1996, 2000, 2002, 2004, and 2008. The declaration contains 35 statements that codify the scientific and ethical beliefs of the members of the WMA and is intended for use by clinicians and researchers alike. The ethical principles adopted in the Helsinki Declaration include but are not limited to:

● First consideration is given to the health of the patient.
● Respect for all humans and protection of their rights.
● Participants shall be given adequate information pertaining to the study in which informed consent to participate can be based on.
● Participation must be voluntary.
● Privacy of personal information must be adequately safeguarded.
● Recognition that ethical, legal, and regulatory norms are dependent on local, regional, and cultural norms. No international or national regulatory body shall reduce principles set forth in the Helsinki Declaration.

To read the entire Helsinki Declaration, use the link provided in Table 12-1 (21).

In 1974, The National Commission for the Protection of Human Subjects of Biomedical and Behavioral Research was created as part of the National Research Act. Largely a response to the gross scientific misconduct that occurred during Tuskegee syphilis study, the commission's main priority was to identify the basic ethical principles under which biomedical and behavioral research involving human participants in the United States is conducted. In 1979, the **Belmont Report** was published and still serves as the cornerstone for the protection of human participants in biomedical and behavioral research (18). For access to the Belmont Report, use the address provided in Table 12-1.

The Belmont Report is instrumental in defining the once vague boundaries between routine healthcare practice and research. Generally, practice is considered the routine and accepted prescription of interventions or therapies for the benefit of well-being of an individual that have reasonable expectations of success. Research, on the other hand, is defined as an activity whereby one tests a hypothesis and draws conclusions. Of course, a lot of generalizable research is needed to know whether a new therapy or intervention will hold clinical benefits for patients. Ultimately, this research will need to comply with the three basic ethical principles established in the Belmont Report (18):

1. Respect for persons: Individuals should be treated autonomously, whereas those who have diminished autonomy are entitled to further protection.
2. Beneficence: Most importantly, research should do no harm. The benefits of research should be maximized, whereas harms should be minimized within the constraints of sound research design.
3. Justice: Design of research should distribute burdens and benefits equitably, and people should be treated fairly.

Finally, the Belmont Report outlines that practices of these principles requires three key considerations for researchers and review committees. First, human participants must provide informed consent about what can and cannot happen to them in the course of participation. To do so, the researchers must provide sufficient information about purposes, procedures, anticipated risk, and the opportunity to ask questions. This requires that the information be presented in an appropriate manner for comprehension. It is important to consider the participant's ability to understand the information provided, and therefore, this information should be presented in the simplest terms and an organized manner. Ultimately, a participant's willingness to participate should be given voluntarily without the presence of coercion or undue influences.

Second, the assessment of risks and benefits should be examined by the investigators, review boards, and participants alike. As an investigator using human participants, you should thoroughly scrutinize your research design to minimize potential harm to your participants. This may mean adopting new techniques to use in your laboratory, acquiring newer and safer material or machinery, or becoming trained or certified in a specific field. Review boards assessing the risks and benefits of proposed research must determine if the potential risks presented to the participants are justified by the benefits. This also means taking into consideration risks and benefits to those other than the participants (*i.e.*, society as a whole). If you are a potential participant in human research, you should take into consideration the potential risks of participating in a particular study when making your final decision to voluntarily provide informed consent.

Lastly, the selection of subjects should not preferentially distribute benefits or burdens to any one social, racial, or cultural class except in cases in which the research is directly investigating these differences as independent and dependent variables. Furthermore, populations already deemed vulnerable (*e.g.*, institutionalized, economically disadvantaged, minorities, pregnant women, or children) may be at a reduced capacity to provide voluntary consent due to their dependent status and should be given further protections.

Institutional Oversight of Human Subjects

Title 45, Part 46 of the Code of Federal Regulations (45 CFR 46), more commonly referred to as the "common rule," was codified into federal law in 1991 by the DHHS. These regulations, specifically Subpart A, make up the federal policy regarding protection of human subjects and are applicable to all research involving human subjects. A human subject is designated as any individual from whom an investigator conducting research obtains data through intervention or interaction with the individual or identifiable private information. At the turn of the new century, the DHHS established the Office of Human Research Protections for oversight of federal policy and compliance to protection of human subjects.

A major initiative of 45 CFR 46 was the establishment of **institutional review boards** (IRB) for review of all research protocols involving human subjects. IRBs are made up of at least five individuals who may or may not be affiliated with the institution and contain the necessary expertise to determine the appropriateness of proposed research with regard to professional conduct, legality, and institutional commitments. At least one of these members will not be affiliated with your university but will represent the community in determining the acceptable research that takes place at the institution.

As you begin to develop your research question, you should become familiar with your institution's IRB policies and the requirements for you as an investigator to submit proposed research studies for review. For instance, many institutions voluntarily participate in the Collaborative Institutional Training Initiative (CITI) at the University of Miami (5). This program provides training courses for the responsible conduct of research in biomedical sciences and other areas for investigators at all stages. Your institution may require you to complete multiple courses in this or other programs before approving you to participate in human research.

You should also become familiar with the term **minimal risk**, which implies that risks associated with the study are no greater than risks that the participants would encounter in daily activities. Depending on the amount of risk associated with participation in the study, the IRB will determine if the proposed study should be reviewed under exempt review, expedited review, or full board review. Figure 12-1 illustrates a typical IRB review process, taking into account that policies and procedures may vary from institution to institution. Following written IRB approval, the proposed research may be performed within the constraints of the approved IRB protocol. Only under circumstances of emergency or immediate danger to participants should any deviation from the approved protocol occur. These instances and events should be immediately reported to the IRB for review. Furthermore, yearly progress and renewal applications to the IRB regarding all approved studies are required.

A major component of ensuring protection of human subjects is obtaining informed consent. **Informed consent** is the process of ensuring that potential research participants are given adequate information about the details of the research study so that they can make an informed decision regarding participation. The first legal establishment of informed consent in the United States came in the 1914 decision of *Schloendorff v. Society of New York Hospital* (13). The plaintiff in this trial, Mary Schloendorff, consented to examination under ether to determine if a previously diagnosed tumor was malignant but did not consent to the removal of the tumor. Upon determining the tumor was malignant, the physician disregarded Schloendorff's decision to not consent to the removal of the tumor and removed it anyway. Schloendorff sued the hospital and in the result decision, Justice Benjamin Cardozo of the New York Court of Appeals wrote:

> *Every human being of adult years and sound mind has a right to determine what shall be done with his own body, and a surgeon who performs an operation without his patient's consent commits an assault for which he is liable in damages. This is true except in cases of emergency where the patient is unconscious and where it is necessary to operate before consent can be obtained (12).*

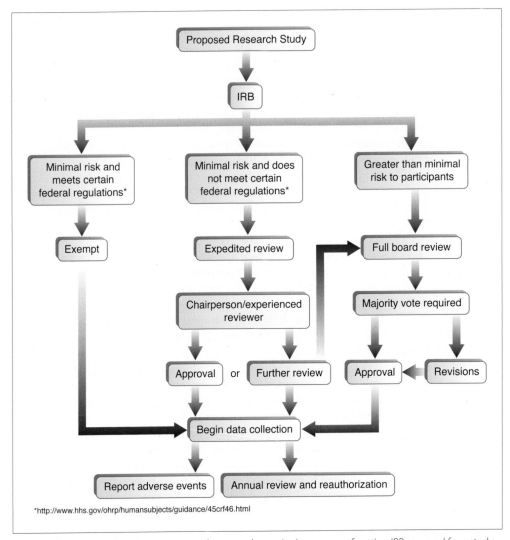

FIGURE 12-1: This flowchart represents the general steps in the process of getting IRB approval for a study. After designing your research approach, you will submit the appropriate IRB documents to the local IRB committee. Once submitted, they will determine the appropriate type of review for your particular protocol based on the assessment of risk associated with it. You cannot begin any study, regardless of review type, until you receive written approval for your protocol.

Despite this ruling, informed consent was not required in human research in the United States until the Belmont Report was published in 1974. Discussed previously, the Belmont Report (18) outlines the criteria for informed consent, and the Code of Federal Regulations (45 CFR 46.116) outlines the requirements for review of informed consent by an IRB. A checklist in Figure 12-2 provides a useful checklist for writing informed consent documents for a proposed research study and you should ask your supervising faculty for examples of previously approved informed consents.

Checklist for Informed Consent Documents

Be sure to include:

☐ A statement of purpose of the research study and the expected duration of participation.
☐ A description of risks and discomforts that may be associated with participation.
☐ A description of the benefits to subjects and others from participation in the study.
☐ A disclosure of advantageous alternate treatments available to participants.
☐ An outline for the maintenance of records for protection of privacy and confidentiality.
☐ A clear description of any compensation awarded for participation.
☐ Contact information for individuals regarding:
　☐ General questions regarding research
　☐ Rights of the participants
　☐ Participation-related injuries
☐ Statement of voluntary participation and the right to withdraw.
　☐ Outline procedures individuals should follow to withdraw.
☐ Any information required or requested by your local IRB.

When appropriate, include statements:

☐ About the possibility of unforeseeable risks associated with participation.
☐ About circumstances in which participation may be terminated by researchers.
☐ About any additional costs to participants as a result of their participation.
☐ About the consequences associated with early withdraw from participation (*i.e.*, loss of benefits).
☐ About disclosure of new findings that may alter willingness to participate.
☐ About the total number of participants being recruited for this study.

FIGURE 12-2:   This is a helpful checklist of required statements and information to be added to informed consent documents. Be sure to contact your local IRB to inquire about any further information that may need to be included. Also, be sure to ask your advisors and other professors for examples of previously approve informed consents to use as a guide.

Lastly, if you are using a population that may be considered vulnerable (*e.g.*, people who are institutionalized, economically disadvantaged, minorities, pregnant, or children), federal guidelines stipulate further protections for these individuals. You should consult your local IRB and become familiar with the federal guidelines (45 CFR 46 Subpart D) concerning special populations so that these protections are included in your research design. Furthermore, if you are using a pediatric population, you are required to acquire **assent**, a statement of agreement to participate, from the child and permission for the child to participate from a parent or legal guardian.

The Institutional Animal Care and Use Committee

Following the articles published in *Sports Illustrated* and *Life* magazine, President Lyndon B. Johnson signed the Animal Welfare Act (AWA) of 1966 into law. This law covered nonhuman primates, dogs, cats, hamsters, guinea pigs, and other warm-blooded animals (alive and dead) for use in research and exhibition. Another major component of the law required animal dealing facilities to be in compliance with federal regulations. Since its passage in 1966, the law has been amended seven times to include more animals and further oversight. Other laws such as the Horse Protection Act (Public Law 91–929; 1970), Marine Mammal Protection Act (Public Law 95–522; 1972), and the Endangered Species Act (Public Law 93–205; 1973) have also been passed to protect animals from certain procedures and experimentation altogether.

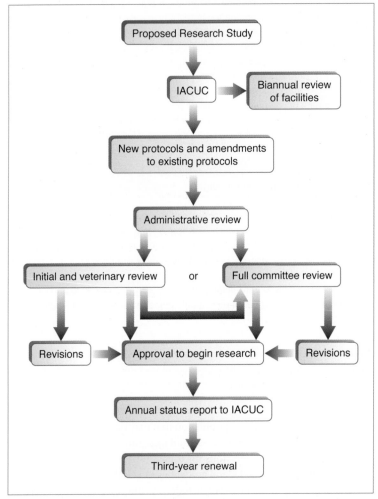

FIGURE 12-3:   This schematic represents the general process for getting IACUC approval for proposed animal research project. After designing your research, you will submit the appropriate documents to your local IACUC where it will be assigned either to a designated reviewer or to full committee review. The IACUC will also conduct biannual inspections of all animal research facilities to ensure compliance with federal regulations.

Prior to 1966, the Animal Care Panel (ACP) was formed in 1961 by a group of veterinarians who would publish "The Guide for the Care and Use of Laboratory Animals" in 1963. That same year, the American Association for the Accreditation of Laboratory Animal Care (ALLAC) was incorporated into the ACP. ALLAC would later change its name to Association for the Assessment and Accreditation of Laboratory Animal Care International. In 1971, the AWA was amended to require institutional accreditation and compliance with the law through an ALLAC accreditation. Prior to this, individual institutions were not regulated, only animal use facilities. In 1979, PHSs began to require each institution involved in animal research to have an animal care committee consisting of at least five members, one of whom is a practicing veterinarian. These committees became known as the **Institutional Animal Care and Use Committee** (IACUC) in a 1986 amendment to the AWA. All institutional IACUCs are responsible for reviewing all research protocols involving animals. Each institutional IACUC process is unique, and Figure 12-3 represents a general outline for the approval process. Note that submitted animal research protocols may be reviewed by an initial (sometimes referred to as a "designated") reviewer and veterinary reviewer, or they may be immediately sent to a full committee review. IACUC is also responsible for a biannual review of facilities where animal research use occurs. In accordance with federal regulation, any issues of non-compliance that result from reviews are reported to the NIH Office of Laboratory Animal Welfare.

As a student, you should become familiar with your institution's IACUC policies before planning to join in a research study involving animals. Similar to CITI training for human research, the local IACUC often provides local training, such as CITI's Animal Care and Use course, that may be required for conducting animal research.

GENERAL ETHICAL CHALLENGES IN HEALTH SCIENCE RESEARCH

Conducting research is a rewarding experience that truly requires a team effort to complete. However, there are some general ethical concerns of which you should be aware. Safeguarding against these ethical dilemmas will be critical not only for IRB or IACUC approval, but it will enable sound research design.

Privacy and Confidentiality

One of the immediate concerns in human research is the protection of an individual's privacy and the maintenance of confidentiality. By collecting personal information on an individual, your records have the potential to expose private information the individual may have otherwise never intended others to know. Here, **privacy** is defined as the individual's or group's right to determine when and the manner in which private information is divulged, which is in agreement with historic definitions of the word (20). **Confidentiality** is the manner in which the personal information gained through participation remains detached from a person's identity.

During the planning of your studies, you should consult your local IRB about acceptable methods for storage and maintenance of your records. Furthermore, the type and amount of information you collect about your participants will have a large influence on the type of IRB review your protocol receives. Greater amounts and detail of information will increase the risk to participants, thus requiring the need for greater scrutiny of procedures. As a researcher, you will also be required to describe and outline your procedures to maintain both privacy and confidentiality to your participants. This will be accomplished through the informed consent documents for your studies. It is important to make sure that the terms and procedures are clearly defined and readily understandable to the layman because a clear understanding of the protections for privacy and confidentiality are a major component of informed consent.

Avoiding Coercion

Another major concern involves the research staff potentially influencing or coercing a potential participant's voluntary decision to become a research participant. Special populations, such as economically disadvantaged individuals, may be influenced by large monetary rewards for participation, thus it is important for research to justify the monetary compensation rewarded (often based on time commitment). On college campuses, students represent the largest population and may be influenced by a professor, responsible for awarding their grades, to participate by offering large amounts of extra credit. If this were a student's only opportunity to receive extra credit, then it would be considered coercive. Lastly, some populations are considered to be especially vulnerable (*e.g.*, children, prisoners, pregnant women, those who are economically disadvantaged, and those who are educationally disadvantaged) to influence and coercion. Thus, 45 CFR 46.111(b) stipulates that extra safeguards be put into place so that informed consent can be obtained without undue influence and coercion.

Ownership of Samples and Data

When subjects consent to being part of a research study, the informed consent generally will state how their biologic samples or other data will be used, and consent is specifically given for that particular study. Data from studies are typically published in journal articles or other publications or used as part of proprietary research such as clinical trials or drug or product development. The privacy of subjects is generally maintained by de-identifying samples and minimizing (and clearly defining) who has access to identifiable records.

However, there are a multitude of ethical problems associated with scientists wanting to use samples for purposes beyond those stated in the original study. One such example is the generation (purposeful or not) of immortalized cells from tissue samples, which are then used in perpetuity in *in vitro* studies. The story of Henrietta Lacks is a good example of an evolving ethical story about sample ownership, and it is detailed in Concept Box 12-1.

Additionally, there are many ethical considerations to biobanking samples for public, private, and/or commercial use. Were public funds used to collect these samples? To whom do they belong? If they are commercialized, does the donor have any rights to compensation beyond any original payments for participation? If a subject consents to DNA testing for a specific purpose (*i.e.*, to test for one disease), is the rest of their genetic code available for exploration? Does any common good coming from projects using

CONCEPT BOX 12-1 Henrietta Lacks and Her Family's Story

Until recent media coverage of a book (14) and court case, most people did not know the name Henrietta Lacks. For decades, Henrietta Lacks provided answers to important questions about how cells work and respond to drugs and various other treatments, although she was not a scientist. Rather, Lacks was a patient at Johns Hopkins Hospital on January 29, 1951, being seen regarding a lump she discovered in her cervix. Upon examination, her physicians obtained a small tissue sample and subsequently diagnosed her with cancer. Until this point, cancer research had always been limited by lack of material with which scientists could test hypotheses. Simply put, human cells were hard to keep alive long enough to do research. However, the tissue obtained from Lacks became a medical oddity when researchers discovered that these cancerous cells could survive and continue to grow outside her body. HeLa (the first two letters of her first and last name) cells were subsequently used in research for decades with hardly anyone

knowing about their origin or the reasoning behind their name. Furthermore, it wasn't until two decades after her death that her surviving family found out that these cells were the centerpiece of large-scale commercialized businesses. In life, Lacks didn't venture far from her birthplace in Roanoke, Virginia, but her cells have been used in research around the world.

At the time of her procedure, consent was not required for researchers to use the cells following collection, and in 1990, the Supreme Court of California determined it was legal to commercialize an individual's discarded tissue (11). Since then, researchers have also published the DNA code of HeLa cells without permission from the Lacks family, potentially exposing the surviving member to a breach of privacy. In August 2013, the National Institutes of Health took the unprecedented step to grant her family some control over the dissemination and use of data from studies that use HeLa cells (7).

biobanked materials outweigh any moral or economic exploitation of the sample donors? These are all issues for which no unifying solution exists. The expansion of biobank creation and their use in modern times should open new dialogues regarding protection of human subjects.

ADAPTING RESEARCH ETHICS IN THE MODERN RESEARCH ERA

Technologic advances have provided many tools for scientists to use to help organize, streamline, and expand their research endeavors. On the surface, many of these advances seem specifically tailored to help accomplish the end goal of research, which is the advancement of knowledge. However, for all the answers and solutions offered by these new tools, new (and old) questions regarding the ethics of their use in human research arise. In the following discussion, we hope to present some of the ethical questions and considerations about the continuing modernization of research methods.

Use of Social Media in Research

The popularity of social networking sites such as Facebook and Twitter provide a very large pool (approximately 1.1 billion and 500 million users, respectively) of potential research participants and readily accessible information. Most people are familiar with the concepts of these social media sites that allow individuals to create personal profiles containing any information they wish to convey and to choose who has access to view this information. Furthermore, these sites provide the opportunity to search for individuals based on interests, affiliations, and keyword searches. What are the potential research uses and ethical dilemmas raised by such a treasure trove of potential information and participants?

Let's say you were interested in physical activity participation on your college campus, and you wanted to determine how many people engage in daily physical activity (structured or unstructured) during the school week. You could easily conceive a study design in which you count the amount of people that enter the local recreational facility on your campus; this study may easily fall under the exempt review category (as decided by the IRB). You could also use a specific set of key words and search refining options built into the social media sites to search them for individuals at your institution who have exercised and readily choose to share this information publicly. Disregarding the potential flaws inherent to each of the designs is one of the previously mentioned observational studies ethically more preferable to the other? It could be argued that by using social media, the individual intended the information for public consumption. However, by identifying that one individual decided to exercise and post to social media, you could subsequently identify that they exercised with two friends, neither of whom posted such information to social media. Is it OK to also count the friends in your observational study? Neither instance elevates the risk to the individual, no personal information is being collected, and both designs would most likely pass an IRB-exempt review. In this instance, it will be essential to clearly define the process and its limits that you intend to use and to strictly adhere to these guidelines so that no inadvertent breach of conduct occurs.

The use of social media in research is a potentially helpful mechanism to relieve some of the costs and time associated with subject recruitment and data collection. As a researcher, you must remain cognizant of any potential breaches of ethical conduct that could easily occur without any intention. For instance, if you are involved in research involving the pediatric population and need to obtain consent from the parent of a child (recalling the age of consent in your state) you have identified through social media, you may inadvertently breach the privacy and confidentiality of the child in doing so (12). You should also keep in mind that although social media sites are excellent communication media, they are often plagued with false and sometimes fraudulent information (8).

Another consideration is the digital footprint you create with the use of social media. The collection and storage of your search history on social media sites and web browsers may leave a trail that could inadvertently become public knowledge and comprise the privacy of your research participants. These and other types of ethical dilemmas should be explored by your research team when formulating your research strategy and submitting your IRB approval documents. Ultimately, the standards for the use of social media in research will need to be determined by your local IRB, any professional organizations of which you are a part, and your research team. Lastly, you should make sure to consult the companies and the user agreements of individual social media sites before planning to use these media, as they may have special instructions for use of their sites.

Electronic Medical Records in Research

In 1996, President Bill Clinton signed into law the Health Insurance Portability and Accountability Act of 1996 (6), better known as "HIPAA." Among the many provisions in this law is the privacy rule that protects an individual's protected health information (PHI). The privacy rule outlines the process under which individual PHI may be disclosed for research purposes (19). This allows researchers access to important medical information for research studies while increasing protections of privacy and confidentiality of patients already established by the common rule. Furthermore, the Health Information Technology for Economic and Clinical Health Act (HITECH Act; Subpart D) (10) was enacted under Title XIII of the American Recovery and Reinvestment Act of 2009 (3). This law provides expanded provisions for the security and privacy policies instituted by HIPAA. The DHHS then went onto publish the Omnibus Final Rule, effective in 2013, in which the modification further describes provisions related to research such as compound authorization, authorization for future research use, and declassification of PHI for deceased persons after a period of time has passed (10). With these guidelines in place, information regarding those that can access electronic medical records and PHI should be clearly stated in all consent forms and carefully controlled.

Sequencing the Human Genome and Ethical Implications

In 1987, The Human Genome Project began with the bold mission to map the entire human genome, and it was completed in 2003 with nearly (99.99%) the entire human genome sequenced. Technologic advances have made large-scale genetic research easier and faster for research labs, enabling genome-wide datasets to be completed routinely. The maturing of the "genomics age" brings along with it its own set of unique ethical implications for biomedical and health science researchers. Today, research on how genetic variations alter an individual's risk of cancer and other chronic diseases holds powerful implications for medicine and personalized treatment plans. This also extends to non-disease models, such as predicting exercise responses or performance variables.

But this information (and the potential misunderstanding of what it means) could significantly impact subjects personally, professionally, and financially. For instance, testing for a genetic variant associated with the risk of developing breast cancer is widely available today (9). The results of such a test could be potentially beneficial in developing preventative treatment plans, but they could also serve to cause emotional distress if not conveyed correctly. Furthermore, if such information were to become public knowledge without the individual's consent, it would be a serious breach of privacy to the individual and family members that may also be affected. In 2008, the United States passed the Genetic Information Nondiscrimination Act (known as "GINA"; H.R. 493) to prevent employers or insurance companies from discriminating against individuals based on any known genetic predispositions. Although GINA helps protect individuals from discrimination by employers and insurance companies, more protections are needed moving forward in research as more genomic sequence data become available.

What does this potentially mean to the field of exercise science and health promotion? As we move forward in determining how and why exercise is beneficial to long-term health and wellness, understanding how an individual's genetic makeup influences that individual's response to exercise will be crucial. This type of information, already being studied and analyzed in the field of exercise science, will help in establishing more personalized approaches to exercise prescription and rehabilitative medicine.

Despite how cutting edge such technology is, the ethical cornerstones to which all research topics adhere do not change. The information that will be gained and how it will be used from these and other types of studies must be clearly explained to the participants, and the privacy and confidentiality of results must be maintained. First, concern for the subjects' health, well-being, privacy, and confidentiality must be maintained.

GLOSSARY

Assent: affirmative agreement of participation in research by a child determined incapable (due to age) of providing informed consent; permission by a parent or legal guardian must also be obtained

Belmont Report: published in 1979 following gross scientific misconduct in the Tuskegee syphilis study; serves as the cornerstone document for protections of human subjects in research in the United States

Confidentiality: the manner in which the personal information gained through participation remains detached from a person's identity

Ethics: the establishment of a set of guidelines for morally acceptable conduct within theoretical framework

Declaration of Helsinki: codified ethical standards of the World Medical Association at the 1966 World Medical Assembly

Informed consent: detailed explanation of the purpose, scope, procedures, risks, and benefits of participation in a research study so that voluntary participation can be determined by the participant

Institutional Animal Care and Use Committee: institutional committee with responsibility to review, approve, and oversee all research and research facilities involving animals in accordance with federal regulations

Institutional Review Board: institutional committee with the responsibility to review, approve, and oversee all research involving human subjects in accordance with federal regulations

Minimal risk: concept that the risk of participation in a research study presents no greater risk than those associated with daily activities

Nuremberg Code: first codified ethical standards for human experimentation published in 1947 as a result of the atrocities of World War II Nazi medical experiments

Nuremberg Trials: name given to the collective trials of 23 Nazi party officials following World War II regarding unethical medical experimentation and genocide

Privacy: an individual's or group's right to determine when and the manner in which private information is divulged

REFERENCES

1. American College of Sports Medicine Web site [Internet]. Code of Ethics. Indianapolis (IN): American College of Sports Medicine; [cited 2013 Sep 23]. Available from: http://www.acsm.org/join-acsm/membership-resources/code-of-ethics
2. American Physiological Society Web site [Internet]. Guiding principles for research involving animals and human beings. Bethesda (MD): American Physiological Society; [cited 23 Sep 2013]. Available from: http://www.the-aps.org/mm/Publications/Info-For-Authors/Animal-and-Human-Research
3. American Recovery and Reinvestment Act of 2009 Pub L No. 111–115, 123 Stat 115.
4. Berger RL. Nazi science—the Dachau hypothermia experiments. *N Engl J Med.* 1990;322(20):1435–1440.
5. CITI Program Web site [Internet]. Miami (FL): Collaborative Institutional Training initiative. Available from: https://www.citiprogram.org/
6. The Health Insurance Portability and Accountability Act of 1996 Pub L No. 104–191, 110 Stat 1963.
7. Hudson KL, Collins FS. Biospecimen policy: family matters. *Nature.* 2013;500(7461):141–142.
8. Keim ME, Noji E. Emergent use of social media: a new age of opportunity for disaster resilience. *Am J Disaster Med.* 2011; 6(1):47–54.
9. Miki Y, Swensen J, Shattuck-Eidens D, et al. A strong candidate for the breast and ovarian cancer susceptibility gene BRCA1. *Science.* 1994;266(5182):66–71.
10. Modifications to the HIPAA privacy, security, enforcement, and breach notification rules under the health information technology for economic and clinical health act and the genetic information nondiscrimination act; other modifications to the HIPAA rules; final rule. January 25, 2013. 45 CFR parts 160 and 164.
11. *Moore v Regents of the University of California*, No. S006987, CA Sup Ct (1990).
12. Moreno MA, Fost NC, Christakis DA. Research ethics in the MySpace era. *Pediatrics.* 2008;121(1):157–161.
13. *Schloendorff v Society of New York Hospital*, 211 NY 125, 105 NE 92 (1914).
14. Skloot R. *The Immortal Life of Henrietta Lacks.* New York (NY): Crown Publishers; 2010. 369 p.
15. Military Legal Resources. *Trials of War Criminals Before the Nuremberg Military Tribunals Under Control Council Law No. 10.* Washington, DC: Military Legal Resources, Federal Research Division; 1949. 181–182 pp. Available from U.S Government Printing Office, Washington.
16. U.S. Department of Health & Human Services Web site [Internet]. The Belmont Report. Washington (DC): U.S. Department of Health & Human Services; [cited 2013 Sep 23]. Available from: http://www.hhs.gov/ohrp/humansubjects/guidance/belmont.html
17. U.S. Department of Health & Human Services Web site [Internet]. Health Information Privacy. Washington (DC): U.S. Department of Health & Human Services; [cited 2013 September 23]. Available from: http://www.hhs.gov/ocr/privacy/hipaa/understanding/special/research/index.html
18. U.S. Department of Health & Human Services Web site [Internet]. Nuremberg Code. Washington (DC): U.S. Department of Health & Human Services; [cited 2013 Sep 23]. Available from: http://www.hhs.gov/ohrp/archive/nurcode.htm
19. U.S. Holocaust Memorial Museum Web site [Internet]. Holocaust Encyclopedia. Washington (DC): U.S. Holocaust Memorial Museum; [cited 2013 Sep 23]. Available from: http://www.ushmm.org/learn/holocaust-encyclopedia
20. Westin AF. *Privacy and Freedom.* 2nd ed. Techlink, Singapore: Ig Publishing; 2015.
21. World Medical Association Web site [Internet]. WMA Declaration of Helsinki—ethical principles for medical research involving human subjects. France: World Medical Association; [cited 2013 Sep 23]. Available from: http://www.wma.net/en/30publications/10policies/b3/

CHAPTER 13

Developing a Funding Base for Your Research

William J. Kraemer, PhD, FACSM, Shawn D. Flanagan, MA, MHA,
Mark T. White, MS, Brett A. Comstock, PhD, and Courtenay Dunn-Lewis, PhD

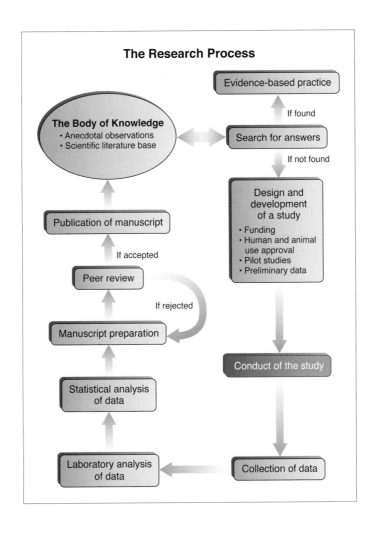

INTRODUCTION

Research can be expensive. The design of the experiment can expand to the point of not being feasible, and therefore, careful attention to the associated costs of the investigation needs to be monitored as one designs a study. As nearly all costs (*e.g.*, materials, assistantships) increase, and molecular or cellular approaches become more common, the cost of conducting research can be prohibitive. This reality forces a principal investigator to spend an increasing proportion of his or her time in search of funding, even for funds to allow graduate students to conduct their own thesis/dissertation research projects. Funding opportunities have in turn become more competitive, even for students, especially in light of larger economic forces that have made funding availability less certain. Thus, designing an experiment that can be completed within the context of the available funding environment is an important consideration. Understanding some of the global issues and aspects of gaining funding for a study, although some of it will be more related to the major advisor, gives the student important perspectives when staring to undertake research.

To overcome these challenges, various funding sources will need to be pursued, including internal or seed grant funds from one's university/entity of employment, public research funding initiatives, and private entities, including foundations, corporations, and professional research societies. It is important to remember that not all student research projects require external funding as many work within the context of the laboratory activities and some are at a "zero dollar" budget and just take research time and effort on the part of the student and laboratory workers. There are many examples (*e.g.*, examining how two different weight training programs in a group of students impact different forms of power testing measures, or analyzing the public available NFL combined data). However, an awareness of current and historical federal funding allocations provides information about a society's research priorities and interests and allows the student a better appreciation of his or her major professors' challenges to keep a laboratory going. This information is also helpful in selecting initiatives that are more likely to be interested in funding your research (Fig. 13-1).

Regardless of a society's interest in funding a given research "category," it is crucial to understand how effective funding efforts are accomplished. A principal investigator must be aware of the potential sources of funds, the availability of funds, and the priorities guiding the decision-making processes of funding organizations. Hence, in addition to designing an effective and compelling research proposal, the investigator must select appropriate and realistic funding sources, especially when working to gain funding for student projects. In such cases, the amount of funding for a project is typically low (*e.g.*, \$1,000 to \$15,000), and again, study designs must be kept in check or spin off of the principal investigators own work. For the student understanding, the principles and characteristics of successful funding efforts can be helpful. One can learn about this through the lens of the research proposal review process.

Like senior investigators, student investigators may wish to pursue research that incorporates a number of costs; a great deal of care is again needed in the design and scope of the study put forth. Here is where working with one's major advisor and

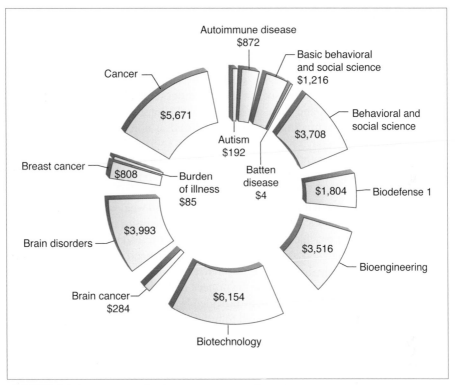

FIGURE 13-1:   2014 NIH funding categories, in millions (3).

senior faculty can give students important context for costs during the experimental design process. Although the sources of funds differ, the basic components of the research proposal are similar. Furthermore, because there will likely be competition for these funds, students, similar to their mentors, must be able to craft clear and persuasive proposals, articulate the importance of a given question, and present a research design that can answer that question sufficiently and ultimately be feasible within the proposed budget.

You may find funding from similar sources as your major advisor. However, you should search for funds to support your project and start to develop an identity for your own area of expertise that can continue into the next phase of your career. This will allow you to pursue an agenda somewhat relevant to your advisor's core competencies while beginning to create a track record of your own research interests. Importantly, this also provides a degree of freedom from the confines of your advisor's current research efforts which may not allow "out of the box" ideas and approaches. Thus, one must then design a project that is of interest. If you are going to need funding due to the nature of the project, then you will need to match your research topic's area of study with an outside funding outlet that has similar interests, missions, and funds such student proposals (*e.g.*, ACSM Student Awards) (1,5).

SELECTING A RESEARCH TOPIC

Practical Considerations

From a more global overview of research in the United States and similar to other national funding agencies around the world, the National Institutes of Health's (NIH) funding allocations reflect larger societal choices about research priorities. However, other funding sources do exist, and these are more probable targets for student-led investigations. But, before potential funding sources are discussed, as noted earlier, it is important to select and match your research topic with the funding source's interests. In this process, make sure that your advisor and committee (if the research is for a thesis or dissertation) have worked with you on the research project's development and experimental design while giving you insights as to the identification of funding sources.

Your research topic should in some way reflect what your advisor and laboratory group interests are. This is important for a number of reasons; namely, your advisor will be better positioned to provide mentorship in an area of research with which he or she is familiar. In addition, the resources available to you will depend on your advisor's basic laboratory's capabilities, help from other research assistants and investigators, institutional review board (IRB) responsibility for the project, and internal funding to contain the costs of the experiment beyond what can be provided by external funding sources.

If your research will be used to fulfill the requirements of a master's thesis or doctoral dissertation, it must also receive approval from your committee. In addition to providing critical support in the development, analysis, and interpretation of your research, committee members can provide constructive criticism that improves your experimental design. The development of the research proposal for your research should occur up front in union with your major advisor and committee and allow for optimal development of the research and position it for successful external funding. Therefore, it is important to consult with these faculty members early in the process as you develop your research proposal.

Finally, if you plan to pursue a career in research, it is wise to, in some way, connect your topic to your desired future pursuits within the scope of your laboratory group. For doctoral students, although tied to the general scope of your advisor's laboratory work, you can in part "spin off" and "branch out" and propose even more high-risk research hypotheses and research questions, as you are not constrained by the scope of your advisor's funded research design and questions. After you leave your degree program and move into a postdoctoral or new position, this research will allow you to gain some independence and develop your own indemnity as an investigator.

Selecting a Reasonable Topic

President Theodore Roosevelt once famously said, "Do what you can, where you are, with what you have!" This mentality is particularly helpful in the search for research funding. The importance of designing an "achievable" proposal that appears feasible given your facilities, equipment, and current skills cannot be overemphasized. In fact, one of the most common reasons for rejecting a research proposal is the perception among review panels that the project cannot be completed or is not technically correct in its design or approach or that it is beyond the student investigator's background and technical skills. The following are many common reasons why grants are not funded:

1. Overall scientific and technical merit of the proposed project was deemed weak.
2. Applicability of proposed research project to the program area is not compatible with its mission or not adequately justified.
3. Expertise and experience in the planned area of research and facilities available was not effectively demonstrated.
4. The proposed cost and budget rationales were not adequately justified.

The reasons for not getting a grant funded are highly variable, but for many students, they are often related to an overly optimistic project timeline, the perception of inadequate experience or laboratory resources, prohibitive costs, or an overly complicated proposal that fails to provide a logical or relatively direct way of answering a question. Any of these conclusions will likely result in an unsuccessful research proposal. Thus, throughout the proposal process, make sure to communicate the importance of your research, show that your design is effective and straightforward, and you have the ability to complete the project successfully with your prior laboratory experiences and institutional support for other needed resources.

DEVELOPING A RESEARCH PROPOSAL

Once the research topic is selected, the focus can be directed toward developing the research proposal. From a global perspective, the process of creating a proposal for the research should be approached from a project management level, keeping the end result in mind at all times (5). As you learned in Chapter 3, the intent of a research study is to contribute to the existing body of knowledge through the findings that are based on a question derived from an identifiable "gap" in current knowledge. As you've previously learned, the answer to the question is the investigator's hypothesis (*i.e.*, predicted outcome), which ultimately establishes the purpose of the study (*i.e.*, statement of purpose) and indicates the impact of the research project on the body of knowledge. In order to find meaningful results, you must develop a research design that includes or accounts for all necessary variables that allow you to answer the question. Next, you have to use this proposal to convince a funding source of the research project's value relative to being worthy of receiving a portion of the sometimes limited funds available. A comprehensive approach to the planning of the research project proposal should originate with a preliminary design sheet that shows the overall impression of the proposed research and its different aspects in brief before one gets into the "gritty" details of its presentation, rationales, and methods; a timeline; and an initial budget estimation to make sure you are not way off in what you will be able to do within the funding limits put forth by the outside agency or funding outlet (1).

Analogous to an architectural blueprint, the design sheet is an outline of the research project. It allows for quick examination of the project, discussions, and quick changes and recalculations of the scope of the project before any "real work" begins on the writing of the proposal. Regardless of the level of investigator (*i.e.*, student level or professional), the design sheet of the research project should include the question/purpose, hypothesis, all independent and dependent variables, experimental design, and the perceived impact of the study. Additionally, the design sheet will help the investigator plan the statistical analysis by seeing the sample sizes, groups, time points, and measures to be used in the project. This allows one to get a feel for what would be needed statistically to test the experimental hypotheses to be put forth in the proposal. The investigator must keep in mind that the process for developing a successful design sheet is dynamic, with a possibility of many revisions before the final product. That is why it only takes up a page or two as one changes and even uses long hand on the printout to make changes to the project ideas and design. Ultimately, the creation of a design sheet can be difficult for a new investigator, because putting an entire research project into figure form may not be intuitive, but using an "old school" approach you can start with a "paper and pencil" and begin to sketch it out prior to formalizing it. A formal figure can then be developed for presentation to your committee and your lab group for further discussion or as part of a research perspective meeting for a thesis or dissertation (Fig. 13-2).

Design Sheet Variable Considerations

As stated previously, the aim or purpose of a research project is to answer a question that either aims to support or expand the current body of knowledge. In order to do so, you must begin with a question that is central to the research proposal. As the design process matures, the question will be further refined, especially as the investigators immerse themselves in the literature review. A review of primary and secondary sources of approximately 10 years in retrospect from the current date is a good rule of thumb for an investigator who is seeking to expand his or her proposed question. As a student-level investigator, the primary sources of peer-reviewed journal articles will likely provide you the most up-to-date information regarding the challenges in the major field of interest, as you learned about in Chapter 4. Additionally, you might consider using secondary sources such as textbooks or review articles as a basis of foundation for the conceptual theory and scientific base of the research topic. As with any source of information, there can be constraints and limitations to the facts the literature you choose presents; however, it is the responsibility of any investigator to glean the important context of its contents to further develop the question and hypothesis.

Once the question has been established, the next logical step in the development of a design sheet is the statement of the research hypothesis or hypotheses (1). The hypothesis relates to the design sheet as its fundamental cornerstone or foundation of the research proposal. Prior to the development of the research question, you have more than likely already established the hypothesis. To assure a solid hypothesis, it is important to soundly incorporate theoretical facts (from secondary sources) and recent findings (from primary sources) in a logical fashion. As a predictor of a research project's results, the hypothesis eventually becomes a specific declaration of the overall construct of the proposal from which all other design sheet variables are delineated.

The remaining design sheet variables that must be well thought-out include (a) the population in question (*i.e.*, subject sample), (b) identification of treatments (*i.e.*, independent variables), (c) measurements (*i.e.*, dependent variables), (d) experimental design, (e) methodology and procedures, and (f) appropriate statistical analyses. Previous chapters have elaborated on these aspects in further detail; now you must think globally as the final

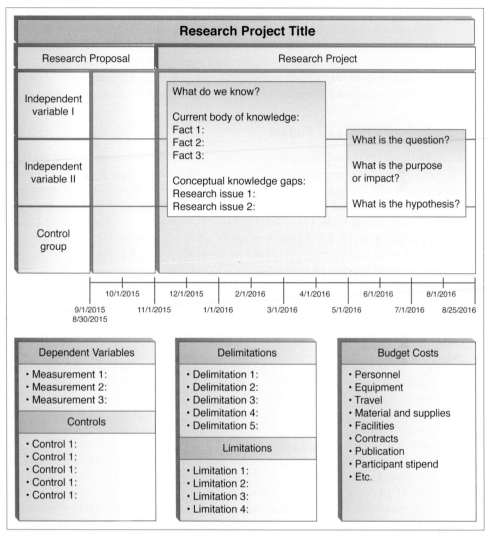

FIGURE 13-2:   Overview of the basic idea of a project from the different perspectives of the investigator. This type of document may act as a blueprint for a grant proposal.

sketch of the design sheet begins to unfold. The first task is to list out all subject groups and levels, the treatments to which each group will be exposed, and the procedural methods to be used to quantify any treatment effect. The final variable connecting all other design sheet variables is time. Once the investigator has considered the timing of the initial research proposal submission, the chronology of all subsequent events on the research timeline (*i.e.*, IRB submission, subject recruitment and testing, organization of data, statistical or biochemical analyses, and manuscript preparation) can be set. Eventually with the question well defined, the hypothesis established, the purpose clearly and concisely stated, the experimental design outlined, and a potential research project timeline drafted, the design sheet nearly develops itself. It is important to keep in mind that the design sheet brings your research proposal to life. This sheet will be how decision-makers (from granting agencies to external funding sources) will visualize and assess your project. Also, this is a useful figure for IRB documents, subject recruitment, and potential manuscripts or presentations, so carefully create your design sheet to be as complete and intuitive as possible.

Research Proposal Budget

The research project design sheet can now be considered a starting point for building the budget for the research proposal. The development of a research proposal budget is intertwined with the research project timeline and the selected methodology needed to achieve the research project outcome (Fig. 13-3). For a professional investigator, the creation of a research project budget for a funding source proposal is a relatively simple task; however, for the student-level investigator, it can be a difficult mission. Hence, the major advisor of the student-level investigator should be integrally involved in the budget proposal process to facilitate learning of basic budgetary terminology and cost categories as they relate to their respective university requirements.

Quite often, the major advisor and the university's Office for Sponsored Programs work in tandem to aid the student-level investigator in understanding the basics of financing a research project (2,7). An investigator needs not be an expert in financial theory to complete a budget, but there are some elemental terms one must have knowledge of, such as **total costs** (TC), **direct costs** (DC), **modified total direct costs** (MTDC), and **facility and administrative** (F&A) **costs** (2). These terms are described in Table 13-1. The research project budget is a detailed, itemized list accounting for every expense required to complete the project. Without serious consideration given to all potential expenses, the inexperienced student-level investigator could easily overestimate or underestimate the cost of the research project (2).

Conveniently, the budgetary terms and definitions from Table 13-1 allow for fitting categorical costs and expenses for the research proposal budget. The breakdown of TC consists of DC with MTDC as a subset of DC and F&A which becomes an itemized list of expenses for the entire research project. The investigator must keep in mind that as the list of itemized expenses is made, it must also be justifiable with regard to the university's or institution's research proposal review process (6,7). Therefore, in planning the budgetary items of the research project, a judicious approach of balancing "wants versus needs" should follow a set of general cost principles: **reasonableness**, **allocability**, **allowability**, and **consistency**. These principles are defined in Table 13-2.

Through an Office of Sponsored Programs, each university has a general format for grouping and categorizing DC, MTDC, and F&A for research proposal budgets (6,7). Table 13-3 is an example of how a university or funding source might define the budget items of DC, MTDC, and F&A. Of course, these budgetary expenses are dependent on the research project timeline, and appropriate adjustments for fiscal or calendar year funding will be crucial in the overall financial management of the project which is the responsibility of the major advisor. One should note in Table 13-3 that items listed under F&A cannot

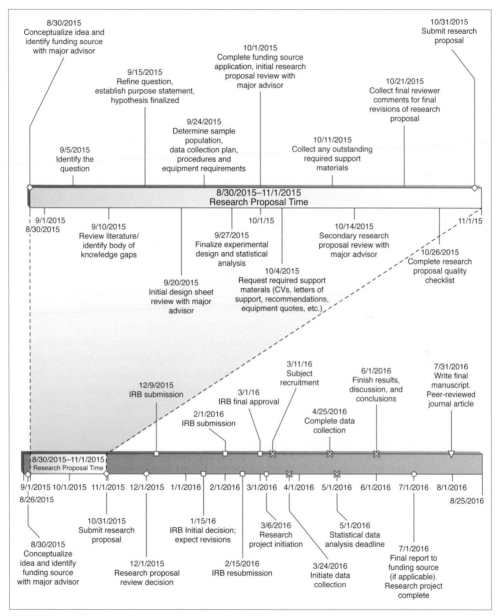

FIGURE 13-3: A sample research project proposal timeline.

Table 13-1 Budgetary Terminology	
Terms	**Definitions**
Total costs (TC)	Total cost of the experimental budget
Direct costs (DC)	Costs that can be identified specifically with conduct of the study related to personnel, supplies, subject stipends, equipment, etc.
Modified total direct costs (MTDC)	Total direct costs minus costs exempted from F&A costs, such as equipment
Facility and administrative (F&A) costs	Synonymous with "indirect or overhead costs"

typically be included in the research project's direct costs because they are deemed "overhead" costs shared university wide.

The final step in the development of a budget for the research proposal should be in review of the expenses (1,2). Thorough and meticulous attention to detail at this juncture is crucial in order to avoid mistakenly forgetting any costs prior to the research proposal submission. A checklist of budget expenses can provide a directed step-by-step analysis of the possible expenses that might be included in the research proposal. Nonetheless, a checklist is only as good as the attention to detail that is given in time toward the review of the budget, so consider the research proposal budget checklist in Table 13-4 as an example that can be modified as necessary for the student-level investigator. Creation of a research proposal budget can be an overwhelming task for student-level investigators, thus requiring guidance from major advisors, university offices, and professional services. The careful preparation of a thorough research budget during the proposal development stage can minimize budget management difficulties later once the research project is funded.

FINDING A REALISTIC FUNDING SOURCE

As the scope of the research project becomes evident in the development of the experimental design, one should start to pay attention to the budget ramifications. To support this developed budget, the investigator must now turn his or her focus toward funding the project. With the scope of the project partially established in the process of designing the experiment, the potential budget needs may well impact the need to "scale back" the project to become more realistic as to the funding level that most advanced graduate

Table 13-2 General Cost Principles	
Terms	**Definitions**
Reasonableness	A cost is considered to be appropriate if the expense and amount reflect sensibleness
Allocability	A cost that is considered beneficial to the research project
Allowability	A cost that is allowed in accordance with general terms and principles of an agreement
Consistency	Reliable, time-after-time treatment of costs incurred for the same purpose under similar conditions

Table 13-3 Total Cost Categorical Expenses

Direct Costs	Facility and Administrative Costs	
Salaries and wages/fringe benefits: Faculty, other professionals, technicians, postdoctoral associates, research associates, and graduate/undergraduate students[a]	**Salaries and wages/fringe benefits:** Clerical and administrative assistants, fiscal manager, secretaries, directors	
Capital equipment: Equipment used for scientific, technical, and research purposes; computers and printers dedicated to a particular project	**Office supplies:** Pens, pencil, paper, staples, ink cartridges, printer paper, word processing and spreadsheet programs	
Travel: Expenses for transportation, lodging, subsistence, and related items incurred by traveling.[a]	**General computer supplies:** Printer paper, word processing and spreadsheet programs	
Other Direct Costs (ODC)	**Materials and supplies:** Medical, scientific pharmaceutical supplies, software/hardware for data collection, and scientific/technical purposes[a]	**Equipment:** General office equipment such as copiers, printers, computers, and fax machines
	Facilities: Project-specific space rental for off-campus facilities from a third party	**Facilities:** Utilities, building use, grounds maintenance, renovations, and alterations
	Publications	**Postage, printing, and photocopying:** U.S. nonpriority or inter-office mail delivery, printing of administrative forms, or photocopying of routine low volume material
	Participant support: Stipends and travel	**Telephone:** Local calls, cell phones, installation, and maintenance
	Professional services[a]	**Maintenance and repairs:** Maintenance and repairs to general purpose equipment, buildings, and grounds
	Advertising: Recruitment of research subjects or for personnel approved for a specific project	**Advertising:** Public relations
	Human subject/animal costs	**Publications:** General
	Freight/delivery costs: Special external courier	**Freight/express deliveries:** Routine internal courier
	Consulting: Project-specific research	**Consulting:** General
	Miscellaneous costs: Subcontract costs, service center charges, and training costs[a]	**Miscellaneous costs:** Dues, memberships, and subscriptions; computer network charges; utilities

[a]**Modified Total Direct Costs (MTDC):** Direct costs to be used in the calculation of F&A.

Table 13-4 Research Proposal Budget Checklist

Direct Costs

Personnel: Salaries and Wages	❑ Principal investigator/project director
	❑ Co-investigators
	❑ Faculty/other senior associates
	❑ Postdoctoral associates
	❑ Other professionals (*e.g.*, technician, programmer)
	❑ Graduate students
	❑ Undergraduate students
Personnel: Fringe Benefits	❑ Faculty/staff fringe benefits rate
	❑ Student fringe benefits rate
Capital Equipment	❑ Any durable equipment that will be expended in short-term use as to items typically costing $5,000 or more
Travel	❑ Personnel
	❑ Conference registration fees
	❑ Transportation (*e.g.*, air, ground, parking)
	❑ Personal vehicle mileage
	❑ Hotel
	❑ Meals
Participant Support	❑ Stipends
	❑ Travel, subsistence
	❑ Advertisement
	❑ Other

Other Direct Costs

Materials/Supplies	❑ Laboratory supplies Animal purchase costs and *per diem* for housing and care
	❑ Instructional supplies
Contractual Services	❑ Consultant services
	❑ Subcontracts
	❑ Lease/rental of equipment
	❑ Service or maintenance contracts
	❑ Professional services, training
	❑ Freight/delivery costs, installation
Publications	❑ Publication/documentation/dissemination

Facility and Administrative Costs

	❑ On-campus
	❑ Off-campus

students are capable of securing in the grant world (*e.g.*, about $10,000). Funding sources might include federal/state/city government funds, private funding agencies, professional organizations, corporations, and/or university scholarships and grants (1). Working with your major advisor and other faculty members on his or her committee is important to help gain perspectives on the project, the experimental design, and potential costs along with where one might secure the necessary funds to conduct the research project.

From a leadership position, the major advisor mentors the senior undergraduate or graduate student in developing the most realistic project that can be completed with the level of funding available for students at their career step. One should always start with a reasonably well-developed and focused research project that requires a smaller level of funding. With experience through subsequent research and collaborations, the maturation process for the junior investigator commences leading into a scientific career after one's doctoral studies. In the field of kinesiology, for example, logical funding sources for undergraduate projects, master's theses, and doctoral dissertations exist within professional organizations such as the American College of Sports Medicine (ACSM) and the National Strength and Conditioning Association (NSCA). On national and regional levels, these professional organizations make grants, endowments, scholarships, and awards available specifically for the student-level investigator.

A student-level investigator and his or her major advisor might fund a thesis/dissertation project from a variety of funding sources. For instance, the major advisor working with departmental accounts might find funds available to support the equipment costs of the research project, as it not only fills an immediate need but can also provide a long-term solution for a laboratory-wide endeavor to use similar scientific instrumentation. Meanwhile, the student-level investigator may complete applications for the ACSM Foundation Doctoral Student Research Grant and NASA Space Physiology Research Grant with the intent of using those funds toward other direct costs (ODCs) such as materials and supplies, recruitment advertisement, and participant support. Final funding for travel, publication expenses, and/or F&A costs may well be provided through university internal funding sources such as faculty or graduate student travel funds and grants. Together, the cumulative funding effort provides scientific data to the expanding body of knowledge, enhances departmental program notoriety and professional growth of the major advisor through mentorship, and provides an unparalleled experience in grantsmanship for the student-level investigator. Refer to Table 13-5 as a sample starting point for the compilation of a research funding source list; one must be mindful of the research proposal scope as it pertains to the size of the project and the selections of appropriate funding sources.

PRINCIPLES OF A SUCCESSFUL FUNDING EFFORT

There exists no single source for locating research funding opportunities; therefore, the responsibility of searching for financial support for a research project rests solely with the investigators. As previously discussed, it is the limited experience of the student investigator that presents the biggest obstacle in development of the research proposal. As more experience is accrued practicing the aforementioned components of research, you will develop the skill and proficiency needed to successfully acquire funds for your research, even as some circumstances dictating funding success may remain completely out of your control.

Table 13-5 Top Funding Sources for Kinesiology

Grants.gov National Research Service Awards	http://www.grants.gov/ http://grants.nih.gov /training/nrsa.htm	Although student grants are not typical for many National Institutes of Health awards, you should be aware that in the United States, federal grants are managed by the Department of Health and Human Services. Grants.gov is an e-government initiative operating under the governance of the Office of Management and Budget with a mission to provide a common website for federal agencies to post discretionary funding opportunities and for grantees to find and apply to them. More appropriate for students, the National Research Service Awards (NRSA) are grants provided by the U.S. National Institutes of Health for doctoral and postdoctoral training investigators in the behavioral sciences and health sciences.
American College of Sports Medicine	http://www.acsm.org/ http://www.acsm .org/find-continuing -education/awards-grants /student-awards	The American College of Sports Medicine (ACSM) invests in the future of sports medicine and exercise science by providing opportunities for students and professionals to apply for grants and awards to offset the rising costs of tuition and travel to support basic and applied science research.
National Strength and Conditioning Association Foundation	http://www.nsca.com /foundation/	The National Strength and Conditioning Association Foundation (NSCAF) mission is to support the NSCA by providing funding for educational and research activities that enhance the practical application of strength and conditioning.
American Physiological Society	http://www.the-aps.org /mm/awards	The American Physiological Society (APS) awards program demonstrates the society's dedication to its members and biomedical research by recognizing the research efforts of outstanding APS members.

A simple internet search using the phrase "successful grant writing tips" would result in a myriad of common sense rules, guidelines, and tips to follow as the investigator makes every effort to guarantee funding for his or her research project. Unfortunately, there is no single recipe, formula, or step-by-step process to guarantee a successful and consistent funding stream. However, it is the major advisor's responsibility to teach the senior undergraduate or graduate student the fundamentals of successful grant writing. Foremost, it is important to seek advice from the university offices (*i.e.*, Office of Sponsored Programs or Research Internal Funding Support) and professional organizations that are responsible for the review and approval of the research proposal. Some of the simplest errors will get the research proposal rejected outright. Not meeting eligibility criteria, missing application deadlines, proposing a project that lacks importance or scientific rationale or does not address the agency's stated priorities, and poor writing are some of the factors that will lead to immediate rejection, resulting in much wasted time and effort.

A strategy to avoid these pitfalls starts with a thorough understanding of the research proposal application process for the university and/or professional organization. Carefully reading the application instructions, eligibility/exclusionary criteria, and deadlines is the first step in submitting a successful proposal. In doing so, the senior undergraduate or

Table 13-6 Research Proposal Preparation Checklist (7)

This proposal checklist will assist you in preparing and double-checking the grant proposal.

To begin the review process:

❏   Internal proposal review form

❏   Budget spreadsheet

❏   Budget justification

❏   Proposal guidelines from sponsoring agency

To complete the review process:

❏   Internal proposal review sheet

❏   Significant financial review form

❏   Proposal cover sheet

❏   Proposal narrative

❏   Electronic application (if required)

❏   Additional items (*e.g.*, bibliography, curriculum vitae, current and pending support, consultant letters)

graduate student can start writing early with the intent of having the major advisor and others review the important documents that comprise the proposal application. By asking questions and seeking reviewer feedback, one can subtly begin the process of networking that can result in research proposal support. As the research proposal progresses through the development process, checklists with interim deadlines should be established to assure timely proposal application submission (an example is provided in Table 13-6). After the final research proposal application is successfully submitted, the major advisor and student-level investigator must wait for a response from the research proposal review board. An understanding of the review process is helpful not only in designing fundable research projects but also in preparing a revised application if the funding agency allows it over different funding cycle deadlines. Table 13-7 lists the components of an effective research proposal.

THE RESEARCH PROPOSAL REVIEW PROCESS

Grant review panels are charged with the difficult task of deciding which research proposals to fund. These panels are typically composed of scientific experts, but in other settings, they may also include relevant decision-makers such as engineers, accountants, lawyers, and executives (1). The importance of review panels in the research funding process warrants discussion on what specific criteria shape their funding decisions.

In order to be objective, grant review panels typically use a scoring sheet. This document allows them to grade each proposal using the same criterion. The NIH scoring

Table 13-7 Top 10 Ingredients for Successful Research Proposals

Research Proposal Ingredient	The Question	Review Criteria	Yes/No
1. The care gap or quality gap	Does the proposal have clear evidence that a gap in quality exists?	Significance Impact	
2. The evidence-based treatment to be implemented	Is the evidence for the program, treatment, or set of services to be implemented demonstrated?	Significance Innovation	
3. Conceptual model and theoretical justification	The proposal delineates a clear conceptual framework/theory/model that informs the design and variables being tested?	Approach Innovation	
4. Stakeholder priorities, engagement in change	Is there a clear engagement process of the stakeholders in place?	Significance Impact Approach Environment	
5. Setting's readiness to adopt new services/treatments/programs	Is there clear information that reflects the setting's readiness, capacity, or appetite for change, specifically around adoption of the proposed evidence-based treatment?	Impact Approach Environment	
6. Implementation strategy/process	Are the strategies to implement the intervention clearly defined and justified conceptually?	Significance Impact Innovation	
7. Team experience with the setting, treatment, and implementation process	Does the proposal detail the team's experience with the study setting, the treatment whose implementation is being studied, and implementation processes?	Approach Investigator team	
8. Feasibility of proposed research design and methods	Does the methods section contain as much detail as possible as well as lay out possible choice junctures and contingencies should methods not work as planned?	Approach Investigator team	
9. Measurement and analysis section	Does the proposal clarify the key constructs to be measured, corresponding to the overarching conceptual model or theory? Is a measurement plan clear for each construct? Does the analysis section demonstrate how relationships between constructs will be tested?	Approach Investigator team	
10. Policy/funding environment; leverage or support for sustaining change	Does the proposal address how the implementation initiative aligns with policy trends?	Impact Significance	

Adapted from Proctor EK, Powell BJ, Baumann AA, Hamilton AM, Santens RL. Writing implementation research grant proposals: ten key ingredients. *Implementation Science* [Internet]. 2012 [cited 2013 Oct 1];7(96). Available from: http://www.implementationscience.com/content/7/1/96. doi:10.1186/1748-5908-7-96.

system is commonly used, but other institutions readily create scoring systems to suit their needs (4). As you design your experiment and write your proposal, you should begin to determine potential funding sources and, during this process, obtain the sources' scoring sheets so each criterion can be addressed as you prepare your application. These sheets are often posted publicly on websites, and they can often be obtained without incident from the funding source itself.

A student can take a lesson in what a grant panel looks at by understanding the current NIH review criteria which are noted in the following text (4). It is important to note that although each review category contributes to the "overall impact" score, individual category scores are not necessarily summed or averaged to produce this score; rather, category scores serve as areas of consideration that are used to form a subjective judgment of overall merit. Once each review panel members submits his or her assessment, each overall impact score is averaged to provide an overall impact score.

- Overall impact. Reviewers will provide an overall impact/priority score to reflect their assessment of the likelihood for the project to exert a sustained, powerful influence on the research field(s) involved, with reference to the following review criteria, and any additional review criteria specific to the project proposed.
    - Scored review criteria. Reviewers will consider each of the review criteria in the following text in the determination of scientific and technical merit and give a separate score for each. An application does not need to be strong in all categories to be judged likely to have major scientific impact (*e.g.*, a project that by its nature is not technologically innovative but may be essential to advance a field).
    - Significance. Does the project address an important problem or a critical barrier to progress in the field? If the aims of the project are achieved, how will scientific knowledge, technical capability, or clinical practice improve? How will successful completion of the aims change the concepts, methods, technologies, treatments, services, or preventative interventions that drive this field?
    - Investigator(s). Are the principal investigators, collaborators, and other investigators well suited to the project? If early-stage investigators or new investigators in the early stages of independent careers, do they have appropriate experience and training? If established, have they demonstrated an ongoing record of accomplishments that have advanced their field(s)? If the project is collaborative, do the investigators have complementary and integrated expertise; are the leadership approach, governance, and organizational structure appropriate for the project?
    - Innovation. Does the application challenge and seek to shift current research or clinical practice paradigms by using novel theoretical concepts, approaches or methodologies, instrumentation, or interventions? Are the concepts, approaches or methodologies, instrumentation, or interventions novel to one field of research or novel in a broad sense? Is a refinement, improvement, or new application of theoretical concepts, approaches or methodologies, instrumentation, or interventions proposed?
    - Approach. Are the overall strategy, methodology, and analyses well-reasoned and appropriate to accomplish the specific aims of the project? Are potential problems, alternative strategies, and benchmarks for success presented? If the project is in the early stages of development, will the strategy establish feasibility and will particularly

risky aspects be managed? If the project involves clinical research, are the plans for (a) protection of human subjects from research risks and (b) inclusion of minorities and members of both sexes/genders, as well as the inclusion of children, justified in terms of the scientific goals and research strategy proposed? If the project involves vertebrate animal research, are the procedures for minimizing pain and distress and criteria for removal from study well specified?

- Environment. Will the scientific environment in which the work will be done contribute to the probability of success? Are the institutional support, equipment, and other physical resources available to the investigators adequate for the project proposed? Will the project benefit from unique features of the scientific environment, subject populations, or collaborative arrangements?

- Additional review criteria. As applicable for the project proposed, reviewers will evaluate the following additional items while determining scientific and technical merit and in providing an overall impact/priority score but will not give separate scores for these items.
  - Protections for human subjects
  - Inclusion of women, minorities, and children
  - Vertebrate animals
  - Biohazards
  - Eligibility for resubmission responsive to reviewer comments
  - Renewal
  - Revision

When you obtain a scoring sheet, you should use it to assess how well your proposal complies with the review criteria. Also, it makes sense to provide this document to your advisor and other reviewers in order to help them provide better consultation. Each grant source will have its own scoring system. In addition, review panels may consider risks and benefits to human and animal subjects and budgetary or period components. These additional items may or may not be individually scored but can be used to help determine the overall impact score.

Why Good Proposals May Often Be Rejected

As discussed earlier, there are a number of common mistakes that lead to the rejection of research proposals. In addition to proposing an impactful and achievable project, it is equally important to follow administrative guidelines, including page limits, font, reference formats, and other instructions. Administrative guidelines may be provided on the application itself or in supplementary materials provided by the funding agency, which are often supplied and explained in further detail on the agency's website.

A good grant "tells a story."

- What is the problem to be solved?
- What is wrong with current approaches?
- Why is your idea *new*?
- What is your technical approach to this idea?
- Why are you (or your team) the one(s) to do it?
- How are you going to show that it works?

SUMMARY

As you will find out, conducting research is more complex than the conception of an idea and a completion of a project. In most instances, the research performed by student investigators must be paid for by a variety of sources. Practical factors such as time, research topic, money, and capability can dictate the project you can complete. Choosing an appropriate funding source to devote time and resources toward applying for external funding is an important decision in the quest to fund your research. Equally important is the development of a clear and complete study design that you communicate to the grant review panel in the form of a research proposal. An important question, a well-formulated design sheet, a practical timeline, and a reasonable budget are all integral parts to increasing your chances to secure funds for your project. Close collaboration with your advisor or advisory committee while understanding what your role is in this process are both important considerations in submitting research proposals. Knowing what the decision-makers are looking for (impact, novelty, cost, etc.) and carefully following submission guidelines can help but cannot guarantee your proposal's acceptance, as the final result is in the hands of the grant review panel.

GLOSSARY

Allocability: a cost that is considered beneficial to the research project

Allowability: a cost that is allowed in accordance with general terms and principles of an agreement

Consistency: reliable, time-after-time treatment of costs incurred for the same purpose under similar conditions

Direct costs: costs that can be identified specifically with a particular sponsored project, an instructional activity, or any other institutional activity or that can be directly assigned to such activities relatively easily with a high degree of accuracy

Facility and administrative costs: costs that are incurred for common or joint objectives and therefore cannot be identified readily and specifically with a particular sponsored project, an instructional activity, or any other institutional activity; synonymous with "indirect or overhead costs"

Modified total direct costs: subset of the direct costs per the university's rate agreement; commonly reflects the total direct cost minus the costs that must be excluded from the facility and administrative costs

Reasonableness: a cost considered to be reasonable if the expense and amount reflect sensibleness

Total costs: cost composed of the allowable direct costs plus the allocable portion of the allowable facilities and administrative costs

REFERENCES

1. Baumgartner T, Hensley L. *Conducting & Reading Research in Kinesiology*. 5th ed. New York (NY): McGraw-Hill; 2012.
2. Higdon J, Topp R. How to develop a budget for a research proposal. *West J Nurs Res*. 2004;26(8):922–929.

3. National Institutes of Health Web site [Internet]. Estimates of Funding for Various Research, Condition, and Disease Categories (RCDC). Bethesda (MD): National Institutes of Health; [cited 2013 Nov 23]. Available from: http://report.nih.gov /categorical_spending.aspx

4. National Institutes of Health Web site [Internet]. Peer review process. Bethesda (MD): National Institutes of Health; [cited 2013 Nov 23]. Available from: http://grants.nih.gov/grants/peer_review_process.htm#Criteria

5. Proctor EK, Powell BJ, Baumann AA, Hamilton AM, Santens RL. Writing implementation research grant proposals: ten key ingredients. *Implementation Science* [Internet]. 2012 [cited 2013 Oct 1];7(96). Available from: http://www .implementationscience.com/content/7/1/96. doi:10.1186/1748-5908-7-96.

6. Texas State University Web site [Internet]. Training Guide: Preparing Research Proposal Budgets. San Marcos (TX): Texas State University; [cited 2013 Oct 1]. Available from: http://www.txstate.edu/research/osp/budget-development/contentParagraph/00 /content_files/file1/Website%20Budget%20Training%20Guide.pdf

7. University of Connecticut Web site [Internet]. Sponsored Program Services: Proposals. Storrs (CT): University of Connecticut; [cited 2013 Oct 1]. Available from: http://research.uconn.edu/sps-proposals/

CHAPTER 14

Conducting a Study: Pilot Testing, Sampling, and Data Collection

Jill M. Slade, PhD

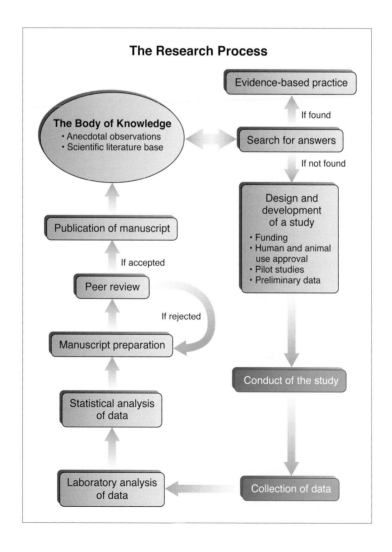

The Research Process

Evidence-based practice

If found

The Body of Knowledge
· Anecdotal observations
· Scientific literature base

Search for answers

If not found

Design and development of a study
· Funding
· Human and animal use approval
· Pilot studies
· Preliminary data

Publication of manuscript

If accepted

Peer review

If rejected

Manuscript preparation

Statistical analysis of data

Conduct of the study

Laboratory analysis of data

Collection of data

INTRODUCTION: STUDY SAMPLE

Once you have designed a sound, ethical study and procured adequate funding, it is time to begin executing your investigation. An important aspect of conducting a study is determining the study sample. In other words, what are the characteristics of the participants to be recruited for the study? Generally, it is not feasible to study the entire population; therefore, a representative subset is "sampled." A sample is a portion of the population that best represents the population on the key variables you learned about in Chapters 7 and 8. From the data collected on a sample, inferences are then made about the population the sample represents. Defining criteria or key variables or "inclusion and exclusion criteria" that describe the population is essential. As you've learned, key variables can include gender, age, health, and body size. In exercise science, health is often a key variable, and the study may require or exclude a number of factors such as cardiovascular disease, metabolic disease, or neurologic disease, among others.

For example, an investigator may be interested in the effects of a walking intervention on blood pressure. The researcher will need to decide if specific key variables can influence the main outcome variable. For example, blood pressure increases with age, is often higher in males, and is increased with the presence of a number of health conditions. Determining key variables that are related to the study outcome is important to increase the homogeneity of the sample. When the variability of the sample is high on a number of factors known to influence the dependent variable, a greater sample size will be required in the study.

SAMPLE SIZE

The size of the **representative sample** or "sample size" should be estimated before a study begins. A study that requires a large sample may require too much time and may be too costly to conduct. On the other extreme, if the study is conducted with too small a sample size, the researcher may not have enough data to accurately test the hypothesis. There is also an ethical reason to consider and plan for an appropriate sample size. A study with too few subjects may expose humans (or animals) to unnecessary risk without advancing knowledge. Likewise, a study with too many subjects will expose more individuals to potential study risks, and in some cases, it could prevent the subjects in a patient population from seeking other alternative treatment. There is a need for a power analysis that allows one to know that the statistical testing performed may have an adequate opportunity to correctly reject the null hypothesis when it is in fact false and therefore accepting the alternative hypothesis that differences do exist.

The sample size is based on the outcomes expected or best predicted outcomes given the available data. The expected outcomes may be based on data from a small number of subjects called a **pilot study**. Alternatively, the expected outcomes can be based on published data from the researcher's lab or published data from other laboratories. Be aware that using other laboratory values could be problematic if there are notable differences in the methods, instruments, or study sample characteristics. The minimum information required for estimating sample size is a measure or estimate of the variability of the main outcome measure. The confidence interval or the standard deviation of the measure may be used in the sample size estimation. A variety of web resources provide software to help calculate an estimated sample size (1,3). In addition, statistical software and graphing software may include a sample size calculator, for example, SigmaPlot.

In robust approaches for calculating sample size, additional information is required related to the study design (4,5). The additional information in "the **power approach**" includes the **effect size**, the **alpha level**, and the **study power**. The effect size is the expected difference between the null hypothesis and the alternative hypothesis. The effect size may be the expected increase following an intervention or the expected differences between groups. For example, a researcher may expect a 10% increase in leg blood flow after an exercise intervention. It is imperative that the effect size be scientifically meaningful or clinically relevant. A study could be powered to statistically reject the null hypothesis but have little application if the group differences or outcomes are not meaningful in the field. For example, a study on the effect of a new training style in elite athletes on 100-m sprint times may use an effect size of 0.1 s; this effect size can be the difference between a gold and silver medal. Using this same effect, size in a sample of sedentary adults would not have the same meaning. (See in-depth coverage of effect size in Chapter 18, p. 331.)

Alpha is the probability of rejecting the null hypothesis when the null hypothesis is true (*i.e.*, no difference between the means). Typically, alpha is set below .05. More liberal alpha levels (greater than $P > .05$) will increase the possibility of a false-positive outcome also called a "type I error." Power is the probability that the selected research method is able to detect a significant difference when a real difference exists. In other words, power is the probability of correctly rejecting the null hypothesis when the alternative hypothesis is true. Power is typically estimated at or above 0.80 (on a scale of 0–1); when power is set at 0.80, if there is an effect present, it will be detected 80% of the time. If the study power is low, sometimes called an "underpowered study," the risk of incorrectly accepting the null hypothesis is increased, leading to a type II error or a false-negative outcome. An investigator would conclude that a treatment had no effect when in fact there is a real difference. Or, he or she may conclude that there is no difference on the dependent variable between two groups when there are differences. It is generally recommended to use the highest variance associated with the measure in order to prevent a study from being underpowered.

STUDY SAMPLING

The random selection of subjects comprising the sample, called "random sampling," should have been addressed in the research design, which you've read about in earlier chapters. After the inclusion and exclusion criteria of the sample have been established, the researcher needs to consider how the sample will be selected or recruited. A random selection is used to ensure that the sample is representative of the population and to eliminate bias in selecting subjects. Improper sampling techniques may lead to results that do not represent the population. The results may then be confined to a narrowly defined portion of the originally intended population. Techniques for randomization were discussed in Chapter 8.

Sampling approaches fall into two main categories: probability and nonprobability sampling. In an ideal situation, probability sampling would be used in selecting subjects. **Probability sampling** allows the potential for all possible subjects in the population to have a random and equal chance of being selected for a study. There are three main categories of probability sampling. In simple random sampling, each person has the same chance of being selected and is not influenced by the selection of other individuals. A random numbers table is most commonly used to select the sample. Each potential subject in the population is assigned a number and then a random numbers table is used to determine which subjects will be selected for the sample. A variety of random numbers tables are available on statistical and graphing software as well as on the web. The table can comprise columns of single digits or columns with many digits, depending on the size of the population. Random numbers tables can also be generated to produce a list of n random numbers—n being the number of samples (Table 14-1). For example, a researcher may be interested in the physical activity time of children in Michigan sixth grades during school hours. There are 400 middle schools, and the researcher would like to sample 50 schools. After assigning each school a number based on the name of the school, the researcher uses a random numbers table like the one shown in Table 14-1.

The systemic sampling approach selects subjects based on a pre-determined manner; for example, every third person to respond to a recruitment letter will be enrolled in the study. In the above example, the researcher may send out surveys to each of the 400 middle schools and choose to sample every third response until they reach the target number of 50. In this approach, additional work is required because the researcher must contact all 400 schools compared to the example with simple random sampling in which the researcher contacts 50 schools. Stratified random sampling creates target subcategories within the recruitment sample. In the Michigan school example, the size of the school may be a subcategory. Other examples of subcategories in research include samples recruited to fulfill groups of age ranges or ethnicities, among others.

Table 14-1 Sample Random Numbers Table

98	26	20	249	193
3	13	102	116	16
154	186	120	126	263
26	355	179	297	141
263	136	333	84	30
363	86	165	202	152
143	108	220	260	51
335	175	208	382	199
109	18	95	34	88
98	203	287	13	352

Fifty random numbers generated from a population of 400 numbers.

Nonprobability sampling is a sampling approach that does not allow for equal probability of participants being selected. Most studies in the field of exercise physiology use nonprobability sampling. The primary reason for this is that human subject research studies require voluntary participation (7). This requires individuals to freely choose to be involved in a study. Individuals who choose to volunteer may be different on a variety of traits compared to individuals who do not volunteer. Researchers may also not have the resources to use probability sampling and may rely on local residents to volunteer for the research. This is true of most laboratory-based studies that require subjects to come into the laboratory for study measurements. However, some qualitative features of probability sampling can be used when selecting participants. For example, unbiased recruiting approaches can be used. Consider a researcher who is interested in studying the effects of interval training on cognitive function in young adults. The researcher may consider posting recruitment advertisements in common areas such as a community center, dining hall, or in a large lecture hall to obtain a sample. In comparison, researchers may choose to only recruit participants from an honors college course. These two recruitment approaches may yield different results because the participants in the latter case may not be representative of the greater population.

Although not generally recommended, researchers may use a sample of convenience. The convenience sample may consist of classmates, friends, or colleagues. Although this approach is often used to reduce the time burden of recruitment, the risk of bias is high, and careful thought should be given to factors that could cause bias or limit the generalizability of the study results. In addition, the ethical impact of convenience samples should be considered. Classmates or friends may feel coerced into participating. In addition, guidelines from the Belmont Report require "fair procedures" to be followed in subject selection (6). Using fair procedures for participant selection includes making the research available for all people who meet the study inclusion criteria such that the benefits and burdens of research are available to all who are interested. Care should be given to balance the feasibility of subject recruitment with ethical issues relating to human subjects research.

Although there are elements of sample selection that may not strictly follow random sampling, the random assignment of participants to different groups within the study is imperative. Each person should have the same chance of being selected for each group, condition, or order of treatments (see Chapter 8). A random numbers table may be appropriate for random assignment or a list of randomized treatments. Random selection can be difficult to implement in research if one group stands to receive a benefit from the research more than another group. For example, exercise intervention studies where one group will be randomly selected to serve as a control or placebo group or a medication study where some individuals receive a placebo treatment. Clear communication is needed for potential subjects to understand the importance of random selection for the research outcomes. In some scenarios, it may be possible to offer other interventions to subjects after completion of a placebo or control group. Alternatively, one may consider an attention control group. For example, the research study includes an intervention of walking for 12 weeks. The control group may be offered a series of seminars or workshops over the 12-week control period. Although this may create additional tasks for the researcher, it may result in fewer dropouts in the control group. In some studies, investigators may also consider using an active control arm in which a well-accepted technique intervention, drug, or test is compared to a novel technique. This research is classified as a **comparative effectiveness trial** (2). The objective of a comparative effectiveness trial can be to determine if a new technique is better, equivalent, or non-inferior depending on the research goals. Trials of equivalence and non-inferiority are justified, as they may reveal a technique that is less expensive, safer, easier to administer, and/or has better reliability. These trials are often performed in clinical trial research but may be used in exercise physiology and related fields.

PILOT TESTING

Pilot testing is performed before the start of the study. Pilot testing involves executing study protocols, collecting data, and analyzing data. It is performed to improve the quality and efficiency of the research study, and it is critical because it may reveal a weak point of the study that could cause the study to fail or otherwise considerably affect the research. Pilot testing can also be used to examine feasibility and timing of the protocols. Its purposes include allowing familiarization or practice for lab personnel and attaining measurement variability. Pilot studies can also reveal whether the length of an intervention or treatment is adequate.

Pilot testing offers an opportunity for all lab personnel to practice data collection protocols. This is important because it can both decrease variance due to measurement error and also provide a positive experience for research volunteers. Volunteer participant comfort and trust will improve if lab personnel are organized and confident with study procedures, the operation of equipment, and lab objectives. Pilot testing can be used to generate written testing protocols or scripts. Detailed protocols will help assure that all lab personnel perform testing in the same way and also can serve as a reminder to lab personnel about subtle but important details that might otherwise be overlooked.

Conducting pilot testing may reveal details that are missing in the protocol as well as details that are not necessary. Even tasks that seem simple, such as taking a participant's height and weight, need practice both to minimize measurement error and to allow the lab personnel to become familiar with the location of equipment and the function of equipment. Lab personnel can also become comfortable with the instructions given to research subjects. Pilot testing can help the researcher evaluate the detailed instructions that are given to research participants. Instructions given to participants should be concise, and time should be given to allow the participant to ask questions. The pilot test may also help determine how long the protocol will take to execute. This includes time to explain testing procedures, time to prepare participants (*e.g.*, any special positioning), as well as how long the procedures themselves will take. Additionally, pilot testing may be conducted to determine the validity and reliability of a research tool or test (see Chapter 10).

A pilot test can also be used to assess the variability of a measurement. The variability of the measure includes the range, the variance, and the standard deviation. The range of the measurement can infer information about the sensitivity of the measurement or test. Pilot testing may allow the researcher to examine floor or ceiling effects; these effects limit the measurement range. A selected instrument or test may not be able to measure extremely low values, which represents a floor effect, or it may not be sensitive to high values, which is called a "ceiling effect." This will result in a skewed distribution of the results; a test that is very easy may be negatively skewed, or a test that is extremely difficult may be positively skewed. As discussed earlier in the chapter, the variability assessed during pilot testing can also be used in part to estimate sample size.

Pilot testing can reduce time and costs associated with research. In particular, if the results from a pilot study show that a planned intervention is not feasible, the study can be redesigned to address problem areas. For example, suppose a researcher wanted to study the influence of increasing ingested antioxidants on vascular function during exercise. The researcher planned to have participants consume 1.5 lb or 3–4 c of blueberries daily for four weeks. After pilot testing, it becomes clear that it is difficult to eat that volume of whole blueberries. In place of the whole blueberries, subjects could alternately consume 2.5 c of blueberry juice and gain the same amount of antioxidants.

Additionally, pilot testing can reveal how much familiarization of the study protocol is necessary for research participants. Familiarization can take place within a single testing session or may be done over several days depending on the experimental requirements. Testing may yield different results if there is a learning effect for the independent variable. In many cases, researchers will want to reduce subject variability by eliminating the effect of practice. This is often best done by allowing research participants to practice a number of trials prior to the actual test. For example, a researcher is interested in examining sex differences in blood flow during low-force contractions done at 10% of maximal voluntary contraction (MVC). The ability of research participants to exactly reach 10% MVC may take practice. The first few times, the participant may give an effort that results in 20%–30% MVC. This is more than twice the expected target level, and in the case of blood flow, it could be the difference in occluding an artery or not. In addition, pilot testing may also show that participants have a hard time maintaining the expected force over time. Is it because the protocol is inducing muscle fatigue, or is it because the subjects do not have enough feedback during the task? All of these details could be controlled and improved upon during pilot testing.

Although it is less common, it is also a possibility that a researcher is interested in initial performance on the selected independent variable prior to improvement that occurs during learning. In this case, pilot testing is extremely important in order to determine if the instructions for the participant are perfectly clear. Otherwise, some participants could benefit from more practice, which could lead to diminished treatment effects. For example, some cognitive tests such as the Stroop test are associated with a large learning effect. The more the person performs the test, the faster and more accurate the performance. In another example, the researcher may be interested in the effects of novel exercise on muscle function. In these research examples, the familiarization may eliminate the effect the researcher is studying. The timing of the outcome measures may also be important. Acute interventions or treatments may have a window of time in which they are effective. For example, acute exercise may increase cognitive function immediately after an exercise bout, but the effect may not persist longer than five minutes.

The results obtained during the pilot testing can be used to prepare data entry and analysis documents. This allows the researcher to determine how the research data will be transferred, saved, and imported and how computations and analyses will be performed on the data (see Chapter 16). Having a data management plan will help with the organization of the study data (see Chapter 17).

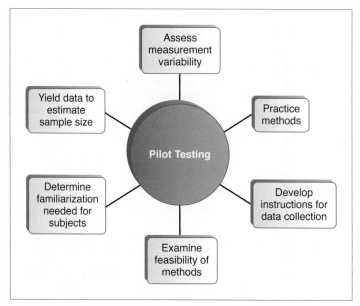

FIGURE 14-1:   Pilot testing may result in a number of outcomes to consider when executing the study itself.

DATA COLLECTION

After completing pilot testing (Fig. 14-1), the data collection period can begin. It is important to plan a timetable for data collection. This will include time to recruit, screen, and schedule research participants. In addition, details related to equipment availability and building access need to be verified. Important details to convey to participants include directions, parking, and laboratory location. If your research participant arrives 20 minutes late because she had the wrong address and when she finally arrived, the building staff did not know how to find you, the subject's disposition could be negatively affected. This may influence the participant's effort, concentration, and performance during data collection. In addition, clear instructions should be given to the participants if the study conditions include details related to recent behavior, such as food and drink intake, medication use, and physical activity. Participants should receive written reminders via text messages or e-mail if these details are important, and adherence should be evaluated by specifically asking the participant about behaviors before data collection begins.

Voluntary informed consent must always precede data collection. Typically, the investigator will overview the study and its procedures, risks, and benefits orally and make sure the content of the informed consent document is clear and the ability to ask questions after reading the consent form is also clear along with their ability to stop participation in the study at any time without prejudice. Oral briefing of subject groups and for each subject individually helps, as sometimes, the potential participant will not read the informed consent document. Additionally, prior to beginning data collection, the condition of the participant should be noted. A designated form or checklist may be helpful. These questions regarding the condition of the patient could include elements related to dietary intake, physical activity, and medication use. For example, a researcher may be interested in the effects of two weeks of interval training on blood pressure and vascular function. The researcher may choose to require that the subject abstain from vigorous exercise and alcohol intake. The researcher may request that participants avoid aspirin, caffeine, and a high-fat meal prior to testing. Standardized protocols should be performed that are consistent across repeated measures and subjects. Even when saving electronic files, a standard routine should be used; this will help keep data organized.

It is important to consider the influence of external factors on the dependent variable. Common external factors include the time of day (diurnal effects), the season of the year, and the phase of the menstrual cycle, among others. The researcher can reduce error variance by considering the influence of external factors and addressing them by including the factors in the study design, for example, completing the testing for each subject at the same time of the day. These factors are easy to address but can create difficulties in planning. Another area to consider is the influence of recent dietary intake, including hydration status, alcohol intake, and meal composition. For example, a researcher is interested in studying the effects of prolonged running on central motor drive. Carbohydrate loading and supplement intake before or during the run may influence the main study outcome. Medication and supplement intake may be important to consider. In some cases, control of a known influential variable can be accounted for in the statistical analyses; for example, an analysis of covariance can be used if the groups differed on an external variable such as body size. It is recommended to consult the literature for information on factors related to outcome measures in your research.

Another important element to consider and for which to plan accordingly is whether participants will be likely to drop out of the study. This is imperative to consider in intervention studies and may be necessary to plan for in short experimental studies, in particular, if a method is associated with any physical or psychologic discomfort. Consult the literature for studies using comparable experiments or interventions for an idea of the expected number of dropouts. If subjects are anticipated to drop out, be sure to include this in the target sample size; the sample size for each group will have to be increased. There are a number of reasons participants may drop out of the study including some reasons related to the study and some reasons unrelated to the study. The person may have an adverse event, for example, a reaction caused by a medication or supplement or an injury during an exercise intervention. The event may be expected (anticipated) or unexpected (unanticipated); expected adverse events may be related to subject dropout and provide direct insight into the dropout number. The person may not feel comfortable with a repeated testing procedure. For example, if testing includes resting metabolic rate or magnetic resonance imaging (MRI) of the head, which both require the subject's head to be enclosed in a small space, the participant may feel too claustrophobic to continue the study. A study participant may also violate specific study guidelines. For example, a researcher is interested in examining the effect of an exercise intervention on lung function. A participant decides to start smoking during the intervention, which was an exclusionary criterion set before starting the study. The participant may also have a change in health, availability, transportation, or motivation. When an individual drops out of the study, note should be taken both for personal records and for reporting to the institutional review board.

Lastly, it is imperative to keep the methods constant for all aspects of the data collection. Any necessary protocol changes should be implemented during pilot testing prior to data collection. Changing approaches or techniques part of the way through a study can introduce bias and certainly will increase the heterogeneity of the dependent variable.

GLOSSARY

Alpha level: the probability of rejecting the null hypothesis when the null is true

Comparative effectiveness trial: a research that compares a new approach/treatment/product to an established approach/treatment/product

Effect size: the expected difference between the null hypothesis and the alternative hypothesis

Nonprobability sampling: a sampling approach that does not allow for equal probability of participants being selected

Pilot study: a small-scale study done to examine study feasibility and methods to improve the quality and efficiency of the research study; may also yield preliminary data

Pilot testing: a small pilot study is conducted before committing to a large-scale investigation. A pilot study costs little and allows evaluation of the experimental design/procedures, instruments, and statistical analyses

Power approach: a statistical method used to estimate expected study sample size that includes the effect size, alpha level, and study power

Probability sampling: a sampling approach that allows the potential for all possible subjects in the population to have a random and equal chance of being selected for a study

Representative sample: a sample of the population that best represents key variables relevant to the research question

Study power: the probability of a statistical test to correctly reject the null hypothesis

REFERENCES

1. Dupont WD, Plummer WD. PS: Power and Sample Size Calculation [computer software]. Nashville (TN): Vanderbilt University Department of Biostatistics; [cited 2013 Sept 24]. Available from: http://biostat.mc.vanderbilt.edu/wiki/Main/PowerSampleSize
2. Grady D, Cummings SR, Hulley SB. Alternative clinical trial designs and implementations issues. In: Hulley SB, Cummings SR, Browner WS, Grady DG, Newman TB, editors. *Designing Clinical Research*. Philadelphia: Lippincott Williams & Wilkins; 2013. p. 151–170.
3. Lenth RV. Java Applets for Power and Sample Size [computer software]. Iowa City (IA): The University of Iowa; [cited 2013 Sept 17]. Available from: http://www.stat.uiowa.edu/~rlenth/Power
4. Lenth RV. Some practical guidelines for effective sample size determination. *Am Stat*. 2001;55:187–193.
5. Lenth RV. Statistical power calculations. *J Anim Sci*. 2007;85:E24–E29.
6. Protection of human subjects; Belmont Report: notice of report for public comment. *Fed Regist*. 1979;44(76):23191–23197.
7. *Trials of War Criminals Before the Nuremberg Military Tribunals Under Control Council Law No. 10*. Washington, DC: U.S. Government Printing Office; 1949.

CHAPTER 15

Instrumentation: Calibration and Standardization

Robert Newton, PhD, FESSA, FNSCA

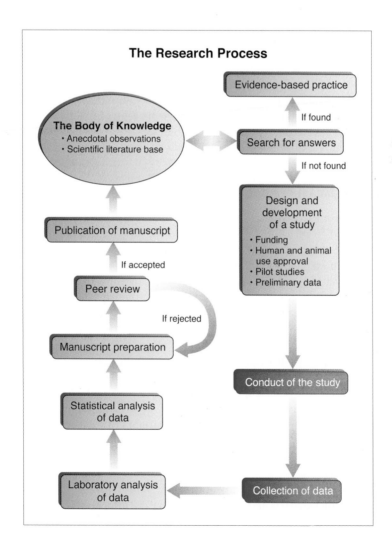

INTRODUCTION: MEASURING PHENOMENA

To pursue research in any discipline of science, a phenomenon must be observed or measured in some way if it is to be described or if changes are to be quantified over time. **Measurement** is a systematic and replicable process by which physical and nonphysical phenomena are quantified. This is usually achieved with the assignment of numerical values. For example, to perform a vertical jump, the human must exert forces onto the ground, and it is these forces which determine all characteristics of the subsequent jump—such characteristics as takeoff velocity and height. To understand how the jump is produced, we have to have some way of measuring these forces and recording them continuously over the duration of the jump. If we then wish to quantify the effects of fatigue or of some training intervention, then we need to be able to measure these forces during the jump but with an intervening period between measurements. This period could be as short as a few minutes or as long as several months or even years. If we are to observe the phenomenon accurately, then what we measure and record must be representative of the phenomenon—physiologic, biomechanical, chemical, etc.—that we are wishing to understand. In our vertical jumping example, the measurements that we are recording must reflect the characteristics of the physical phenomenon that is the force being applied to the ground. To observe and compare the characteristics of force during vertical jumps performed at different times, the measurements must faithfully reproduce the same values for a given force applied. Just as your research design must be valid and reliable (see Chapter 10), so must the measurements you take.

Validity of Measurement

Validity of a measurement is the degree of success in describing or quantifying what it is designed to measure (5). In other words, how faithfully does the measurement represent the true nature of the phenomenon being examined? For many decades, researchers in exercise science measured body composition using underwater weighing, which involved submerging the subject in water (adding known weight if needed) and measuring their weight force (7). Equations were then applied to estimate residual lung volume because this would greatly affect buoyancy. Underwater weighing is no longer used because the validity of measurement was poor due to errors in predicting air volume in the lungs, totally ignoring air in other body cavities, variance in bone density, and the fact that it was fairly unpleasant for the subject. There were also validity problems because prediction equations had to be applied to convert body density into estimates of fat and muscle mass, and these equations had limitations (1). As you can see, for a whole range of reasons, the validity of the measurement was compromised, and the test did not faithfully measure the variable of interest—body fat percentage. More modern methods include dual-energy x-ray absorptiometry (DEXA), which uses low-dose x-ray to image areas of fat and muscle, is a more direct method, and has greater validity.

Validity of a test or measurement is highly important if you are to describe the phenomenon correctly, so it is necessary to pay special attention to this aspect. Validity is usually verified by comparison to some "gold standard." In the example earlier, DEXA is sometimes compared to cadaver analysis, in which the dead human body is scanned by DEXA and then dissected and chemically analyzed into fat, muscle, and bone components.

Reliability of Measurement

Reliability is the degree to which a measurement technique or system can produce consistent results each time it is used (5). This is often determined by taking repeated measures of the same parameter over time. For example, to determine the reliability of a set of weighing scales, a series of weights would be measured and recorded. The process would be repeated later in the day and the two sets of results compared. This provides a measure of the intra-day reliability. However, this does not assess the variation of measurement of the device over longer periods of time, so the process can be repeated with one or more days intervening and the results compared again. This gives an indication of the inter-day reliability of the measurement system. Reliability is evaluated using a number of statistical methods. Two of the most common are the **intraclass correlation coefficient** (ICC) and the **coefficient of variation** (CV).

Intraclass Correlation Coefficient

ICC is actually a modification of the interclass correlation (**Pearson correlation**) with which most people are more familiar. ICC is calculated slightly differently to take account of the fact that it is a measure of reproducibility of measuring the same quantity (8). Calculation of the ICC is beyond the scope of this chapter, but it is included in any statistics package.

Coefficient of Variation

The CV is often calculated as a quality control indicator of a particular measurement. This is an easy measurement to calculate. It is the standard deviation of the measurements expressed as a percentage of the mean. It tells the reader when the same quantity is repeatedly measured how much this measurement varies around the mean (9).

Technical Error of Measurement

All instruments and measurement systems have inherent imprecisions, and when human action is involved in taking the measurement (*e.g.*, skinfolds), additional inconsistencies are introduced; this means that measurements are never totally free of error. Technical error of measurement is the variability encountered when the same phenomenon or quantity is measured multiple times. The **technical error of measurement** (TEM) is a random error distributed normally around the true value (10). Quality measurement techniques, procedures, and systems aim to minimize TEM so that this error does not influence the results or study outcomes. If the TEM is greater than the change in the underlying phenomena you are trying to measure, then the outcome of interest will be lost in the noise. As an example, the TEM of modern DEXA machines for measuring bone density is 1%–2% and so it is not possible to detect changes in bone over short periods of time. TEM can be quantified by taking repeated measurements of the same object or phenomenon with a greater number of repeated measures, providing a better assessment of the variability. TEM can be expressed as an absolute measure, for instance, fat mass in grams or as a percentage of the mean.

Minimal Detectable Change

Minimal detectable change (MDC) is the smallest amount of change beyond TEM that is a true change between two time points (2). This is usually applied to a noticeable change in the physical ability of a participant or some change in the status of a patient. In the example earlier for the DEXA measurement of bone density, the MDC would be $\pm$ 2%.

Minimal Worthwhile Effect

Minimal worthwhile effect (MWE) is also termed "smallest worthwhile effect," "minimal worthwhile change," "minimally important difference" (MID), "minimal clinically important difference" (MCID), and even "minimum worthwhile incremental advantage," but all these terms refer to the same parameter; they are just being applied to different situations (2). In terms of human performance, because this is the smallest change in a measure, for example, maximum oxygen uptake that could be deemed meaningful in terms of outcome performance, say in 5-km time. Modern systems for measuring oxygen consumption have accuracy of only a few milliliters per kilogram per minute, but changes of at least 5% are often considered MWE for recreational athletes. In medical research, MWE of a drug, therapy, or exercise is linked to observable improvements in health or symptoms, which would be clinically useful.

STANDARD MEASURES

Due to their development over the many different parts of the world, there are numerous measurement standards, such as the U.S. imperial system. However, the standard measurement system used in science is the **International System** (SI) of measurement for units. This provides a standard measure for all physical phenomena such as length (meter), mass (kilogram), and time (seconds). These standard measures are precisely known; for example, 1 m is the distance traveled by light in vacuum in 1/299,792,458 s, and a second is currently defined based on the radiation wave period from an unstable atom.

COMPONENTS OF A MEASUREMENT SYSTEM

There is a vast array of measurement systems ranging from the simplest, such as a tape measure, to the most complex, such as a three-dimensional motion capture system. In the past, instruments and measurement systems were **analog**. The final number or measurement would be read from a chart or gauge and then recorded by hand. All contemporary measurement systems and instruments including even the simple weighing scale are now **digital**, meaning the measurement is converted to an actual number that is displayed and recorded.

The most common measurement systems (Fig. 15-1) include the following:

1. Sensor which detects changes in a signal or transducer which converts one form of energy to another form of energy (*e.g.*, a physical phenomenon such as sound or light into an electrical signal or vice versa)

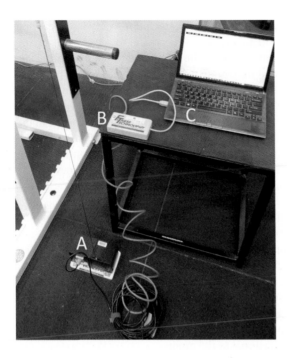

FIGURE 15-1: Typical measurement system with AD conversion taking an input signal and converting to a stream of digital data. **A.** Transducer which in this case converts linear displacement of the cable to an analog voltage. **B.** AD converter. **C.** Computer receiving data stream via the USB port for analysis, display, and recording.

2. Amplifier which magnifies the signal so that it is an appropriate range for input to the analog to digital (AD) converter
3. AD converter which takes the electrical signal (usually a fluctuating voltage) and converts the input into an integer (whole number) value, which can then be processed by computer and software
4. Computer and software that convert these integer values into real-world numbers representing the magnitude of the physical phenomenon being measured (*e.g.*, force in Newtons); the computer and software are then used to perform various analyses and visualizations (*e.g.*, graphs) of the physical phenomenon being observed

Sensors

The range of **sensors** (also termed "transducers") available is enormous simply because there are so many different phenomena that need to be measured, and each will require a specific type of sensor. The general function of a sensor is to receive the physical quantity being measured and convert it to an electrical signal, most often a varying voltage. There are sensors to measure mechanical quantities such as force, pressure, and torque. Other common sensors used in exercise and sports science measure temperature, concentration of a solution, electrical conductivity, or the concentration of gases such as carbon dioxide and oxygen in the expired breath of a patient or athlete. There are some key terminologies important to sensor performance for measurement:

- **Range:** Every sensor is designed and constructed so that it will work effectively and reliably over a particular range of input. These design ranges are usually fixed and a part of the mechanical or electronic design. Usually if the range of the sensor is exceeded, it will result in an alteration on how the sensor operates, permanent damage, or possibly even destruction of the sensor. For this reason, it is critical to select a sensor specific to the range of input that is to be measured. It should also be noted that most sensors are less accurate at the minimum and maximum extremes of their range. This is usually due to nonlinearity at inputs less than 10% and greater than 90% of maximum range. Selection of the sensor should allow measurement within its most accurate range.

- **Sensitivity**: The change in the output of the sensor for each unit change in the parameter being measured is termed as "sensitivity." This factor is usually constant over the range of the sensor, meaning it is linear and generally easier to calibrate and use. However, some parameters cannot be measured in this way, and the required sensors may be nonlinear, requiring slightly more complex calibration curves.

- **Resolution**: The smallest change that can be detected by a sensor is termed as "resolution." This is most often a limitation of the AD converter to be discussed shortly, but it can also be a factor of the sensor itself.

- **Response**: This is a performance quality of the sensor with regard to how quickly the sensor produces its output when subjected to a given change in the input; this is also termed the "response time." In practical terms, however, this is usually expressed by how consistently the sensor responds to a range of frequencies of changes in the input. This is termed the **frequency response**, and it specifies that if the sensor is subjected to a sinusoidally oscillating input of constant amplitude, the output will accurately reproduce another output signal proportional to the input.

- **Cross-sensitivity**: Some sensors are affected by changes in the ambient conditions other than purely by the input parameter. This is because the sensor is not only sensitive to the input signal but also to other phenomena. An example is a force transducer which will be influenced by changes in temperature as well as changes in force applied. Most modern force transducers, however, are temperature-compensated to overcome cross-sensitivity. Another example that is more difficult to deal with is sensors for electromyography (EMG) from a given muscle potentially picking up electrical signals from other muscles nearby. This is also termed "cross-talk."

Amplifiers

Most sensors output very low voltage signals, which must be amplified (multiplied) before they can be sent to the AD converter. For example, the electrocardiogram (ECG) signal measured at the chest by the sensors (electrodes) has an amplitude of only 1–2 mV. This signal is amplified electronically by approximately 1,000 times so that the output signal from the amplifier is of the order of 1–2 V, which fits well with the range of common AD converters. The gain (slope) and zero offset, both of which are discussed below, can often be electronically adjusted within the amplifier. However, with the development of modern AD measurement systems, most contemporary amplifiers have fixed gain and zero offset.

Analog to Digital Conversion

Practically all measurement now uses AD conversion to get the information into a form that we can readily use. Even a simple weighing scale for bodyweight will have an AD converter built into its electronics to convert the weight force of the person standing on it into an easily read and understood digital display, converting mass in kilograms. This is fine for observing a phenomenon which is fairly static such as body mass, but a mechanical quantity such as force is usually constantly changing and at a rate far too quick to read and record manually. For this, electrical signals which are changing in direct relationship to changes in what we are measuring require very rapid AD conversion. Then it requires some system by which this data can be recorded for later analysis.

An AD converter is an electronic device which may consist of only a single electronic component or a separate interface device that can take an electrical signal, which is usually a varying voltage, and convert it into an integer (a whole number). This process is all based on binary arithmetic.

Analog to Digital Resolution

AD converters are manufactured with a range of resolutions which is based on how many bits or binary numbers into which it can convert the input voltage (Table 15-1). Modern AD systems are usually 16-bit which gives a very high resolution, and it is likely that the noise in the signal is actually greater than the effective resolution, so having a higher bit conversion resolution is not of any benefit. The input voltage will vary depending on the transducer and the nature of the real-world phenomenon being measured, but it is generally 0 to 5 V, 0 to 10 V, -5 to $+5$ V, or -10 to $+10$ V.

It is important to recognize that AD conversion does not result in a continuous set of numbers representing the quantity being measured but rather integer or whole number approximations of the actual quantity. This results in a staircase-like representation of what is, in reality, a much smoother and continuous stream of data. As a result, the AD conversion process can result in high-frequency noise in the resulting data stream, the frequency of which is exactly equal to the sample rate and may need to be considered in our discussion of noise sources later in this chapter.

Sampling Rate

All AD converters will have a specified **sampling rate**, which is how many discrete measurements they can convert and transmit to the recording device each second. Sampling rate is

Table 15-1 Range of Values and Effective Voltage Resolution of Analog to Digital Converters of Increasing Bit Range

Analog to Digital Converter, Number of Bits	Range of Values	Effective Resolution for a 0–10 V Input Signal
8-bit	0–255	0.039 V
10-bit	0–1,023	0.0098 V
12-bit	0–4,095	0.0024 V
14-bit	0–16,383	0.00061 V
16-bit	0–65,535	0.00015 V

expressed in units of samples per second or Hz and can range widely depending on the cost and application of the measurement system. Measurement of some phenomena does not require high speed because changes occur relatively slowly. For example, when measuring postural sway, the data is usually recorded at 20–50 Hz because that is all that is required to capture the nature of these relatively slow and subtle movements. Foot impact during sprinting occurs over only 80 ms, and some of the forces of interest are changing very rapidly, so even to measure the time period of foot impact requires a sampling frequency of 1,000 Hz or higher to be able to measure these very quick events with an accuracy of 1%–2%.

The AD conversion process produces a stream of data which is then stored, usually on the hard drive of a computer. For some measurement systems, only a single variable or "channel" is recorded, but for other applications, multiple inputs will be recorded simultaneously, producing multiple streams of data all synchronized in time. For example, a typical metabolic system for measuring oxygen consumption and carbon dioxide production will simultaneously record channels for ventilation flow, oxygen concentration, carbon dioxide concentration, and possibly an additional channel for heart rate.

Sample Period

The time between two consecutive samples is called the **sample period** and can be calculated as the inverse of the frequency, in other words, 1 divided by the sample frequency. For example, if the sampling frequency is 100 Hz, then the sample period is 0.01 s, and for 200 Hz, the sample period would be 0.05 s. The sample rate, and therefore sample period, is timed with high accuracy to ensure that there is exactly the same time between consecutive samples.

Wireless or Wired

Traditionally, the components of the measurement system have been hardwired between the subject and the various components and then into the computer. For example, an EMG system would consist of electrodes wired into an amplifier with the resulting signal input to the computer, usually via an AD interface card installed in the computer. Modern wired systems do not require modification of the computer but use the universal serial bus (USB) interface with the amplifier and AD converter contained in a small interface box plugged into a USB port. However, such hardware attached to the subject may limit mobility and movement of wires, and components can interfere with accurate measurement. To solve these issues, many measurement systems now use wireless data transmission at some or even all stages of the process. For example, EMG systems can now use small battery-powered electrodes which amplify the signal and then transmit wirelessly and usually digitally to a receiver, which then interfaces to the computer via USB. Most modern computers have several digital wireless interfaces such as Bluetooth or wireless ethernet built in. With inexpensive USB interfaces, other wireless technologies such as ZigBee can be added. The result is that an increasing number of measurement systems are being controlled wirelessly and can transmit data directly to the host computer wirelessly, eliminating hardwired connections. Although providing greatly increased mobility and smaller sizes, these "wearable" sensors are limited by battery life and transmission bandwidth. Depending on the technology, the amount of data and thus sampling frequency that can be moved between the sensor and the computer is limited by wireless technology. For measuring heart rate, this is not a problem, but wireless recording of EMG becomes a challenge.

CALIBRATION

It is not meaningful to have a whole stream of numbers unless we can relate them back to the standard measure of the phenomenon we are examining. Expressing and trying to analyze force, for example, when it is in the raw number coming out of the AD converter is not possible, so we must get it back into standard units, which in the case of force is the Newton. We do this through a process called **calibration**, which involves measuring known quantities and recording the output from the AD converter. In other words, calibration is a process of measuring the output of a sensor in response to an accurately known input. To provide an accurately known input, devices or phenomenon of known quantity are applied, and these are called "calibration standards." Coming back to our force plate example, we could place highly accurate known weights on the plate, record the digital readings, and then work out the relationship between them, which is usually a straight line.

The calibration function can be described by a linear equation of the form: $y = mx + b$, where:

$$y = \text{input } (e.g., \text{force})$$
$$m = \text{slope (span adjustment)}$$
$$x = \text{output (AD reading)}$$
$$b = \text{zero adjustment}$$

This equation can then be used to calculate the actual force being applied given an AD reading. For the example in Figure 15-2, if the AD reading is 12,345, then the actual force being applied is 744.9 N. That is:

$$744.9 = 0.059(12,345) + 16.546$$

Two Versus Multiple Calibration Points

As a minimum, this process requires the setting of at least two points of calibration. Also, it is good practice that these points be at the expected minimum and maximum of the quantity to be measured. A more rigorous method is to use multiple inputs, and then it can be determined as to whether and to what degree the relationship between the input signal and the output measurement is in fact linear. For most modern measurement systems, the linearity of measurement is extremely high, but this was not always the case. Technology has made measurement much easier for the scientist.

Most equipment manufacturers will provide detailed information on how linear their measurement systems are, but when buying new equipment, and in particular for rigorous research, a multiple-point calibration should be completed to confirm this and also to ensure that there are no faults in the system.

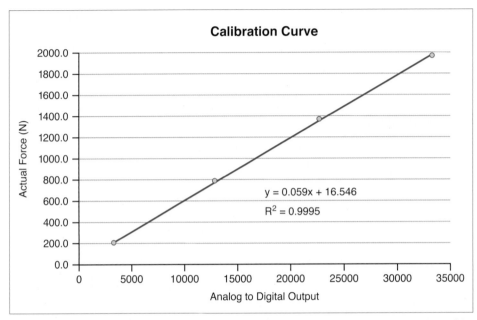

FIGURE 15-2:   Line graph to calculate the equation of the instrument calibration line. The slope of the line is 0.059 and the zero offset is 16.546 N. The measurement system is highly linear with an $R^2 = 0.9995$.

Zero Offset and Span

To reiterate, most measurement systems are highly linear in the relationship between the magnitude of the phenomenon being measured and the numbers produced from the AD converter. This relationship can be expressed in the form of an equation of a straight line. The rate of change of the input relative to the output is the slope of the line (m), and this is also termed "span," which is a carry-over from the past, when measurement systems were purely electronic rather than computer-based.

So to fully describe the relationship between the input and output, we not only need the slope of the line but also the "y" intercept, or what is known as the **zero offset**. To be of practical use when making a measurement, it is necessary to start at a known datum, which is a standard reference point. For example, the temperature at which water freezes at normal atmospheric pressure is 0°C, but this corresponds to 273° Kelvin on the absolute temperature scale. The zero point is therefore a value ascribed to some defined point in the measured range. Another example is measurement of height for a vertical jump in which standing upright is usually set as the zero point.

This can be determined by placing a zero input quantity (*e.g.*, no weight force on the plate) and recording the output measure. This is the zero offset. This assumes that the relationship is perfectly linear, so a more rigorous procedure for determining the zero offset is to record the output measurement over the full range of input quantities, use these x and y coordinates to calculate the line of best fit, and the calculated "y" intercept will be a more accurate measure of the zero offset. This can be done relatively easily using Excel; an example of the resulting line graph is given in Figure 15-2. Once the equation of the calibration line is known, it is relatively straightforward to convert any AD output number into a value representing the quantity of the phenomenon being measured.

Zero drift can be a problem in some measurement systems. The signal level may vary from its set zero value over time, and this is usually due to alterations within the sensor. This introduces an error into the measurement equal to the amount of variation, or "drift," as it is usually termed. Examples of environmental conditions that may cause zero drift include changes of temperature, electronics stabilizing, and/or physical stress or aging of the transducer or electronic components.

Range Over Which to Calibrate

Any measurement system should be calibrated over the full range of input signals that it can record. However, this may not be possible or desirable in some situations. For example, most force plates for measuring human movement have a range from 0 up to 10,000 or more Newtons, which is around 14 times the average bodyweight of an adult human. The forces produced during a vertical jump range only two to three times bodyweight, so it can be justified to calibrate the system using a series of input weights from zero to perhaps four or five times bodyweight to assure upper limits of performance. This is easier than moving very large amounts of weight on and off the force plate, but more important, you are calibrating over the range of interest for your measurements, so the calibration slope and zero offset will likely give you more representative values.

When to Recalibrate

Most important, any new measurement system should be calibrated once it has been unpacked and placed in the position where it will be located. This is part of the commissioning of any new piece of equipment, and even if calibration values are provided by the manufacturer, it is important to confirm that these are correct, have not changed as a result of transport and/or the new location, or that a fault has developed in the system.

Following this initial calibration, for research purposes, any measurement system should be calibrated before and after each testing session. The reason for calibrating both before and after taking your measurements of interest is to check that the calibration has not changed over the measurement session because some systems will be affected more or less by the phenomenon that is being measured. In addition, measurement systems can be affected by changes in the environment such as temperature, electrical supply, and atmospheric pressure, so this should be checked using the post-calibration to see if there has been any drift in the calibration factors. If there have been any changes, then there are mathematical methods to adjust for this.

Whenever there are changes in the measurement system such as moving location, or swapping any components, even powering down and restarting, the system should be recalibrated.

Bench Calibration and Field Calibration

Some measurement systems are used solely within the confines of a laboratory and may spend many years never being moved. However, many measurement systems are used in the field or are constantly being moved from site to site, and this requires special considerations. The physical movement of a measurement system can cause changes in the calibration factors. As mentioned earlier, changes in environmental conditions such as temperature and pressure can also impact the relationship between the input phenomenon and the measured output. For this reason, measurement systems which are used in the field should undergo both bench and field calibration procedures. **Bench calibration** is completed in the controlled conditions of the laboratory where the measurement system is calibrated using highly accurate input parameters. For example, a portable force plate system could be placed on a larger and more accurate laboratory force measuring system and then weights of very high accuracy used in the calibration process. This would be the bench calibration. Measurements from the portable system can be directly compared to the fixed force plate as well as the standard weights. When the portable force plate is then out in the field, for example, on a basketball court or in the weight room, a simple **field calibration** can be completed to check that there are no problems with the system and that the calibration has not drifted. In our force plate example, this could be as simple as placing a single known weight (*e.g.*, the tester's bodyweight) on the force plate and checking that it accurately measures this input parameter.

Sources of Error

With rigorous calibration procedures and regular checking of measurement accuracy, errors will be quite minimal, but they can still occur. It is important to apply sound scientific method, incorporating a set sequence of equipment setup, calibration, and testing to minimize the chance of errors of measurement.

Span Error

Span error is when the calibration slope (m) is not correct either because the calibration was not performed correctly or the relationship between the input signal and output values has changed due to moving the system or environmental factors. If the span error is detected and accurately quantified by recalibrating the system, then the erroneous measurements can be corrected simply by applying a scaling factor (Fig. 15-3).

Zero Error

Zero error occurs when the "y" intercept (zero offset) is not determined correctly during calibration or has drifted. All of the outcome measures will be shifted up or down depending on the direction of the error. If the zero error is detected and accurately quantified by recalibrating the system, then the erroneous measurements can be corrected simply by subtracting or adding the error to the erroneous measurements (see Fig. 15-3).

Combined Zero and Span Error

When both span error and zero error are combined, the data can be corrected, but it is more difficult. If the correct calibration factors can be determined, then the same corrections outlined earlier can be applied to rescue the data (see Fig. 15-3).

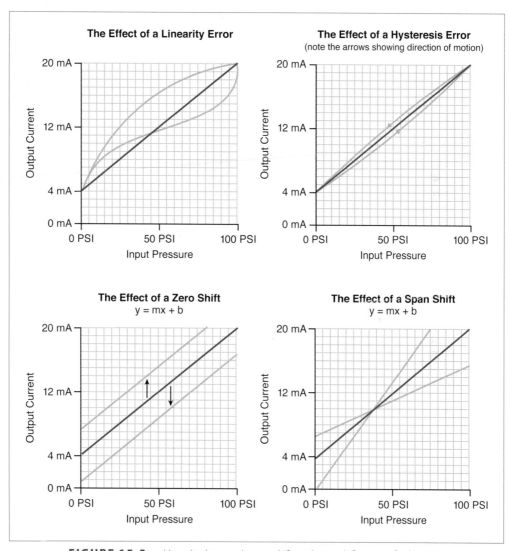

FIGURE 15-3: Linearity, hysteresis, zero shift, and span shift errors of calibration.

Linearization Errors

As outlined earlier, most modern measurement systems are highly linear with correlation coefficients between the input and output measures being as high as 0.999 and with coefficients of variation much less than 1%. However, some phenomena are more difficult to measure on a linear scale, and these errors need to be quantified and understood. As a general rule, most measurement systems are designed to be highly linear through the midrange of their measurement and can become curvilinear near the maximum and minimum values that they can quantify (see Fig. 15-3).

Hysteresis Errors

Again it is rare to see hysteresis errors in modern measurement systems, but it still can occur. As the input phenomenon is increasing (*e.g.*, force) the output increases, but as the input then returns back to lower values, the descending output does not track exactly on the ascending output. To overcome this requires calibration of the system over both increasing and decreasing input values with separate calibration curves being calculated (see Fig. 15-3).

Establishing and Maintaining a Calibration Log

A most critical part of rigorous research practice is to maintain a "research logbook" to record notes and observations from the research and also calibration information on any measurement systems that you are using. At a bare minimum, this should include the date and time, name of the device, the calibration slope (m or span), and the "y" intercept (b or zero offset). Then each time you calibrate the device, you will be able to check whether there is much drift from previous calibrations. If the calibration factors have been very consistent and you see a marked change, then this could indicate you have not calibrated correctly or that you have an equipment fault. The calibration log is also invaluable when you later find inconsistencies in your data and try to go back to forensically determine the problem. You may even be able to rescue your data if you can determine when and what the problem was with the calibration.

SYSTEMATIC ERRORS

Systematic errors include the span error and zero offset error described earlier. These errors affect all measurement equally and are relatively easy to address if you have accurate knowledge of the type and quantity of the calibration error (3).

RANDOM ERRORS

As the name suggests, **random errors** affect measurements in different directions and with different magnitude and are much more difficult to remove from your data (3). Sources of these errors can be due to:

1. "Noise" in the input phenomena (*e.g.*, vibration of the building due to a passing truck is appearing on the force plate measurements)
2. "Noise" in the electronic components of the measurement system (*e.g.*, the large electric motor in the air conditioning unit of the laboratory is emitting electromagnetic radiation which is affecting measurement electronics)
3. "Noise" due to the AD conversion process (*e.g.*, particularly in lower resolution AD converters, the discrete integer measurements can create a staircase appearance on the output data)

Apart from implementing rigorous scientific method design, including checking all equipment and removing all extraneous sources of noise, digital filtering or smoothing can be applied to reduce random errors.

DIGITAL FILTERING (SMOOTHING)

Often signals from force, acceleration, or displacement transducers will contain random noise. For example, force data measured from a force plate may contain very small oscillations superimposed on the actual force signal due to vibrations of the floor or the plate. This random noise is generally of very small amplitude and may not even be visible on a graph of the data. As such, it is not generally a problem when just observing and taking measures from these raw signals. However, when additional signal processing is applied such as integration or differentiation, these small amplitude random errors are greatly magnified and can result in data which is practically unusable (4). In the past, filters would be hardwired into the measurement system. These would be electronic circuits which would filter out or "smooth" the electrical signal without distorting the signal of interest. However, with the ready availability of inexpensive AD measurement systems combined with powerful personal computers, such digital filtering is usually done in software being applied to the digital data stream. It is important to know that neither the older "analog" electronic filters nor the latest digital filters can completely remove all noise without some alteration to the actual signal of interest that is to be recorded and analyzed. Therefore, it is important to consider the type of filter used and particularly the cutoff frequency that is selected. The closer the cutoff frequency of the digital filter to the frequency of the signal of interest, the greater will be the distortion that occurs, and this can result in spurious measurement.

High Pass Filter

A **high pass digital filter** is designed to allow any frequencies above the filter cutoff to pass through to the smoothed dataset. Any frequencies in the signal or dataset below the frequency cutoffs are removed. A common application of a high pass digital filter is the measurement and recording of the electromyographic signal from the muscle. Most of the volume or "energy" in the EMG signal is between 50 and 250 Hz. However, EMG is normally measured during human movement, and this can induce fairly large amplitude but very low frequency (6–10 Hz) "movement artifact" into the electrical signal being measured. Because the frequency of the movement artifact and the actual EMG signal of interest are quite different, a high pass digital filter with a cutoff of say 20 Hz is usually effective for removing this low-frequency noise while retaining all of the higher frequency EMG signals of interest.

Low Pass Filter

A **low pass digital filter** is designed to remove frequencies above the filter cutoff while allowing lower frequencies of interest to pass through and be retained in the resulting dataset. A common application of a low pass digital filter in exercise and sports science is the smoothing of the displacement data from a linear potentiometer to remove high-frequency noise such as electrical interference and vibration, leaving the lower frequency component which is the actual change in displacement of the object being tracked, for example, movement of the barbell during weight lifting. An example of a low pass digital

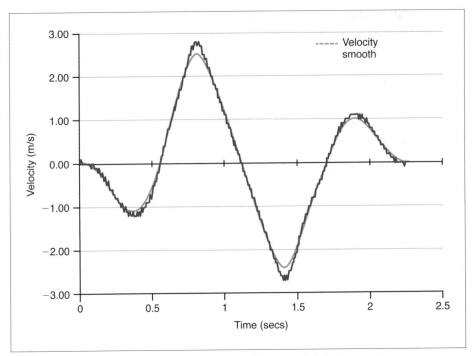

FIGURE 15-4:   Example of a low pass (10 Hz cutoff frequency) digital filter applied to displacement-time data with subsequent calculation of velocity-time data. The unfiltered dataset is also shown for comparison. Note that the maximum and minimum values are attenuated, illustrating that no filter is perfect at removing all noise without some distortion of the true signal.

filter applied to displacement-time data with subsequent calculation of velocity-time data is presented in Figure 15-4.

Band Pass Filter

A band pass filter is a combination of high and low pass filters such that frequencies above and below the two cutoff frequencies are removed, leaving only signal frequencies in the resulting output dataset that are within the band of interest. Again, this is commonly applied in EMG to remove high-frequency noise due to AD sampling approximation and low frequency movement artifact.

Notch Filter

A notch filter is used to remove a very narrow band or even a single frequency from the dataset. Where this is most commonly applied is for removal of electrical "hum," which is the noise that can occur in measurement systems due to the alternating current (AC) electricity which is powering the equipment, lights, air conditioning, etc. Depending on country of location, this will be either 50 or 60 Hz. Although there are filters to remove such electrical noise, it is better scientific procedure to remove as many sources of this electro-magnetic interference as possible. Modern measurement systems are well shielded against this noise source, but when measuring extremely small electrical signals such as EMG or electroencephalogram (EEG), it is best to take precautions to minimize the problem. This might mean turning off lights, as fluorescent lights in particular are noisy, air conditioning units, and fans, which generate considerable electrical noise. It is also prudent to ensure that no cables, transducers, or even the subject are in contact or close to electrical cables carrying AC power.

NYQUIST SAMPLING THEOREM

More correctly termed "Nyquist-Shannon sampling theorem" (6) but most often stated simply as Nyquist sampling theorem or "the sampling theorem," this theorem states that the minimum sampling frequency must be at least twice the highest frequency of interest in the signal. This is well illustrated with an example. The electrical activity in muscles when they are activated has a maximum frequency of around 250 Hz, so to accurately measure the EMG signal, it must be sampled at 500 Hz or more. In reality, it is better to choose a sampling frequency that is four to five times the frequency of the phenomenon of interest. With modern data collection systems, this is easily achievable for all movement and electrical signals such as ECG or EMG. As another example, the maximum frequency of movement of the hands and fingers is around 10 Hz, so a video camera recording at 30 Hz is theoretically capable of accurately measuring this movement, but we get a far more accurate recording with cameras capable of 100 Hz or more.

DATA PROCESSING

Once a set of data has been collected, there is usually some amount of post-processing to be completed to derive new measures or summary variables. There are numerous methods of doing this, and it depends on what is to be measured and how it is to be quantified. However, there are a few common methods of data processing in exercise and sports science which should be briefly described.

Differentiation

Differentiation is a measure of the rate of change of the variable with respect to time. Probably one of the most common is the calculation of velocity based on the displacement of an object. Another example is the calculation of rate of force development which is a common measure to assess a human's ability to rapidly apply muscular force. In this case, the force-time data series is differentiated.

Integration

Integration is also usually determined with respect to time. It is the area under the curve for the data series. The simplest way to calculate this is the value at that time point multiplied by the time between samples, which is the period. This creates a fairly rough approximation, although it can be reasonably accurate at high sample rates. It is preferable to use a more sophisticated integration method such as the **trapezoid** or Simpson's method. An example of integration is when the force recorded during a vertical jump is integrated with respect to time to derive a dataset which is the change in velocity with time or acceleration.

Area Under the Curve

Although integration is in fact calculation of area under the curve (AUC), in some areas of exercise and sports science, AUC is applied for particular data processing. A common application is to determine the "exposure" of the body to a particular hormone quantified by the AUC. In this case, the concentration of the hormone, for instance testosterone, at each time point is measured and multiplied by the time since the previous sample, and these blocks or areas are summed to give an overall indication of testosterone exposure (11).

Normalization

In exercise and sports science, it is often useful to express a particular measure relative to some base or benchmark. This is often done by expressing the measurement as a percentage or ratio. One common application is the quantification of the EMG measured from a muscle. Because the EMG signal varies markedly from individual to individual and also changes over time, absolute measures may not be particularly informative. In EMG analysis, a maximum contraction of the muscle can be measured and then all subsequent measures of EMG are expressed relative to this volitional maximal isometric muscle activation. This process is called **normalization**.

REPORTING MEASUREMENT PROCEDURES IN SCIENTIFIC PAPERS

The measurement system used in research, its characteristics, how it has been set up, and how the data is subsequently processed and quantified will have an impact on the resulting measurements that are reported. The equipment used must be named, including the model, manufacturer, city, and country of origin. For this reason, it is important to accurately describe how the particular parameter was measured. Here is an example describing the measurement of force during a vertical jump:

> *Vertical ground reaction force was measured using a portable force plate (Model 400S, Fitness Technology, Adelaide, Australia) sampling at 600 Hz using 16-bit AD conversion. Force data was filtered using a low pass Butterworth 4th Order digital filter at a cutoff frequency of 100 Hz and subsequently integrated using the trapezoid method to derive velocity data. Power was calculated as the product of force by velocity at each time point. Force and power measures were normalized by expressing relative to bodyweight. In our laboratory, the ICC (CV) are 0.98 (1.2%), 0.95 (2.2%), and 0.91 (3.6%) for peak measures of force, velocity, and power, respectively. The force plate system was calibrated immediately before and after each testing session using two accurately known weights of 20 and 200 kg.*

GLOSSARY

Analog: a continuous signal which varies in time, usually referring to an electrical signal of voltage, current, or frequency

Bench calibration: calibration completed in controlled conditions of a laboratory where the measurement system is calibrated using highly accurate input parameters

Calibration: process of measuring known quantities and recording the output from the AD converter for the purpose of converting digital values to physical quantities

Coefficient of variation: measure of dispersion of measurements about the mean calculated as standard deviation of the measurements expressed as a percentage of the mean

Cross-sensitivity: characteristic of how to influence the sensor is by changes in the environment other than the signal for which it is designed to measure

Differentiation: measure of the rate of change of a variable with respect to another, usually time

Digital: a physical (analog) signal represented as a sequence of discrete values

Field calibration: calibration done in the environment where the actual measurements are to be recorded using known input parameters

Frequency response: indication of how faithfully a measurement system will reflect the input signal across the full range of frequencies

High pass digital filter: mathematical processing of the data which allows frequencies in the signal above the filter cutoff to pass through and removes frequencies below this cutoff to produce the smoothed dataset

International System: abbreviated SI from the French "Le Système International d'Unités"; this is the latest metric system and most widely used system of measurement in the world

Intraclass correlation coefficient: descriptive statistic which describes how strongly measurements, items, or members of the same group or sample resemble each other

Low pass digital filter: mathematical processing of the data which allows frequencies in the signal below the filter cutoff to pass through and removes frequencies above this cutoff to produce the smoothed dataset

Measurement: a systematic and replicable process by which physical and nonphysical phenomena are quantified

Minimal detectable change: smallest amount of change beyond TEM that is a true change between two time points

Minimal worthwhile effect: smallest change in a measure that could be deemed meaningful in terms of outcome performance or health or symptoms which would be clinically useful

Normalization: mathematical process of expressing a particular measure relative to some base or benchmark

Pearson correlation: measure of linear correlation (dependence) between two variables

Random errors: errors or noise in the output data affecting the measurements in different directions and with different magnitude

Range: difference between maximum and minimum values that a system can reliably measure

Reliability: degree to which a measurement technique or system can produce consistent results each time it is used

Resolution: smallest change that can be detected by a sensor or measurement system

Response: how quickly a sensor produces its output when subjected to a given change in input; also termed the *response time*

Sample period: time between two consecutive samples

Sampling rate: how many discrete measurements per second that a measurement system can sample and record

Sensitivity: change in output of the sensor for each unit change in the parameter being measured

Sensor: hardware device which converts a physical phenomenon into an electrical signal

Technical error of measurement: random error distributed normally around the true value indicative of the accuracy or resolution of the measurement system

Trapezoid: method of integrating a dataset to determine the AUC

Validity: degree of success of a measurement in describing or quantifying what it is designed to measure

Zero offset: y intercept of the calibration relationship between the input signal and output measurements which is effectively the value from the AD conversion corresponding to the relative zero of the phenomenon being measured

REFERENCES

1. Clasey JL, Kanaley JA, Wideman L, et al. Validity of methods of body composition assessment in young and older men and women. *J Appl Physiol*. 1999;86(5):1728–1738.
2. de Vet HC, Terwee CB, Ostelo RW, Beckerman H, Knol DL, Bouter LM. Minimal changes in health status questionnaires: distinction between minimally detectable change and minimally important change. *Health Qual Life Outcomes*. 2006;4:54.
3. Evans MD, Goldie PA, Hill KD. Systematic and random error in repeated measurements of temporal and distance parameters of gait after stroke. *Arch Phys Med Rehabil*. 1997;78(7):725–729. doi:10.1016/S0003-9993(97)90080-0.
4. Giakas G, Baltzopoulos V. Optimal digital filtering requires a different cut-off frequency strategy for the determination of the higher derivatives. *J Biomech*. 1997;30(8):851–855. doi:10.1016/S0021-9290(97)00043-2.
5. Hammersley M. Some notes on the terms "validity" and "reliability." *Br Educ Res J*. 1987;13(1):73–82. doi:10.1080/0141192870130107.
6. Jerri AJ. The Shannon sampling theorem—its various extensions and applications: a tutorial review. *Proc IEEE*. 1977;65(11):1565–1596. doi:10.1109/PROC.1977.10771.
7. Katch F, Michael ED, Horvath SM. Estimation of body volume by underwater weighing: description of a sample method. *J Appl Physiol*. 1967;23(5):811–813.
8. Koch Gary G. Intraclass correlation coefficient. In: Kotz S, Balakrishnan N, Read C, Vidakovic B, editors. *Encyclopedia of Statistical Sciences*. New York (NY): John Wiley & Sons; 2005.
9. Lovie P. Coefficient of variation. In: Eviritt BS, Howell D, editors. *Encyclopedia of Statistics in Behavioral Science*. Hoboken (NJ): Wiley; 2005.
10. Perini TA, Oliveira LO, Ornellas JS, Oliveira FP. Cálculo do erro técnico de medição em antropometria. Cálculo do erro técnico de medição em antropometria. *Revista Brasileira de Medicina do Esporte*. 2005;11:81–85.
11. Pruessner JC, Kirschbaum C, Meinlschmid G, Hellhammer DH. Two formulas for computation of the area under the curve represent measures of total hormone concentration versus time-dependent change. *Psychoneuroendocrinology*. 2003;28(7):916–931. doi:10.1016/S0306-4530(02)00108-7.

First Analyses After Data Collection

Elaine C. Lee, PhD, and Kathrine R. Weeks, PhD

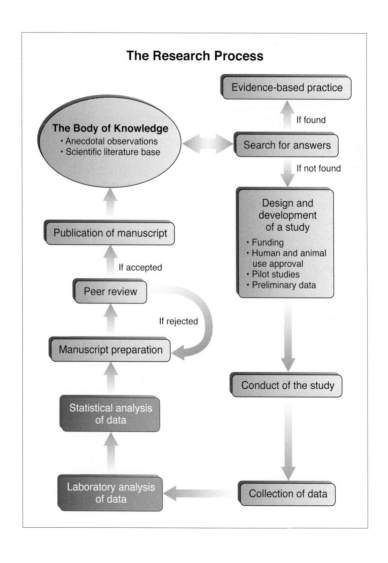

INTRODUCTION: GENERAL APPROACHES TO FIRST DATA ANALYSES

First data organization, quality control checks, and first analyses follow the successful execution of a well-designed study based on an informed hypothesis. Different types of experimental approaches generate different types of data and thus require distinct approaches to handling first data analyses. Nonetheless, the first steps in any analyses after initial data collection include the following: (a) revisiting details of the experiments, (b) assessing quality of experiment conducted, (c) organizing data, (d) grouping data (*e.g.*, based on time point or other grouping variable), (e) assessing quality of data (accuracy, precision, and reproducibility), (f) making decisions about data to include based on objective and standard criteria, (g) making decisions about analyses to run, (h) initial analyses, and (i) contextualization of data to understanding of physiology and function. First data analysis is a thoughtful, organized, systematic, and somewhat nuanced process depending on the type of data. In this chapter, we provide practice examples for applying these and other aspects of decision-making in first data analyses in two very common biochemical assays used in exercise science research, enzyme-linked immunosorbent assay (ELISA) and Western blot. We also summarize common themes independent of assay-specific considerations.

ENZYME-LINKED IMMUNOSORBENT ASSAYS

Background

In the study of exercise, many different assays techniques are used to assess a host of different variables. The biologic assays (called "bioassays") that were used prior to the development of current immunoassay techniques are even now taking on renewed importance to gain a greater understanding of the measured variable (*e.g.*, growth hormone as bioassay gives a different answer compared to immunoassay). But common to so many variables measured in the blood to evaluate exercise stress, adaptations to exercise programs, or recovery from exercise stress, immunoassays have become a popular tool. Immunoassay kits come in a variety of arrays from individual tubes to 96-well plates replacing a tube with a well. So each assay kit will have specific instructions and approaches. It is important that each investigator understands the theory and use of these assay tools or mistakes can be made in their conduct and interpretation. Although companies designed such kits to be helpful tools and make analyses easier with less prep time, they were not meant to replace the fundamental knowledge needed from chemistry, organic chemistry, biochemistry, clinical chemistry, and cell biology to work with the construct of the assay and its theoretical basis for their conduct.

Radioimmunoassays (RIA), enzyme immunoassays (EIA), and ELISA were developed by separate groups in the 1960s and 1970s and use distinct methods of detection, but fundamental features of each of these protein detection methods are the same. The first of these three to be published was the RIA, in 1960, by Yalow and Berson who used the RIA technique to measure human insulin concentrations in blood plasma (15). About a decade later, two independent groups, Anton Schuurs (principal investigator [PI]) and Bauke van Weemen (13) at the Research Laboratories of NV Organon (Oss, Netherlands) and Peter Perlmann (PI) and Eva Engvall (7) at Stockholm University (Stockholm, Sweden), published the EIA and ELISA methods, respectively. Since then, these immunoassay approaches have become ubiquitous in multiple areas of research; protein-level analyses in thousands of papers (8) would not exist without them. Newer developments have focused on increased sensitivity, microbead-based formats, new methods of detection including luminescence and fluorescence (in addition to radioactivity and colorimetric enzyme-substrate detection), and even multiplexing to allow for measurement of multiple proteins simultaneously. The analysis approach for these methods is similar.

There are many variations and formats of ELISAs (and similar assays), but the basic principles are illustrated in Figure 16-1. Two features define these assays: (a) **Specificity** of recognition is achieved by engineering an antibody-antigen (Ab-Ag) system in which an **antibody** is made to recognize a specific **epitope** on an **antigen**. For measuring endogenous

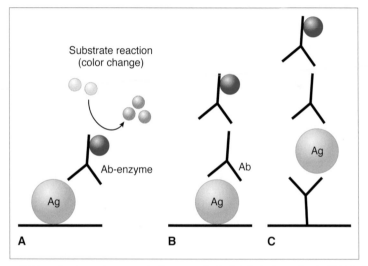

FIGURE 16-1: ELISA methods vary in approach. The general principle includes antibody (Ab) binding to specific epitopes on proteins of interest or antigens (Ag). Secondary antibodies conjugated to functional enzymes (Ab-enzyme) recognize bound primary antibody and allow us to indirectly quantify the amount of protein in a given sample. Enzymes act on substrate to promote a reaction that usually generates a product that may have a different or newly detectable color. Color can be detected using spectrophotometry. **A.** Direct ELISA approaches typically use one antibody conjugated to a functional enzyme. The antibody recognizes the protein of interest directly, and the enzyme conjugated to the antibody acts of a substrate that is provided. The substrate undergoes a reaction catalyzed by the conjugated enzyme and changes into a product that generates a measurable color. **B.** Indirect ELISA uses a system of antibodies to detect a protein of interest. A primary, unconjugated antibody recognizes the protein of interest and binds an epitope with specificity. A secondary antibody conjugated to an enzyme then is added and recognizes the primary antibody. The enzyme functions as described for a direct ELISA assay, and the color change reaction is a quantifiable indirect measurement of the amount of protein present in a solution. **C.** Sandwich ELISAs may use three separate antibodies to detect a protein of interest. A capture antibody is adsorbed or attached to a surface and is used to capture proteins of interest at their specifically recognized epitopes. The bound antigen or protein of interest is recognized then by a primary unconjugated antibody that also has specificity for the protein at a different epitope. Finally, a detection antibody, an Ab-enzyme, is added to permit the color-generating, or chromogenic, response that will be an indirect measure of the amount of protein present in a given sample.

proteins, the "antigen" in this reaction is merely a specific protein of interest. (b) **Sensitivity** of detection typically depends on an enzyme, which is chemically conjugated to an antibody that either directly or indirectly binds the antigen or protein of interest. The enzyme functions normally and changes a substrate that is provided. In this example, the enzymatic reaction may result in a substrate change that causes a colorimetric change, detectable on some arbitrary scale of either **spectrophotometric absorbance** or color intensity.

Standard Curves and Interpolation

Figure 16-2 illustrates how an example ELISA may be used to indirectly determine the amount of a specific protein in a biologic sample. Standards are samples which contain a known amount of the protein of interest. Often these are made by adding **recombinant protein**, or protein artificially made in mass quantities in a laboratory-based system and to known volumes of buffer. In this way, a researcher can obtain samples that have an exact known concentration of a protein of interest. In the example shown, the highest concentration of the known standards is 100 pg $\cdot$ mL^{-1}. There are six total known concentrations of proteins ready for assay in this example. "Standards" are named as such because they will be test cases for which the binding of antibody to the proteins present in solution, and the subsequent detection of this binding will give an indication of how much protein is present in an unknown sample. Figure 16-2 illustrates how different concentrations of protein might give different color results, depicted as different variations of gray and denoted by arbitrary units.

Once a number of standards are assayed to give a colorimetric result for each known value, a standard curve may be generated by graphing respective concentrations (x values) and color results (y values) on a scatter plot. In this example, six standards have six different proportional color results, and the graph resembles the shape of a line with the formula $y = mx + b$. Figure 16-2 shows three samples that may have been obtained in an experiment; these samples have unknown concentration of our protein of interest but have been assayed in an ELISA and show some color result. The equation for the line is used to calculate protein concentrations in the three separate tubes based on their color indicator measurements and comparisons to our known standards. However, it is also clear qualitatively, using the logic of a standard comparison approach, that the first standard with color measurement of 10 contains likely close to 100 pg $\cdot$ mL^{-1}. Similarly, the second unknown sample likely contains very close to 0 pg $\cdot$ mL^{-1}, and the third unknown sample likely has protein concentration between 12.5 and 25 pg $\cdot$ mL^{-1}, although for this sample, determining the exact protein concentration is an estimate or prediction. Using a standard curve to estimate values for unknown samples is a common practice in many biochemical and molecular approaches. First data analyses of these assays require some of the following steps demonstrated in the example dataset below.

Example Data: Testosterone Enzyme-Linked Immunosorbent Assay

Organizing and Considering Experimental Notes

An example dataset is provided in Table 16-1. The data provided are example absorbance values (a measure of color intensity at a certain wavelength [in this case, $\lambda = 540$ nm] following an Ab-enzyme conjugated reaction on chromogenic substrate TMB [3,3′,5,5′-tetramethylbenzidine])

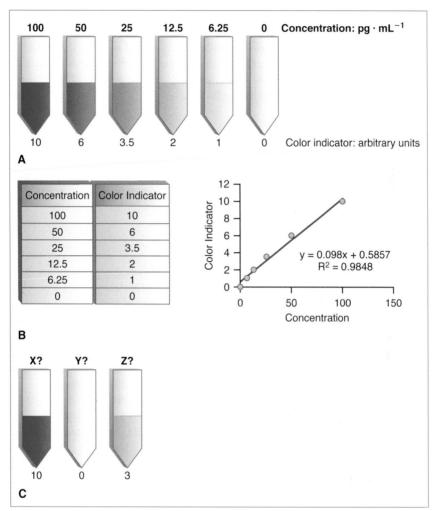

FIGURE 16-2:   In a typical ELISA, direct measurements of samples with known concentrations of protein and their respective enzymatic color reactions are used to estimate the amount of unknown protein in a set of samples. **A.** Six standards with concentrations 100, 50, 25, 12.5, 6.25, and 0 pg · mL^{-1} were assayed in a colorimetric ELISA. Example results for the color intensity are shown as "color indicator" in arbitrary units. The highest concentration standard in this example has the darkest color, which in the arbitrary units has a value of "10." **B.** Standard curves are generated by plotting color indicator values (y-axis, dependent variable) versus protein concentration in pg · mL^{-1} (x-axis, independent variable). The mathematic relationship between these two plotted variables can be determined by software; in this case, we used Microsoft Excel to determine that there is a good linear relationship between the two variables, characterized by the equation $y = 0.098x + 0.5857$ ($R^2 = 0.9848$). Using this equation, it is possible to predict concentrations for measurements of any color on this continuous line. **C.** Example unknown samples are presented here. The concentration for these samples might be unknown, but the samples have theoretically been assayed via ELISA and give the color results shown. Unknown samples X, Y, and Z thus have color results of 10, 0, and 3, respectively. Using these color indicators and comparing to our measured standards in **(A)**, it is logical that samples X, Y, and Z likely have protein concentration values close to 100, 0, and between 12.5 and 25 pg · mL^{-1}. You can also directly use the equation provided in **(B)** to calculate the unknown x value in the $y = mx + b$ linear equation.

from an ELISA used to measure testosterone levels in human blood plasma. Data are for eight standards, each with known concentration of testosterone, and eight samples with unknown concentrations of testosterone; each sample was measured in triplicate, meaning that each sample was assayed three times in the same assay to account for assay differences from tube to tube. Table 16-1, Panel B, defines the identity of each of the samples for which values are shown in Table 16-1, Panel A. Often, preparing a database or table of data similar to Table 16-1 requires revisiting the experiment details. Details may be in a detailed lab notebook or the assay insert with kit instructions. If assays are done in a 96-well plate or individual tubes, there may have been experimental exceptions or notes on mistakes and things to note about quality or nature of the samples from the day the assay was performed. These should be noted and revisited in first data analyses. Organizing data and either decoding subject samples before or after analyses in a logical database is critical to data analysis. Often, data analysis requires revision and multiple check steps; being able to go back to raw data and the initial quality check steps and clearly understand the database organization ensures the accuracy of the final calculations and conclusions before statistical analyses.

A specific example of how proper lab notes and organized data can help in accurate first data analysis is provided in Table 16-1, Panel A, with the value shown in well A6. On first data analysis, it is clear that this value of 0.27 is different from the other two sample repeats in A4 and A5 (1.40 and 1.30, respectively). Being able to go back to a lab notebook might clarify this discrepancy. An organized experimental lab notebook for this experiment made note that the sample assayed three times in wells A4, A5, and A6 was more viscous than the other samples. There was a question about whether the full volume of sample was aliquoted into well A6 during the assay. Having these kinds of organized records allows us to make a well-informed decision to eliminate this value from calculations.

Many times, data analysis involves making challenging decisions. Organized assay notes and a careful scan of the database prior to actual calculations are critical; they allow scientists to make choices that yield the most accurate data possible. In this instance, if the incorrect value had been included in the calculation for sample 1, the mean of the triplicate values would have been 0.99. When it is correctly omitted, the mean value for sample 1 absorbance is 1.35 and the testosterone concentration is 2.2 ng · mL^{-1}. With the incorrect value, the **interpolated** testosterone value is 100% higher (4.3 ng · mL^{-1}). The example provided here is a clear case in which one value stands out. Without organized notes, it is not correct to arbitrarily exclude specific values. In truly ambiguous cases, it is better to rerun the assay for questionable samples. In extreme cases, it may be necessary to rerun the entire experiment.

Assessing Accuracy and Precision of Your Data: Controls and Intra-Assay Coefficients of Variation

There are also approaches that allow you to effectively scan large amounts of data. Although we will not discuss all approaches in detail here, you should understand that there are some key quantitative measures that can provide information about the quality of your data. One simple test of whether your assay is accurately detecting protein concentrations sufficiently is the results from control patient samples used during the assay. **Quality control samples** are different from known standard sample preparations. Standards prepared for a standard curve are often known concentrations of protein prepared from recombinant protein diluted

Table 16-1 Data from Example Testosterone Enzyme-Linked Immunosorbent Assays

Panel A

	1	2	3	4	5	6
A	3.03	2.78	2.89	1.40	1.30	0.27
B	2.59	2.49	2.50	1.10	1.11	1.09
C	1.99	2.09	2.06	0.64	0.51	0.60
D	1.54	1.43	1.48	0.84	0.79	0.82
E	0.79	0.83	0.80	1.19	1.20	1.14
F	0.25	0.26	0.25	1.23	1.16	1.15
G	0.17	0.16	0.17	1.61	1.43	1.57
H	0.06	0.07	0.04	1.15	1.19	1.17

Panel B

	1	2	3	4	5	6
A	std 1	std 1	std 1	1	1	1
B	std 2	std 2	std 2	2	2	2
C	std 3	std 3	std 3	3	3	3
D	std 4	std 4	std 4	4	4	4
E	std 5	std 5	std 5	5	5	5
F	std 6	std 6	std 6	6	6	6
G	std 7	std 7	std 7	7	7	7
H	std 8	std 8	std 8	8	8	8

Panel C

	1	2	3	Mean	SD	CV	%CV
A	3.03	2.78	2.89	2.90	0.13	0.04	4.32
B	2.59	2.49	2.50	2.53	0.06	0.02	2.18
C	1.99	2.09	2.06	2.05	0.05	0.03	2.51
D	1.54	1.43	1.48	1.48	0.06	0.04	3.71
E	0.79	0.83	0.80	0.81	0.02	0.03	2.58
F	0.25	0.26	0.25	0.25	0.01	0.02	2.28
G	0.17	0.16	0.17	0.17	0.01	0.03	3.46
H	0.06	0.07	0.04	0.06	0.02	0.27	**26.96**

Continued

Table 16-1 Data from Example Testosterone Enzyme-Linked Immunosorbent Assays *(Continued)*

	4	5	6	Mean	SD	CV	%CV
~~A~~	~~1.40~~	~~1.30~~	~~0.27~~	~~0.99~~	~~0.63~~	~~0.63~~	~~63.19~~
A	1.40	1.30		1.35	0.07[a]	0.05[a]	5.24[a]
B	1.10	1.11	1.09	1.10	0.01	0.01	0.91
C	0.64	0.51	0.60	0.58	0.07	0.11	**11.41**
D	0.84	0.79	0.82	0.82	0.03	0.03	3.08
E	1.19	1.20	1.14	1.18	0.03	0.03	2.73
F	1.23	1.16	1.15	1.18	0.04	0.04	3.69
G	1.61	1.43	1.57	1.54	0.09	0.06	**6.15**
H	1.15	1.19	1.17	1.17	0.02	0.02	1.71

Data from example testosterone ELISAs illustrate the use of standard curves and unknown sample measurements in triplicate measure. Panel A. Table rows A–H represent distinct samples. Table columns 1–3 show triplicate measurements for each respective standard sample with known concentrations. Table columns 4–6 show triplicate measurements for each respective patient sample with unknown concentration. Data point present in row A, column 6 (value = 0.27) is in strikeout font because it represents a value that suggests a bench-top error and should be eliminated from analyses. Panel B. IDs for the samples shown in panel A. Concentrations for standards 1–8 are 0, 0.1, 0.5, 2.0, 6.0, 18.0, 21.0, and 26.0 ng · mL^{-1}, respectively. Panel C. The means and standard deviations for each set of triplicates is shown in respectively labeled columns. Intra-assay CV is shown for each set of triplicate values. The values are calculated by dividing each standard deviation of three repeats for each sample by the mean of those three samples. To calculate %CV or CV as a percent value, the CV column is multiplied by 100. Five percent or less is acceptable for a CV within an assay. Hatched wells indicate wells in which the CV is high and questionable. In first data analysis, one must carefully address these issues. The values for wells A4–A6 were recalculated after eliminating the third of the repeats in A6 because of experimental error as noted in the text. This corrects the intra-assay CV issues and provides an example of how a large CV and organized lab notes may help in first steps in data quality control.
[a]It is important to note that calculating standard deviations with only two values and thus the CV calculations from this do not represent the most ideal scenario for truly evaluating variance. This example is provided to illustrate a general concept about easily identifying quality control issues in first data analysis.
std, standard; SD, standard deviation; CV, coefficient of variation; %CV, percent coefficient of variation.

in assay-suitable buffer. Biologic samples (patient samples, blood serum or plasma, tissue lysates, experimental cultured tissue/cell lysates or supernatant, etc.) are complex. Unknown proteins, molecules, compounds, and salts in actual experimental samples may complicate the kinetics of any assay's detection methods. For this reason, sometimes standard curves with known concentrations may follow a predictable mathematically definable pattern, but samples spiked with standards may not. Some assays circumvent this issue by asking you to perform a standard curve calculation in samples spiked with known amounts of recombinant protein.

In cases in which this is not part of the protocol, it is important to have patient control samples. Known positive and negative controls, in other words, in which amounts of a protein of interest (testosterone in our example here) are known to be high and low, can be used in the assay to determine if the assay can detect the difference in complex biologic experimental samples. For this assay, we ran two controls, or patient samples, that were known to be high and low in testosterone. The low patient control had an average absorbance value of 0.07, and the high patient control had an average absorbance of 3.00. Using the standard curve generated and explained in the next sections, the low control had 0.06 ng · mL^{-1} and the high control had 25.47 ng · mL^{-1}. Using two patient samples like this in an ELISA assay can demonstrate that the standard curve can be used to reliably predict protein concentrations in complex biologic samples. Biologic samples are complex matrices of proteins, salts, and molecules that may give different results from provided or prepared standards dissolved in simple buffer solutions. It is useful to include patient or biologic sample controls in addition to prepared comparative standards in these types of indirect assays, and first data analysis should certainly include control validation.

Among the many quality control steps in first data analysis is a simple calculation of **coefficients of variation** (CV). If you run each sample three times in a 96-well plate format, each set of three values should be either the same or fairly close to each other. The measure of how variable the repeats are from each other when run in the same assay conditions is **intra-assay CV** and is calculated by taking the standard deviation of the repeats for each sample and dividing by the mean for those three samples (6). The percent CV (%CV) is calculated by multiplying this ratio by 100. An intra-assay CV of 5% or less is typically acceptable and means that in your assay, when a sample was assayed multiple times (in this case, three times), the assay was reliable enough to give a similar value for that sample over and over again.

Table 16-1C shows the mean standard deviation and CV calculations for the example testosterone data. Larger and boldfaced font shows CVs higher than 5%. These values could easily be found in a large database by using a sort or search function to find all values above the threshold of 5%. In this way, you can easily spot where potential errors in accuracy or precision might have occurred and begin your data analysis by more closely examining these values. Samples that have high intra-assay CV are problematic because it is difficult to determine which of the replicate measures is accurate. High intra-assay CVs for multiple samples suggest an assay that lacks precision. It is important to note that low intra-assay CVs for an assay do not guarantee accuracy, although this observation does support the precision of the assay itself. You can choose to rerun questionable samples in a separate assay to determine the correct concentration. You can also go back to the notes and see if there is a single value among the three repeats that might have led to the variation. As previously discussed, we had rationale to eliminate the value in A6. Table 16-1C shows the CV calculations with and without the third value, although keep in mind that calculating a standard deviation and CVs with only duplicate values is not considered entirely useful or correct. Having within-assay controls and paying attention to precision of your multiple measurements per sample can help you make decisions to clean up your data before you begin formal analysis and interpolation as discussed in later sections.

Assessing Accuracy and Precision of Your Data: Inter-Assay Coefficients of Variation

Before moving on to the first calculations on quality-checked data, we should discuss the importance of **inter-assay CV**. In studies with many samples, it is unlikely that you will be able to run all samples in one assay with a controlled single set of conditions. This is also not wise, given that many of these assays require careful attention to each sample, and the greater the number of samples you attempt to run in a single assay, the greater likelihood of errors and variability at multiple steps. Thus, many times, samples are run in batches. Each time you run an assay, you must include a standard curve because standard curves can vary slightly from run to run. However, it is difficult to tell if one assay run on a given day is comparable to another run on another separate day. Inter-assay CV is a calculation that can tell you whether your multiple assays are relatable to each other.

Table 16-2, Panel A, provides an example of how you might run 60 samples when you have limited space or research technicians and need to spread the assays over three separate days. The most reliable experimental setup will include standards, high- and low-quality control samples, and, if possible, a subset of experimental samples run each day. Before you begin interpolation, you should verify using inter-assay CVs that the values that should be the same among the three days are reasonably close. Table 16-2, Panel B, illustrates how

Table 16-2 Calculating Inter-Assay Variation

Panel A

	Day 1	Day 2	Day 3
Common Samples Each Day (in duplicate or triplicate)	Standards 1–10	Standards 1–10	Standards 1–10
	High-quality control	High-quality control	High-quality control
	Low-quality control	Low-quality control	Low-quality control
	Patient sample 1	Patient sample 1	Patient sample 1
	Patient sample 2	Patient sample 2	Patient sample 2
Experimental Samples Unique to Each Assay (in duplicate or triplicate)	Patient samples 3–20	Patient samples 21–40	Patient samples 41–60

Panel B

	Absorbance Values for Sample 1		
	Day 1	Day 2	Day 3
	1.35	1.37	1.46
	1.42	1.38	1.42
	1.40	1.45	1.40
Mean of Triplicate Values	1.39	1.40	1.43
Standard Deviation of Triplicate Values	0.036	0.044	0.031
Mean of All Days (mean of means)	1.41		
Standard Deviation of All Means	0.019		
Inter-Assay CV	$0.109 \div 1.41 = 0.013$		
%CV	$0.013 \times 100 = 1.3\%$		

Calculating inter-assay variation based on running repeat samples every assay will provide a first quality control check. Panel A. This provides an example of how a researcher might plan to run repeat samples on each of three days for many samples that cannot be run in one single assay run or day or by the same person. Panel B. Even for the same samples run on separate days, there will be slight variability in the observed absorbance values for an ELISA. One of the first steps in data analysis is to calculate the inter-assay CVs to ensure that the same sample results in a similar calculated concentration each time the assay is run. An example calculation is shown.
CV, coefficient of variation; %CV, percent coefficient of variation.

you might calculate the inter-assay CV for one sample only. Like the intra-assay CVs, the inter-assay CVs should be less than 5% in the most conservative ideal situation. Inter-assay CVs above 5% for specific samples raise questions about the accuracy of any given sample concentration from your repeat runs. Inter-assay CVs above 5% for a large number of samples suggest that the assay you have selected is not precise for repeat runs on separate days. Again, it is important to note that inter-assay CVs that are less than 5% do not guarantee that an assay is accurate. To test for accuracy, one can use a variety of approaches including, spiking samples, using appropriate standards, and incorporating known control test samples in each of your runs.

Example First Data Analyses

Once you have verified the experimental controls, it is then possible to work with the pared-down data to calculate standard curves and interpolate the unknown sample concentrations. Following the approach provided in Figure 16-2, we first averaged the triplicate values for each respective standard. For example, the average of wells A1, A2, and A3 was 2.90 and this corresponded to the first standard, which was a sample with known concentration of 0 ng · mL^{-1}. The other standards were analyzed in the same way and graphed to determine the relationship between measured absorbance values and known testosterone concentrations (Fig. 16-3A). This example data illustrates a standard curve that is mathematically more complex than the simple linear relationship shown in Figure 16-2. Although many different types of mathematical equations or relationships will define a curvilinear shape that fits almost all the standard curve points, in first data analysis, we should also consult our understanding of the enzymatic detection reaction and perhaps the kit or assay components will come with detailed instructions on what type of kinetics the color-generating reactions typically follow. In this example, a parabolic or quadratic equation shape and a natural log equation can be generated to fit almost all of the points. You could use these equations to calculate what the testosterone concentrations of unknown samples might be from their observed absorbances. However, this assay came with instructions that suggested a special type of equation called a "five-parameter logistic equation." The calculations based on this standard curve will be used to determine all the unknown experimental sample concentrations. Thus, it is important to carefully consider what the most appropriate mathematical equation is to fit to the standard curve.

Once you determine the equation that the standard samples best fit, you can use that equation to estimate the protein concentration of the unknown samples. In our example Figure 16-3B, we have also used these standards to first calculate the high and low control samples as part of the quality check discussed already. Figure 16-3C shows the sample absorbances measured during the experiment, which were entered into the equation generated in Figure 16-3B. You also see the final result for the testosterone concentrations finally calculated to provide our final values for statistical analyses. In this case, because the equation was more complicated, we used statistical software to interpolate the unknown concentrations from the standard equations. There are a variety of software packages that are user-friendly and allow you to efficiently do these types of calculations for large datasets.

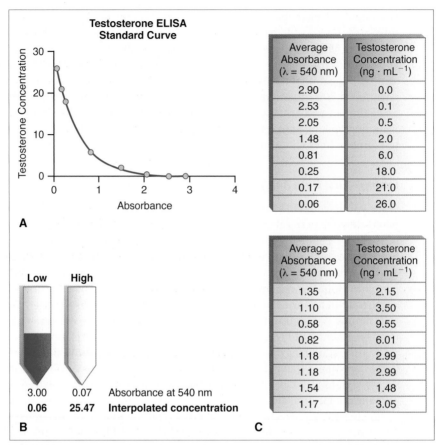

FIGURE 16-3:   A standard curve generated by plotting known testosterone concentrations vs. observed absorbances can be used to estimate the concentration of samples with unknown amounts of testosterone. **A.** Eight testosterone standards with concentrations 0, 0.1, 0.5, 2.0, 6.0, 18.0, 21.0, and 26.0 ng · mL^{-1} were measured by ELISA. Standard curve was calculated using GraphPad Prism 6.0. A five-parameter logistic equation best fit the curve plotted by graphing known testosterone concentrations vs. mean absorbance (triplicate). **B.** This equation was used to determine the concentration of two quality control samples (high and low). **C.** The same equation was also used to calculate the testosterone concentrations (ng · mL^{-1}) of eight unknown samples. The absorbances shown are the average of the observed repeat values for each sample.

Other Considerations

Often, novice researchers will stop here and consider the first data analyses complete. First data analysis includes organized and trimmed databases, careful lab notebook documentation for decision-making, assessment of variability within replicates and between assays to assess precision, quality control checking to ensure reasonable accuracy of the standard curve, and equations for interpolating unknown concentrations. However, before statistical analysis, this process is not complete. You must assess the concentrations with a critical mind, especially in the case of human or patient samples where there are many known reference ranges and clinical thresholds for what is physiologically normal and if not normal, then possible. Evaluating many published and peer-reviewed sources that provide normal and pathologic testosterone concentrations in serum/plasma give us confidence that our values are in a realistic physiologic range (1–4,14). It is a useful exercise to go and look in the literature for the reported testosterone concentrations in plasma and serum. Consider the variability, the different units of concentration presented, and the context of each study you find.

WESTERN BLOTTING

Background

Another commonly used assay technique in the study of exercise is the Western blot analysis that is used to detect the presence, molecular weight, relative abundance, and/or modified state (*i.e.*, phosphorylation) of a specific protein. These aspects of protein changes in an exercise science research protocol are not detectable with ELISA. Western blotting is typically more expensive than ELISA but provides more information about protein changes occurring in exercise protocols. The Western blotting method was developed independently by three separate groups in 1979. Renart, Reiser, and Stark (10) at Stanford University were the first to publish, whereas Harry Towbin's group (12) in Basel, Switzerland, published the method most closely followed today. Simultaneously, W. Neal Burnette in Robert Nowinski's lab at the Fred Hutchinson Cancer Research Center developed a similar method and gave the Western blot its name (5) (after the Southern blot invented by Edwin Southern [11] to detect DNA).

Western blot analysis comprises five steps: (a) sample preparation and total protein determination, (b) separation of proteins through **electrophoresis**, (c) transfer of the proteins from a gel to a solid membrane (blotting), (d) probing with antibodies, and (e) visualization and data analysis. These steps are illustrated in Figure 16-4. Samples are prepared by homogenizing tissue or lysing tissue/cell suspensions and then extracting protein fractions from these lysates. Protein extraction allows you to collect almost all cytosolic protein and should take place under cold conditions along with a protease inhibitor to prevent the proteins from being denatured. Total protein concentration is usually determined using a spectrophotometer. A color change occurs when a dye such as Coomassie blue binds to proteins in a sample extract or standard. The concentration is calculated from the spectrophotometric absorbance reading (see sample calculations of protein concentration from "Enzyme-Linked Immunosorbent Assays" section earlier).

Knowing the extract's concentration is important for determining the amount of protein to load, or what volume is needed to load each sample onto the gel during electrophoresis to ensure that the same amount of protein is being compared across lanes. Once sample concentration is determined, a known volume is diluted with a loading buffer containing a dye such as bromophenol blue (for visualizing the sample as it runs through the gel) and glycerol (for ensuring the sample sinks into the well). The solution is then heated, which denatures the proteins' three-dimensional structures to reveal their negatively charged regions. (The proteins' exposed negatively charged regions cause them to move through the

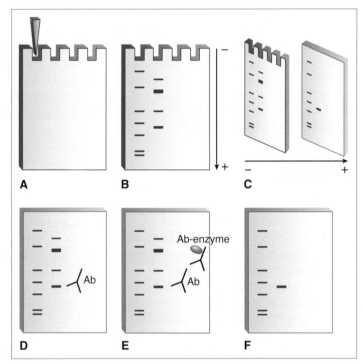

FIGURE 16-4:   Western blotting involves a number of independent steps. **A.** Samples are mixed with a loading buffer containing dye and glycerol, heated, and loaded into a well of a polyacrylamide gel submerged in a buffer. **B.** An electric current is applied to the system, which causes the proteins to migrate through the gel from the anode to the cathode. **C.** The proteins are then blotted onto a solid membrane by applying another electric current. The membrane is sandwiched between the gel and the cathode. **D.** The membrane is treated with a blocking agent, washed, and incubated with a primary antibody which recognizes the protein of interest. **E.** The membrane is washed to remove the excess primary antibody then incubated with a secondary antibody that binds to the primary antibody and emits a signal. **F.** The protein of interest is detected by film or a fluorescence detection box which captures a digital image of the fluorescing secondary antibody. The intensity of the fluorescent signal can be quantified by various programs.

electric field applied during electrophoresis.) The sample is loaded into a lane on an agarose and polyacrylamide gel (Fig. 16-4A). Gels can be prepared in the lab or purchased from a manufacturer. Gels vary in acrylamide concentration, which affects the size of the pores in the gel and are used for different applications. Gels are formed in a mold and designed with small wells for loading samples (see Fig. 16-4).

During electrophoresis, an electric current is applied to the gel which is oriented between two electrodes in a buffer. Proteins migrate through the gel away from the **anode** (negative electrode) and toward the **cathode** (positive electrode) at different rates according to charge and molecular weight (Fig. 16-4B). Smaller proteins travel more easily and therefore faster through the porous membrane than large proteins.

Once proteins are separated by electrophoresis, they are transferred or "blotted" onto a solid membrane (composed of nitrocellulose or polyvinylidene difluoride [PVDF]), also using an electric current which is run perpendicular to the original current to mobilize proteins out of the porous gel and onto the solid state membrane (Fig. 16-4C). It is important that the membrane is sandwiched between the gel and the cathode causing the proteins to migrate out of the gel and onto the membrane.

After electrophoresis and blotting, the proteins must be visualized for analysis. Visualization uses fluorescently tagged antibodies that bind to proteins of interest while emitting fluorescent light. The membrane is washed in a buffer (phosphate buffered saline [PBS] or tris-buffered saline with Tween 20 [TBST]) and then incubated in a solution of generic protein such as non-fat dried milk or 5% bovine serum albumin (BSA) diluted in wash buffer. This step "blocks" the antibodies from binding non-specifically to the membrane. Next, the membrane is incubated in wash buffer containing the primary antibody which binds to the protein of interest (Fig. 16-4D). The concentration of antibody depends on the manufacturer's suggestion and trial and error by the researcher. Excess primary antibody is thoroughly rinsed from the membrane through subsequent washing steps. Buffers such as PBS or TBST are used to wash the membrane, which is important to minimize non-specific staining that causes high background. The membrane is then incubated in secondary protein which is labeled with an enzyme such as horseradish peroxidase (HRP) or a fluorescent tag (Fig. 16-4E). The membrane is gently washed again, and the secondary enzyme is detected by the signal it emits. Secondary antibodies containing enzymes that require a reaction to emit light are incubated with its substrate according to manufacturer's directions. Secondary antibodies that are fluorescently tagged emit light when excited by high-intensity light sources such as lasers. This light is captured on film or by various detection boxes that turn the signal into a digital image for analysis. Only the protein of interest bound first by the primary antibody (see Fig. 16-4D) and then detected by the secondary reporter antibody (see Fig. 16-4E) will result in a detectable band on the final blot (Fig. 16-4F). How far this single amount of protein or "band" has traveled indicates the relative size to other proteins that have traveled through the gel. How dark or bright the band is indicates how much protein is present.

Quality Controls

First analysis will also reveal the purity of the protein extract or homogenate. Lanes that appear as one smear, blurred, or wavy may indicate contaminated or poorly prepared samples. Western blotting is a complex technique with many steps that require troubleshooting including sample preparation; gel selection; and antibody specificity, quality, concentrations, and incubation times. A number of controls, somewhat similar to those discussed for ELISA techniques, are critical to first data assessment.

Among the many quality controls, you must load a positive control from a source containing the protein of interest along with a negative control from a null cell line or tissue extract. The positive control is used to confirm the identity of the protein in question and the activity of the antibody you have chosen for your detection method. The negative control allows you to verify that antibody staining is specific and will not detect other proteins. In first data analysis in Western blotting, you must verify the presence of a band in your positive control sample and the lack of a band in a negative control sample. If the results for controls are not as expected, then you must revisit the experimental conditions, reagents, and most importantly, the antibody that you chose that should have specificity for the protein of interest. There may be some critical experimental error if your positive and negative controls do not yield expected results. This aspect of quality control in first data analysis is relatively straightforward. The assessment can be qualitative or a simple check of whether the bands are present or not by visual inspection.

In addition to positive and negative controls, it is critical that you load a standardized protein ladder solution composed of proteins with known molecular weight onto the gel alongside actual samples as a comparison. Protein ladders are available commercially and provide a range of different molecular weights. In Figure 16-4, a representation of the protein ladder is in the far left column of the gel and blots. As you can see, the protein ladder has a number of bands that correspond to known molecular weights and often has color indicators to distinguish between bands. The location of the band that is measured in your sample in the second column of the gels and blots shown in Figure 16-4 will give you an indication of how large your detected protein is. It should match up with known information about your protein of interest. If the molecular weight position of your band does not correspond to the known molecular weight of your protein of interest, again, it is critical to revisit the experimental design and antibody specificity. It may also be necessary to explore whether other forms of your protein exist in multimers or complexes as well as in pre- or pro-forms prior to post-translational processing.

Finally, the most ideal Western blot assay includes a standard curve run simultaneously on the gel as described in a recent publication (9). Much like ELISAs, using standard curves and positive and negative controls and repeating similar samples across multiple separate gel runs or Western blot assays allows for the first quality control steps to ensuring accurate and precise protein concentration determination.

Example First Data Analyses

Once you have verified the quality of your Western blot experiment by assessing all the controls similarly to the way you would in an ELISA, you can begin first quantitative data analysis. Data acquired from Western blot analysis is considered semi-quantitative. In other words, it provides a relative comparison of the amount of protein present in each sample. Loading of the samples and the blotting process vary between each blot, making exact quantification of protein concentration difficult. Also, the signal emitted from secondary antibodies is not linear across the concentration range of samples, so it should not be used as a precise quantification of protein concentration. Programs such as Quantity One (BIO-RAD) and Image J (National Institutes of Health [NIH], Bethesda, Maryland) are available for analyzing blots. These programs allow researchers to manipulate and analyze images without changing the properties of the original image. They quantify the relative intensity of fluorescent bands by assigning an arbitrary value to pixel intensity, an indication of protein concentration.

An example of Western blot and its quantified data are shown in Figure 16-5. These blots measure the amount of phosphorylated FoxO1 (P-FoxO1) protein from mice fed different diets (Fig. 16-5A). Actin bands are shown as a comparison of the amount of total protein added to each sample lane. The intensity of the bands was measured by a program that quantifies pixel intensity, and the data were plotted (Fig. 16-5B). The data in

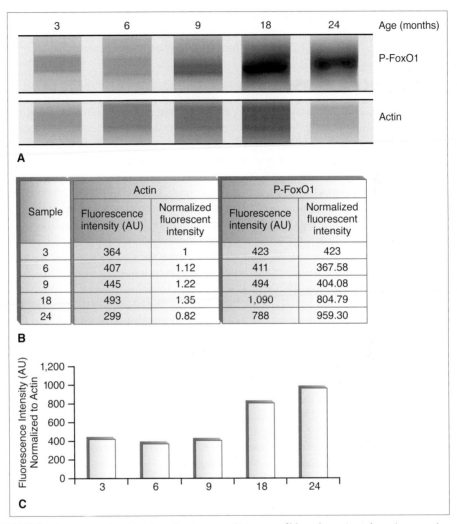

FIGURE 16-5:   Western blot data allows you to take images of blotted protein and acquire approximate relative protein concentration from pixel intensity. **A.** Example blots of protein extracts livers of B6 mice. Mouse livers were collected at 3, 6, 9, 18, and 24 months. Protein extracts were prepared from liver sections and used for Western blot analysis. Membranes were probed with antibodies against P-FoxO1 and actin. Visualization of the secondary antibodies revealed bands at the expected molecular weights. **B.** Pixel intensity for each P-FoxO1 band was analyzed using Image J and normalized to the pixel intensity for the actin bands. **C.** Bar graph showing the fluorescence intensity of P-FoxO1 normalized to actin levels.

Figure 16-5 provide an example of how visual blot data may be quantified for comparison between groups or treatments. This approach should be used for repeat measurements of the same sample, which should be relatively precise (intra-assay CV) and for repeat measurements across multiple blots (inter-assay CV). The assessment of repeat measurements as an indication of how precise your experiments along with quality control checks and standard curves to ensure the accuracy of your measurements are similar to those described previously for ELISA data analysis. In the next section, we describe image-based data and how first analysis might vary slightly for microscopy experiments.

FLUORESCENCE MICROSCOPY

Fluorescence microscopy is used to image specimens tagged with a **fluorophore**. These fluorophores are genetic modifications to proteins (such as green fluorescent protein [GFP] isolated from the jellyfish *Aequorea victoria*) or fluorescently tagged antibodies bound to proteins of interest (**immunohistochemistry**). A fluorescence microscope uses a high-intensity light source such as a mercury or xenon arc-discharge lamp to excite the fluorophore attached to a protein of interest. The fluorophore's electrons are excited to a high-energy state, and when they relax, they emit lower energy light. Filters in the microscope only let through light of the specific wavelength of the fluorophore of interest, giving researchers a clearer picture of a very specific area of a sample (Fig. 16-6). Fluorescent labeling of specimens is a useful tool for determining the presence and location of specific proteins in a sample tissue or cells. Fluorescence microscopy can be used to capture a variety of data including the presence or absence of the fluorescent signal, intensity of the signal, or the location of the signal (*e.g.*, in the cytoplasm vs. the nucleus). In exercise science, fluorescence microscopy is a powerful tool to not only assess specific protein level changes in tissue but also add information about the localization, trafficking, and tissue-specific abundance of proteins. Fluorescence microscopy can also be used to ask questions about cell types that change in a particular tissue. Furthermore, the newest techniques in fluorescence microscopy allow researchers to ask questions about small molecules, DNA, or metabolite changes with exercise; any fluorescent or taggable unit can be studied. These types of information cannot be acquired from ELISAs or Western blotting in which samples are either in suspension or homogenates and inquiry is based on antibody binding a specific region of a large protein. One particularly powerful use of fluorescence microscopy in exercise science is to explore muscle cell and tissue level changes.

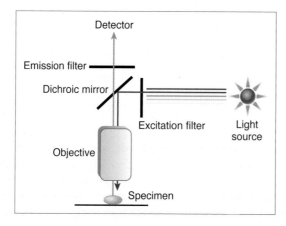

FIGURE 16-6: Fluorescence microscopy is based on excitation–emission patterns of specific fluorophores. High-intensity light emitted from a mercury or xenon arc-discharge lamp is filtered by the excitation filter and directed toward the sample by a dichroic mirror. This light excites the fluorophore attached to a protein of interest. When the fluorophore's electrons relax, they emit lower energy light. The emission filter only lets light of the specific wavelength of the fluorophore of interest through to the detector.

First analysis of captured images should be of control samples. Despite the different types of data acquired with microscopy versus biochemical assays, it is still important to have positive and negative controls. These controls, as discussed previously, will depend on what you are measuring. If your experimental model allows it, a positive control would be a tissue sample in which your fluorescent protein is guaranteed to be present and provide a detectable fluorescent signal. A negative control might, for example, be a tissue sample in which the genes responsible for production of that protein are knocked down or out and the detection of your fluorescent protein sample is impossible because production of that protein is entirely inhibited. In your negative control, it is an important first data analysis step to also verify that your tissue sample does have detectable protein in it, just not your protein of interest. This type of step, like in ELISA or Western blot, or any technique based on specificity of antibody binding and detection, is critical because these data provide the validation that your antibody is detecting the protein in which you are interested, and that in samples that should not express the protein of interest, there is no false-positive signal.

Additionally, in microscopy experiments involving treatments which can include not only exercise but also diet, supplements, or drugs with and without exercise, it is important to analyze the data of controls simultaneously and assess relative expression between control and treatment tissues. We provide an example of fluorescent protein changes with drug treatment for simplicity's sake, but the treatment can be anything more complex than a simple drug administration. An exercise bout or period of exercise training can certainly be the treatment itself. If you are measuring the expression or intensity of the fluorescently tagged protein in response to a drug or other treatment, have a sample that is treated with vehicle (no drug) as a control. To determine whether the drug truly had an effect on the presence of a fluorescently labeled protein, you can compare the microscopy images from a drug-treated sample versus a sample not treated with drug. The difference in fluorescent signal will define whether you make a conclusion that the drug treatment can be associated with a discernible difference in fluorescence intensity. In Figure 16-7, we have example data showing comparison between "fed" and "starved" tissue side by side. We also have two comparison groups, "B6" and "B6TR," side by side. Because there is variation in microscopy settings; technique; antibody binding; and fluorescent signal with user, time, equipment, and many other variables, it is important to have control and experimental groups treated within the same assay or experimental conditions.

Another general qualitative step in first data analysis of fluorescent images is to determine whether you have high-background fluorescence or not. If so, during image acquisition (while using the microscope), it is possible to adjust the filters in the microscope, the exposure times, or rerun the experimental preparing samples in a manner that reduces background (*i.e.*, increase wash times after antibody staining if you are performing immunohistochemistry). If you are attempting to reduce background following image acquisition, you may have to include some image optimization using software during your first data analysis. It is important that you are careful not to alter the image inappropriately or misrepresent the true results of an experiment in this process.

Finally, in acquiring images and doing final quantitative analysis on images, sometimes it is important to select random regions of interest (ROI) in your captured image for analysis. Computer programs such as NIH Image J have powerful tools for selecting ROI, measuring pixel intensity, adjusting thresholds (to minimize background fluorescence)

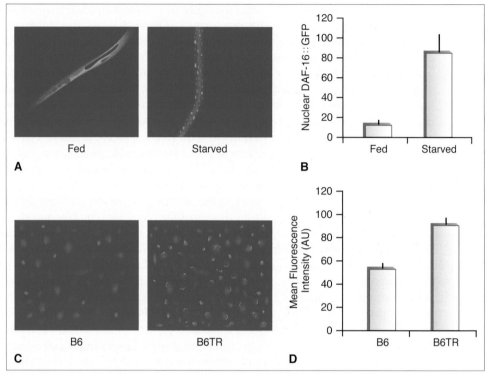

FIGURE 16-7: Fluorescence microscopy allows you to gather quantitative data about localization in tissues. **A.** *Caenorhabditis elegans* expressing GFP-tagged DAF-16 (DAF-16::GFP) protein were fed or starved for eight hours. Upon starvation, DAF-16::GFP leaves the cytoplasm and localizes to the nucleus. **B.** Quantified DAF-16::GFP localization. The data was generated based on the ratio of fluorescence intensity in the nuclei compared to the intensity in the adjacent cytoplasm. **C.** Mouse liver sections from a control mouse (B6) and a transgenic mouse that over-expresses FoxO1A (B6TR) stained for FoxO1A using immunohistochemistry. **D.** Quantified fluorescence intensity of FoxO1A.

as well as many other useful tools for manipulating and analyzing fluorescence microscope images without altering the raw data. Some examples of fluorescence microscopy data are outlined in Figure 16-7, and the corresponding quantitative data are shown in panels 16-7B and 16-7D. Again, as with any type of assay or experiment, there should be repeatability, and you must capture multiple images and make measurements on multiple samples. The intra-assay and inter-assay CV analysis is still important first data to collect in making your final summary conclusions.

SUMMARY

We have discussed three different types of experiments in which the format and precision of data acquired from each is slightly different. There are many other types of assays that cannot be covered here and that should be studied individually before planning an experiment when it comes to proper experimental design and first data analyses. However, there are a number of common themes in first data analyses, regardless of the type of assay you acquire your raw data from. The specific questions were presented in the chapter outline, so it is a useful exercise to revisit those questions now and use them as a guide to follow the example data provided. No matter the type of data you have, it is important to have organized experimental notes and annotated raw data that remains untouched. A copy of data can be used for analysis but having a raw copy as a backup is always good practice. Having quality controls (positive/negative controls and known standards for comparison) ensures that you can trust your data and results. Assessing the variability in your repeat measurements will give an indication of the precision of your data. The accuracy of your data will be determined by controls for the assay itself as repeatability does not prove accuracy. Thus, your assays must have assay accuracy and validity as well as being repeatable in order to be an effective measure. Finally, as you interpret and make conclusions about your results, it is important to keep the perspective of what is biologically or physiologically realistic. Many times a biochemical assay or a microscope image will result in data that came from an undetected human or mechanical error. Evaluating whether the data you have represents something rational and logical in the context of your hypothesis and working research model will help you make informed decisions about first data analysis.

GLOSSARY

Anode: in electrophoresis, refers to the positive terminal toward which anions or negative charges flow

Antibody: an immunoglobulin protein that recognizes specific antigens or regions of other proteins and has the ability to bind these specific regions

Antigen: a substance that produces an immune response

Cathode: in electrophoresis, refers to the negative terminal away from which anions or negative charges flow

Coefficient of variation: ratio of the standard deviation to the mean of a set of repeat values and may be used to determine the precision of repeated measurements

Electrophoresis: a method of separating molecules or proteins based on charge and size

Epitope: part of an antigen that is recognized by antibodies

Fluorophore: compound that can absorb energy and emit fluorescent light that is often used as a detection method in biochemistry and molecular biology

Immunohistochemistry: the art of detecting proteins in tissues by using antibodies that bind to the specific protein targets of interest

Inter-assay CV: the coefficient of variation among multiple independent experiments or assays

Interpolate: to estimate the value of an unknown based on the results from known comparison values

Intra-assay CV: the coefficient of variation within one experiment on repeated samples tested in a single assay run

Quality control samples: various types of samples run to validate the results and reliability of an experiment

Recombinant protein: proteins generated from expressing protein from engineered DNA expressed in living cells; these are proteins that are produced artificially

Sensitivity: the measure of how well a test can detect whether a target is present or not or the ability to detect true positives

Specificity: the measure of how well a test can avoid detecting false positives or the ability to avoid giving false positives

Spectrophotometric absorbance: quantitative measure of a material's ability to absorb light of a certain wavelength or a precise, quantitative measure of color

REFERENCES

1. Bardin CW, Hembree WC, Lipsett MB. Suppression of testosterone and androstenedine production rates with dexamethasone in women with idiopathic hirsutism and polycystic overies. *J Clin Endocrinol Metab*. 1968;28(9):1300–1306.
2. Bardin CW, Lipsett MB. Estimation of testosterone and androstenedione in human peripheral plasma. *Steroids*. 1967;9(1):71–84.
3. Bardin CW, Lipsett MB, French AM. Testosterone and androstenedione production rates in patients with metastatic adrenal cortical carcinoma. *J Clin Endocrinol Metab*. 1968;28(2):215–220.
4. Bhasin S, Cunningham GR, Hayes FJ, et al. Testosterone therapy in men with androgen deficiency syndromes: an Endocrine Society clinical practice guideline. *J Clin Endocrinol Metab*. 2010;95(6):2536–2559.
5. Burnette WN. "Western blotting": electrophoretic transfer of proteins from dodecyl sulfate-polyacrylamide gels to unmodified nitrocellulose and radiographic detection with antibody and radioiodinated protein A. *Anal Biochem*. 1981;112(2):195–203.
6. Diamandis EP, Christopoulos TK, editors. *Immunoassay*. San Diego (CA): Academic Press; 1996.
7. Engvall E, Perlmann P. Enzyme-linked immunosorbent assay (ELISA). Quantitative assay of immunoglobulin G. *Immunochemistry*. 1971;8(9):871–874.
8. Lequin RM. Enzyme immunoassay (EIA)/enzyme-linked immunosorbent assay (ELISA). *Clin Chem*. 2005;51(12):2415–2418.
9. Murphy RM, Lamb GD. Important considerations for protein analyses using based techniques: down-sizing Western blotting up-sizes outcomes. *J Physiol*. 2013;591(pt 23):5823–5831.
10. Renart J, Reiser J, Stark GR. Transfer of proteins from gels to diazobenzyloxymethyl-paper and detection with antisera: a method for studying antibody specificity and antigen structure. *Proc Natl Acad Sci U S A*. 1979;76(7):3116–3120.
11. Southern EM. Detection of specific sequences among DNA fragments separated by gel electrophoresis. *J Mol Biol*. 1975;98(3):503–517.
12. Towbin H, Staehelin T, Gordon J. Electrophoretic transfer of proteins from polyacrylamide gels to nitrocellulose sheets: procedure and some applications. *Proc Natl Acad Sci U S A*. 1979;76(9):4350–4354.
13. Van Weemen BK, Schuurs AH. Immunoassay using antigen-enzyme conjugates. *FEBS Lett*. 1971;15(3)232–236.
14. Vermeulen A, Verdonck L, Kaufman JM. A critical evaluation of simple methods for the estimation of free testosterone in serum. *J Clin Endocrinol Metab*. 1999;84(10): 3666–3672.
15. Yalow RS, Berson SA. Immunoassay of endogenous plasma insulin in man. *J Clin Invest*. 1960;39:1157–1175.

Database Development and Management

Beth A. Taylor, PhD, Baylah Tessier-Sherman, MPH, and
Linda S. Pescatello, PhD, FACSM, FAHA

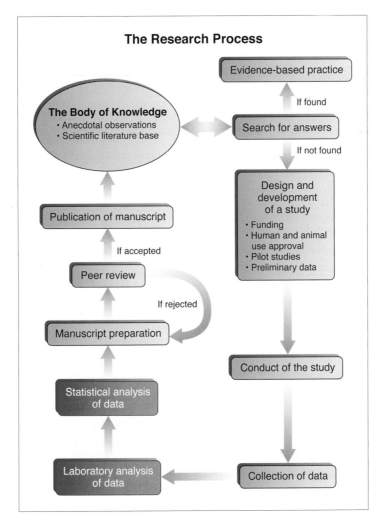

INTRODUCTION

Designing a research study may be one of the most grueling tasks a researcher will undertake, as you may have gathered while reading previous chapters. The time involved in idea conception, study logistics, estimating power calculations, conducting statistical analyses, and troubleshooting alternative hypotheses can be daunting to even the most experienced researchers. However, it has been the authors' experience that considering how to store and access data is an unexpectedly difficult and often over-looked aspect of study management. Most investigators currently use an electronic database to enter, store, and extract study data. An effective database can exponentially increase data use and facilitate ease of analysis. By contrast, a poorly designed database will at best cause needless delays in data management and use and at worst lead to data mismanagement, error, and even loss. Therefore, the purpose of this chapter is to describe the considerations for database design and management from data collection and entry to data retrieval and security. The chapter is structured around the authors' experience with a recent clinical trial, the effect of statins on skeletal muscle function and performance (STOMP) study (10,16) which will be referenced repeatedly so as to provide readers with concrete examples of the various suggested considerations and methodologies.

The Effect of Statins on Skeletal Muscle Function and Performance Study: Description

Hydroxy-methylglutaryl (HMG) CoA reductase inhibitors, or **statins**, are the most effective medications for reducing elevated concentrations of low-density lipoprotein cholesterol (LDL-C) and are the most widely prescribed drugs in the United States and the rest of the world. Statins have been extremely well tolerated in controlled clini-cal trials, but statins can produce a skeletal myopathy with symptoms ranging from mild complaints such as myalgia (muscle pain), cramps, and weakness to rhabdomy-olysis with renal failure. Although rhabdomyolysis is rare (14), the frequency of the less serious muscle side effects has not been well defined because these muscle symptoms are rarely reported in clinical trials (15). Muscle weakness can also occur with statin therapy, but weakness and muscle performance in general again have not been carefully examined. These muscle side effects have no documented serious sequelae, but they do compromise medication compliance and may also reduce physical activity and muscle performance. Therefore, better understanding of the frequency of muscle side effects as well as their effects on aerobic performance and muscle strength and endurance is of critical importance for clinicians weighing the costs and benefits of statin therapy, particularly in physically active individuals and/or older adults at risk for sarcopenia or reduced muscle strength.

Consequently, the **STOMP** study was a randomized, double-blind clinical trial con-ducted from 2007 to 2011, designed to assess the incidence of statin-associated muscle side effects in healthy adults using a rigorous study definition of myalgia. It also ad-dressed the direct effects of statins on aerobic exercise performance (maximal oxygen uptake) and skeletal muscle strength and endurance. The study recruited approximately

420 men and women older than 20 at three clinical sites (Hartford Hospital, University of Massachusetts, and University of Connecticut) over five years. Baseline lipid, liver, kidney, thyroid, and creatine kinase measurements were obtained. Subjects completed a baseline muscle symptom questionnaire and underwent baseline exercise testing including a maximal exercise test with gas analysis; hand grip, elbow flexor, and knee extensor strength testing; and a knee extensor endurance exercise test. Subjects were then randomly assigned to identical placebo or atorvastatin 80 mg daily in a double-blind fashion. Subjects were called twice monthly to ascertain symptoms and undergo a safety assessment including creatine kinase values and liver function testing after three months of treatment. Subjects underwent repeat testing after six months of treatment or after they developed muscle symptoms meeting the study's definition of statin-induced myopathy (new and unexplained muscle pain that abated on study drug cessation and was reproduced upon reintroduction of the study drug). The study schematic has been included (Fig. 17-1) so that readers may appreciate the complexity of the study design as well as the multiple measurements and considerations for database design necessary to store and use STOMP study data.

DATABASE DESIGN AND MANAGEMENT

When designing a research database, it is helpful for investigators to take a moment to assess their data needs from three viewpoints: data entry, storage, and analysis. When considering these viewpoints, incorporate the following points:

Type of Data Collected

Quantitative and qualitative data have quite different requirements with respect to database management. Quantitative data must be considered in terms of units of measurement, the standard number of significant digits reported for each variable, the accepted practice associated with rounding up or down, and the mode in which the investigator will seek to analyze data. An example of these considerations is blood pressure, which can be assessed as systolic blood pressure, diastolic blood pressure, and mean arterial pressure. Blood pressure is taken to the units position, so the relevant significant figure is one beyond the unit of measure (the 10th position). Researchers who enter blood pressure into the database as the standard clinical expression (*e.g.*, systolic/diastolic blood pressure, or 140/90 mm Hg) may be confounded by consequently attempting to analyze data which will be retrieved from the database as a decimal (140/90 or 1.56) rather than two distinct numbers (140 mm Hg and 90 mm Hg).

Qualitative data also require substantial planning for data entry because responses may be open-ended or limited to certain answers such as "some of the time, all of the time, none of the time," etc. Investigators then must determine whether such data are better entered from a drop-down list (which limits data entry to pre-selected responses) or in text boxes, which can be prohibitive for data analysis if uniform language is not used.

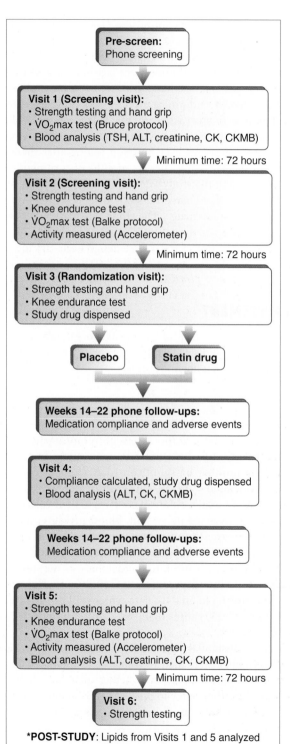

FIGURE 17-1: A schematic representing aspects of the STOMP study data collection.

Data Coding

Both quantitative and qualitative data are often coded to protect subject identity, categorize responses, and determine trends in otherwise continuous or non-numerical data. It is critical that investigators determine these codes prior to setting up a database because retroactively adding codes to a database often requires that data be reentered or altered using the new coding schematic. Moreover, institutional review boards (IRBs) will require language in the original application stating that subjects be given a unique identifier, no subject names or initials should be used, and the coding sheet be kept in a locked physical or electronic location available only to research personnel. Thus, it is beneficial for researchers to develop a **data coding scheme** prior to beginning data collection and use it consistently throughout the study.

Type of Data Collection

Researchers must also consider the type of data collection that will be used for the study. Will it be online, electronic, in-person, or through self-administered questionnaires? Electronic means of data collection can often be coupled with data entry such that subjects' information can be directly inputted into a database from online forms or electronic data submission. By contrast, if data are recorded by an observer (*i.e.*, a research technician) on paper or electronic forms, they will then be manually entered into the database, which will require a series of controls and safety checks to ensure reliable, safe, and accurate data management.

Size of Study Population

The sample size of the planned study (as well as the size of the proposed dataset) will drive the type of database necessary to store and manage study data. Small datasets can be managed with software programs such as Microsoft Excel and Access (Microsoft, Inc., Redmond, Washington) and FileMaker for Mac users (FileMaker, Inc., Santa Clara, California) where relatively few variables can be stored and accessed easily. By contrast, large datasets, such as those maintained by the government in health surveys (*e.g.*, National Health and Nutrition Examination Survey [NHANES] available at http://www.cdc.gov/nchs/nhanes.htm) require sophisticated data management systems that can be accessed securely by multiple investigators across multiple sites. A popular data management system that meets federal requirements for data security is Research Electronic Data Capture (**REDCap**), a secure web application designed exclusively to support data capture for research studies (3). The REDCap application allows users to build and manage online databases. REDCap software and support are available at no charge to institutional partners and is currently in production use for more than 81,000 projects (REDCap database: http://project-redcap.org/).

Number and Type of Confounding Variables to Consider

It is typical that researchers consider the main study outcomes they want to analyze when designing the database only to discover after data collection and entry is complete—and data analysis has begun—that new confounding variables should be considered in the analysis. Therefore, it is helpful for researchers to make a comprehensive list of *all* study data collected in the study and design a database that can facilitate entry and retrieval of these data. Nontraditional data such as changes in subject medication, new or unexpected life stressors, and dates of study visits may end up being critical in study analyses. Thus, researchers should be prepared to design a database that can store descriptive and supplementary data collected across multiple study visits as well as a database that includes the dependent and independent variables and covariates or any other confounding variables that will be examined.

Plasticity of the Database

Investigators might also consider how the proposed database for the current study could be used in the future and across multiple studies. For example, a well-designed database can be accessed repeatedly to merge and fluidly retrieve data from multiple studies, follow-up investigations, and even meta-analyses. Therefore, researchers who design databases with enough plasticity to hold data from a myriad of potential subject encounters of different types and purposes may find themselves with databases rigorous enough to answer questions far different and more complex than those originally planned.

Given the complexity of designing a study database, the authors of this chapter recommend that researchers develop a sample questionnaire prior to designing a database such as that shown in Table 17-1. This questionnaire can help the researcher better clarify some of the considerations described earlier and initiate new ideas regarding planned analyses and data sharing among multiple sites.

The Effect of Statins on Skeletal Muscle Function and Performance Study: Database Considerations

In the original grant application for the STOMP study, the plan for data management and storage was written as follows: "Paper recording forms will be developed for each measurement session and clinical encounter. Data from these forms will be entered into an Excel spreadsheet by the study personnel at each site and checked for completeness, inconsistencies, and aberrant values by the database manager at Hartford Hospital." Clearly, with a six-month clinical trial consisting of screening visits, biweekly phone calls, and six study visits, the proposed data management scheme was resultantly far more complex than originally described. STOMP data outcomes included anthropometrics, serologic results, physical performance tests, self-reported medical and social histories, questionnaires, and physical activity assessments.

Moreover, these data were collected repeatedly at multiple time points and across multiple sites. After approximately one year of data collection, STOMP investigators brought in a database design team—an independent contractor from a local software and database design company—to develop a database rigorous enough to facilitate data storage and analysis. The design team systematically examined all of the study source documents and recording forms by reviewing data from completed subjects (which were coded with unique identifiers) to better understand the types and quantities of data collected. The resulting database was a web-based data entry system (Microsoft SQL Database) that could

Table 17-1 Pre-Study Database Design Questionnaire

Question	Considerations
What type of data will be collected?	Researchers should provide a brief overview of the study including major outcomes as well as potential covariates and supplementary research questions.
What type of files will be used to store and use the data?	Options might include statistical analysis data files (SPSS, SAS) or Microsoft products (Excel, Access).
How will the data be collected?	Will the data be collected in surveys, interviews, self-report, online, lab tests, study visits, etc.?
What type of data will you be working with?	Researchers should consider quantitative and/or qualitative data; if qualitative, will the data be fully descriptive or limited to pre-selected answers?
What is the content of the data collected?	Researchers should list the broad range of measurements, such as anthropometrics, vital signs, demographics, screening data, survey responses, questionnaire scores, follow-up and longitudinal tracking data, dropout characteristics, etc. For each measurement, researchers should define acceptable units and whether a number is a whole number or integer and number of significant digits allowed by convention.
How many participants will be in the study/dataset?	Researchers will benefit from including subjects at all stages of the study: screenings, inclusion/exclusion, enrollment, and study completion. This allows for easy monitoring and reporting throughout the study.
What is the description and setting of the participants and study?	Researchers should think about the how, when, why, what, where, and who of a study to aid in fully understanding the scope of data collected and the ways in which the database can be structured to optimize planned and new analyses.
What is the data collection period?	Researchers should plan for the duration of data collection, and it will be beneficial to consider how best to track time and date in order to analyze temporal trends and their effect on outcomes.
Will the data be coded? If so, how?	If data will be coded, it is to the benefit of researchers to design these codes prior to initiating database entry.
How many people will have access to the data? Will there be multiple sites? How will the database be managed?	Answers to these questions provide the researcher with the impetus to consider how best to manage data security as well as to track data entry and management across multiple sites.

be accessed online from the multiple study sites. Each data technician was coded by identity and location so that data entry could be later examined by site and research assistants.

In retrospect, the most challenging problems with designing the STOMP study database were inherent in the volume and heterogeneity of data collected. Because the database had not been designed prior to starting data collection, the first year of study data from subjects included many responses to open-ended questions on the medical history and current well-being questionnaires and the physical performance tests that could not easily be coded for data entry.

Moreover, subjects who experienced adverse muscle events were entered into a complex myalgia network of human participants which required extensive reporting, testing, and subjective description of pain symptoms. After all these data related to myalgia were entered into the database, investigators repeatedly added coding schematics to the database to better quantify certain descriptors of muscle pain and statin side effects. These efforts were time-consuming and frustrating. This example highlights that it is imperative for researchers to thoroughly think through data collection and planned statistical analyses in entirety at the beginning of the research study prior to any data collection in order to design a database that is fully operational and functional for all data entered and used. This can be accomplished by setting up meetings between the key members of the research team and the statistician on the project to list primary outcomes and related independent and dependent variables and then working with the database manager to conceptualize how best to capture these data in the database.

CHARACTERISTICS AND DESIGN ASPECTS OF DATABASES

Options for Data Entry

Choosing a particular database to support your research depends largely on the method of data collection. For single users, Microsoft Excel and Access are the simplest and most accessible options. Although limited by its original design as a spreadsheet program, Excel does not require technical expertise for data input and storage. Microsoft Access is a **relational database** program that allows the user to input data in either a spreadsheet view similar to Excel or using customized forms. A relational database is a collection of tables, which are called "relations," with each table comprising a tabular format consisting of columns and rows. The rows contain the data or the data instances, with one value per cell. This type of database is termed "relational" because there are relationships within tables and between tables. Consequently, custom queries create reports for aggregate or sliced data in a variety of user-friendly formats.

For multiple users, REDCap is a relational database program that is web-based, making it practical for multi-site data gathering. As mentioned earlier, REDCap is free for institutional use and can be used to design surveys and databases (either via an online designer or a template file in Microsoft Excel). REDCap also tracks data manipulation and user activity and provides automated export procedures for seamless data downloads to Excel, PDF, and common statistical packages (SPSS, SAS, Stata, R). A backend (data storage) database managed by REDCap eliminates the need for the researcher to create a dedicated server as the primary repository for all user data. REDCap can also be used on mobile devices such as tablets. Microsoft Access has similar capabilities for multiple users but would require connection to a central server.

Database and Data Security

Creating a strategy for protecting data is typically done when writing IRB protocol. Please see comments made earlier in the "Data Coding" section about creating a subject unique identifier. Two primary aspects need to be addressed: **data at rest** (the physical storage of data) and **data in motion** (the transmission of data). Data at rest can take the form of paper surveys, databases on a computer, or files on a thumb drive. Security of subject information is critical and legally mandated according to the Health Insurance Portability and Accountability Act (HIPAA), which provides standards and security procedures for protection of a patient's health information (17). Therefore, a database must be secured with password protection and information coded when entered into the database by the subject's unique study identifier. Electronic communication with outside collaborators must involve only unidentifiable information. All study-approved electronic data must meet the security demands of the institution at which they are registered, which tend to be more strict in healthcare than academic settings. Data collected in paper form must be collected and recorded into the subject's source document folder, and all source documents should be kept in a locked office in one location at the study site. Only study staff, investigators, and monitors should have access to information.

Where protected health information is present, computers and accessory electronic storage drives must be encrypted using one of several forms of **cryptographic protocols**. Microsoft Excel and Access allow users to password-protect files with the option of adding encryption. The majority of external drives come with an optional encryption protocol. A computer's entire storage system can also be encrypted; however, it is often more efficient to protect only those files with vulnerable data as whole-system encryption can markedly slow down a system. The standard method of encryption is known as "Advanced Encryption Standard" (AES) 256-bit encryption (2) and is available on most devices in the form of several competing programs.

Data in motion refers to data being sent across a computer network, either hardwired or wirelessly. In order to secure data being sent, encryption should be done prior to the transmission to protect data from being intercepted. The file transfer protocol (FTP) standard does not provide end-to-end encryption. Although it can be configured to require authentication, this is not the same as encryption. The secure FTP (SFTP) protocol uses secure shell (SSH) to enforce end-to-end encryption and is preferred. There are several open-source FTP products available, although most academic institutions prefer affiliated researchers to use the FTP product supported by their information technology department. A properly configured SFTP server is also required.

COLLECTING AND ENTERING STUDY DATA

Certainly, the cornerstone of data management is the development of a standardized, secure, robust data collection technique that can be reproduced across multiple sites and future studies if necessary. Ideally, investigators will use the time between the initial award of funding and the approval by the IRB (which typically takes a few months) to finalize all aspects of data collection and management and develop electronic or paper forms that can be used for reference and subject contact. Finalizing data collection and management methods for each subject encounter usually requires pilot data collection and practice sessions to determine how best to streamline and standardize various procedures.

Data Collection and Standardization

Most large clinical trials use two techniques with which to address the standardization of study procedures (5). The first is the creation of documents that outline the **standard operating procedures** (SOPs) of a study. SOPs are typically manuals developed for every aspect of data collection and patient contact. They will include recruitment scripts, lists of prohibited medications for study participants, detailed checklists for inclusion/exclusion criteria, and comprehensive instructions for performing physiologic assessments, administering questionnaires, and other study procedures. Once they have been developed, they should be tested by having research technicians familiar with the project, but not involved in the production of the SOPs, perform a series of pilot or trial studies to determine how effective the SOPs are at reducing measurement error and variability in study techniques.

The second necessary recording form for standardization of study procedures is the **source document**, which is developed for every measurement and participant contact, again to ensure standardization of data collection. Source documents traditionally have been paper-based, thus being stored in a binder referenced by the research subject's study identification number. However, increasingly, source documents are becoming digitized such that research technicians can enter data in realtime via a laptop, smartphone, or tablet. The benefit of electronic recording forms is that they can be synchronized with a database such that data are automatically entered into the database at each subject contact rather than transferred from paper recording forms to the database at a later date.

Data Entry

As noted earlier, data entry can take two forms: recording study data on paper forms and transferring it to an electronic database at a later date and entering data electronically such that it automatically inputs (or can be transferred) into the study database. There are pros and cons to each method.

Using paper recording forms is still standard in many laboratories and research studies because it is far cheaper relative to the cost of upgrading to a completely digitized data collection system. This paper-based approach also allows investigators discretion and flexibility to record thoughts, comments, observations, and insights not directly included in the source documents. Paper recording forms can also allow student technicians or interns not directly trained with a specific study software to gain experience recording study data without an extensive preparatory time requirement. And finally, benefits of a paper recording form include the safety and reassurance of having a hard copy of study data that can be referenced without any dependence on electronics and online databases.

However, there are drawbacks to the use of paper recording forms. The most obvious is the potential for error associated with recording data twice (once on paper and once again electronically) as investigators move from data collection to data analysis and entry. Therefore, strict methodologic protocols should be put in place, consisting of a series of checks and balances to ensure that data entry from paper recording forms is accurate, valid, and reliable. In addition, paper recording forms can be damaged or destroyed by a variety of substances, and handwriting may be hard to decipher. Therefore, data stored on paper forms should not be considered secure, and every effort should be made to transfer paper-based data into the electronic database as soon as possible after the study visit.

Entering data electronically confers some obvious benefits for study investigators (5). The first and most obvious is efficiency, as data that are entered electronically can be available for analysis almost immediately. Electronic data entry allows investigators to easily generate the necessary reports on participant dropouts, subject characteristics, and data safety and monitoring often required by large granting agencies. It is far more cost-effective from an employee time perspective to require study technicians to enter data only once rather than record it on paper and then again in the database. Additionally, realtime data entry can often allow more complex and thorough data entry. Investigators are more likely to include supplementary data (*e.g.*, breath-by-breath oxygen uptake measurements rather than just peak oxygen uptake calculations) in a database if these data do not have to be entered manually and can be transferred from an electronic recording device. Moreover, electronic data collection improves uniformity and standardization of data input, as data collection by paper forms is more likely to include nonstandardized entries that are difficult to interpret. For example, investigators using paper entries more likely note responses and outcomes in descriptive sentences that can be open to interpretation when entering into a database.

However, the drawbacks of electronic recording of study data can be substantial. Research technicians must be trained in the recording software, and there needs to be a backup recording plan should the electronic device used for data entry fail. Also, there are no paper forms that contain raw data in the case of data corruption or massive database failure, and there is not an easy manner with which to check the accuracy of data recorded electronically. Furthermore, as only one study technician can enter data electronically (rather than multiple study technicians observing and using paper source documents throughout the study visit), then the study technician charged with data entry needs to be able to focus on this task and be mature, trustworthy, well-trained, and reliable.

Finally, when data are collected electronically, they are instantaneously available for analysis. This can tempt investigators to analyze data at multiple time points throughout the study, a practice which increases the likelihood of type I error (7). For example, significance set at $P < .05$ indicates that the probability of an effect occurring randomly (by chance) will occur five out of 100 times. Therefore, conducting repeated analyses of the data throughout the study simply increases the likelihood that findings will be artifactual as multiple looks at the data augment the chances of a random event. Repeated analyses throughout the study may also bias ongoing study data entry if study outcomes appear different than expected or show considerable variability. It is therefore common practice that the plan for data analysis be fixed prior to beginning the study, with outcomes being measured at pre-selected time points according to costs and benefits of continuing versus stopping the study. The ease with which electronic data entry permits analysis to occur should not alter this statistically robust practice.

Accuracy, Validity, and Reliability Methodology

A plan for repeatedly overseeing data collection and entry should be developed prior to initiating data collection, and study investigators should plan to report the results of these accuracy and reliability assessments at regular study meetings and to personnel (institutional, regulatory, and/or fiduciary) overseeing the research. A data review schedule should also be created so that investigators develop a routine plan for quality control checks on the data in a recurring and timely manner. Table 17-2 provides an example quality review schedule. Individuals designated to supervise data collection (the principal or co-investigator, study manager, and/or laboratory manager) should review all data collection forms on an ongoing basis for data completeness and accuracy as well as protocol compliance.

Table 17-2 Example Quality Review Schedule		
Data Type	**Frequency of Review**	**Reviewer**
Subject accrual (adherence to protocol regarding demographics, inclusion/exclusion)	Biweekly	Principal investigator and co-investigators
	Biannually	Data Safety Monitoring Board
Adverse event rates (excluding serious adverse events, which must be reported immediately)	Monthly	Principal investigator and co-investigators
	Biannually	Data Safety Monitoring Board
Compliance to treatment	Quarterly	Principal investigator and co-investigators
	Biannually	Data Safety Monitoring Board
Out of range (non-clinically significant) laboratory data	Yearly	Principal investigator and co-investigators
	Yearly	Data Safety Monitoring Board

Collected data can be verified with the following methods. Study staff should perform routine quality assurance checks and calibrations on equipment to calculate coefficients of variation for within-subject and between-tester variation (9). If paper recording forms are used, then study personnel should also randomly select patient binders to audit for completeness and accuracy. Study personnel may also choose to audit all patient information collected after each subject has completed the study to check for aberrant values and missing data. This is especially good practice because IRBs frequently audit studies (especially federally funded studies), and study personnel should be vigilant about making sure study records are accurate and orderly on a prospective rather than retrospective basis. All paper and electronic source documents should include the date of testing and initials of staff who performed the procedures so that any questions regarding data can be referred to the individual who performed the data collection. In the case of data collection involving physiologic samples, such as tissue or blood, samples can be archived to verify aberrant values. This latter procedure is useful given that funding for additional analyses is typically not available in the original grant application, so the archived samples serve not only as a backup for current data collection but also a databank for future investigations.

Checking for Outliers and Measurement Errors

Outliers (extreme data points) can arise from either measurement error or inherent physiologic variability. Outliers can reduce the statistical power of many tests and increase the probability of a type I or type II error (9). Moreover, outliers that arise from measurement error are of particular concern because they introduce variance into a dataset associated with methodology rather than physiologic outcomes, and thus, identifying and assessing potential explanations for outliers is a critical aspect of data collection and analysis. There are many common methods with which to assess a dataset for outliers and other measurement errors (*e.g.*, zero values or input errors) and many proposed solutions for dealing with outliers and errors once they have been identified (1,11).

The most frequently used solution in physiology for continuous dependent variables involves calculating and standardizing residuals (the difference between the individual data point and the mean of the dataset normalized to the standard deviation); outliers are then detected as values that exceed a pre-selected threshold (4). However, there are multiple other methods with which to detect outliers, and statistical software packages identify outliers through a variety of modalities. Moreover, genetic studies use different approaches to statistical analyses involving heterogeneity of data, given that variations in single nucleotide polymorphisms are not easily classified within a standardized normative range (13). The most important principle is to determine the appropriate methods to be used prior to initiating data collection and then apply a systematic and uniform technique with which to treat all data. Should outliers be detected, the original source documents and/or testing output (if they exist) should be checked for accuracy and to determine whether testing or sampling error indicates that the data should be excluded from analyses. Given the ethical considerations associated with manipulating or removing any data from a dataset, it is of critical importance that work with outliers (or other data deemed inaccurate) be disclosed to the study team and any individuals overseeing the project so as to maintain data integrity and transparency.

Problem Solving for Potential Data Integrity Issues

Independent of methodologic data problems (*i.e.*, outliers, data inaccuracies, measurement errors), it is possible that other data integrity issues may arise during the routine use of the database. These problems include instances of missing or nonsensical data, difficulties retrieving qualitative data, and unexpected transformation of data between data entry and data retrieval (*e.g.*, data that are entered as a decimal but retrieved as a whole number).

Troubleshooting these data issues can be frustrating and time-consuming. Therefore, it is advised that the database design and maintenance be treated as any other initial startup step of the study: with collaborative discussion, thorough planning, and substantial pilot work. The initial database design phase should also include defining and programming accepted variable input. For example, defining an input field as a number will prevent inadvertent text from being entered in that field. In addition, several subjects should be entered initially and data accessed and retrieved to ensure functionality. The importance of this step cannot be overemphasized given the time that will be invested throughout the study in data entry.

Moreover, the database manager (or study manager) should maintain the data through a series of routine checks, which may consist of running subject demographics, conducting quality control checks, assessing accuracy of one particular variable over a period of time, and cross-checking research technician reports of data entry with database input and output. In addition, when problems with the database do arise, the database manager should approach the problem by making a comprehensive list of steps and tasks to troubleshoot. It is possible that one or more errors in the process of data collection and analysis have combined to create data inaccuracies, and therefore, working through a checklist of potential data integrity issues will ensure that any database problems are thoroughly addressed.

The Effect of Statins on Skeletal Muscle Function and Performance Study: Data Collection, Entry, and Accuracy

The STOMP study used paper recording forms to ensure that all subject encounters were uniform between the three study sites. The study manager visited the three sites routinely to check study binders to ensure synonymous data management between the sites. Any questions about data collection, entry, or accuracy were addressed at biweekly study meetings conducted at the principal investigator's institution. Once the database was created and data entry began, each research technician was given a unique database identifier so that the database manager could track data entry at each site and for each individual. Completed and entered study binders were sent to the principal investigator's institution to be stored so that any questions on data accuracy could be addressed quickly and by the same individual (the database manager).

As data entry progressed, the database manager used the database for generation of routine safety data and subject demographics. This process allowed the database manager to assess whether the weekly reports generated from each site on the number of subjects entered into the database matched the subject data being retrieved from the database. The database manager also retrieved subject data on multiple variables (from a pre-determined list) to assess whether data were being entered and stored accurately. This procedure allowed him or her to catch potential data inaccuracies attributable to data entry or database design. For example, certain serologic variables, if measured below a certain level, were reported by the laboratory as "below the detectable limit of the assay." The study team determined that no value would be entered for these subjects. However, when data were retrieved from the database, a zero value was (unexpectedly) automatically generated to fill the spot of the missing data. Because this erroneous entry created an artifact in the dataset, the database manager was able to catch the error and work with the database designers to change the default retrieval function. Other systematic mistakes in data entry were also caught in this manner and included slight discrepancies between sights in entering qualitative descriptive data or coding social data from dropdown boxes. In STOMP, constant analysis of study variables on a routine basis by generating lists from the database served to quickly identify omissions and errors in data entry that could substantially impact data analysis.

STATISTICAL SOFTWARE USED FOR ANALYSIS

Table 17-3 provides a summary of the most common data management and statistical analysis software programs used by exercise, health, and social science researchers. A researcher's favored program is typically a function of what graduate program he or she attended as opposed to what functionality is most needed. However, understanding the strengths and limitations of these programs is essential, and the most productive researchers will likely use a variety of programs to serve different needs. Because data come in all formats and data collection often originates in Microsoft Excel or Access, data transformation software is a valuable tool for most researchers. For example, StatTransfer (Circle Systems, Seattle, Washington) allows researchers to choose the input and output format of their data, alter variable types, and create subsets of data. StatTransfer uses a menu-driven interface and is available on all operating systems.

Table 17-3 Common Statistical Analysis Software Programs Used in Health and Social Science Research

Statistical Software	Overview	Benefits	Limitations
R (Institute of Statistics and Mathematics; Vienna, Austria) http://www.r-project.org/	R is a free, multi-platform programming language increasing in popularity due to expanding functions. The core package is enhanced by thousands of user-created packages all available online.	Open-source abundant list serves for reference; new add-on capabilities created regularly; superior graphing.	Large number of add-on packages can be difficult to navigate; steep learning curve; historically not good for big data.
SAS (SAS Institute, Inc., Cary, North Carolina) http://www.sas.com/	SAS has long been considered the standard in statistical computing, and it excels at data manipulation and analysis of large datasets.	Exceptional interactive list serve run by SAS; supports advanced hierarchical modeling techniques; wide user audience allows for an abundance of online manuals.	Poor graphing abilities; expensive and annual licenses required; not currently supported on Mac unless using a virtual Windows operating system.
SPSS (SPSS, Inc., Armonk, New York) www.ibm.com/software/analytics/spss/	SPSS is the most user-friendly package, offering both menu-driven and command-line interfaces. Wizards available for common functions.	More intuitive to use given the point-and-click design; multi-platform support; variety of graphing capabilities; readable program manuals make for an easy learning curve.	Easy to make mistakes and not have a record of commands without intentionally reading and saving command outputs; as the program has expanded into more advanced capabilities, they are now sold separately from the base program; typically lags in incorporating emerging statistics.
Stata (StataCorp, LC, College Station, Texas) http://www.stata.com/	Stata is another full-service data management and statistical analysis program that originally used only a command-line interface. It has since incorporated a menu-driven interface that allows a more user-friendly environment.	Use of the menu and dialogue boxes will automatically create and display a log of the command code created; multi-platform support; excellent online support community; supports hierarchical modeling techniques.	Poor graphing abilities; less efficient at processing very large datasets than SAS.

OTHER CONSIDERATIONS FOR DATABASE MANAGEMENT

There are several other important decisions that can substantially impact the management of the database and should be considered thoughtfully prior to initiating database design and data entry. These decisions include the pivotal question of the individual who will be designated to oversee and manage the database. Ideally, this individual will be a senior research technician with database experience who has committed to staying with the institution for the duration of the study. He or she should be involved in the initial database design because the database manager often provides a unique perspective that is more functional and utilitarian than theoretical. Moreover, the individual overseeing the database should be fully familiar with study procedures and variables collected. Familiarity with study data and techniques ensures that the database manager is able to catch problems and troubleshoot them more easily than an untrained technician. It is also helpful if the database manager understands and is able to work with some of the proposed statistical methods and software programs earmarked for data analysis. This familiarity will allow the study team to more easily transition between data entry and storage and data analysis because an effective database manager will be preparing data retrieval for the format necessary for analysis. And finally, the database manager must be able to understand basic reporting requirements necessary for IRBs, granting agencies, and data and safety monitoring boards. Understanding these requirements will allow the individual a level of autonomy in managing study data necessary for routine reporting.

Although it is ideal to find a database manager and research team that will be employed for the duration of the research study (and a period of time thereafter), it is highly unlikely that the research team will remain wholly the same for the proposed study period. Thus, it is imperative for the principal investigator and/or study manager to cross-train multiple individuals on the various steps of data entry, management, storage, and retrieval.

Moreover, creating an SOP for all study procedures related to the database can ensure that unexpected staff turnover doesn't temporarily impede database use. A plan for developing the database manual and cross-training research staff routinely should be created at the beginning of data collection.

Additionally, the research team must consider the sustainability of long-term storage and data retrieval using the study database. For example, if the database is stored on an institutional server that can be accessed on multiple sites, it may eventually need to be moved to a permanent location so as not to take up server space indefinitely at the original institution. Or, the principal investigator may move institutions and wish to take the database to another facility. Therefore, the database design should take into account how flexible the investigators wish to be in moving the database and where the long-term storage of the data will take place. Moreover, the software programs used for any of the steps in data entry, storage, and retrieval should be considered with respect to longevity and use with other programs. For example, if the database is built using proprietary software, long-term maintenance may be difficult, as upgrades may occur outside of the length of the original contract. Moreover, proprietary software may not synchronize well with other mainstream statistical programs. Therefore, investigators are urged to consult with other research teams who have used similar data tools to determine the best combination of programs and designs for the anticipated needs of the study both in the short and long terms.

Another consideration is how widely available the dataset will be to other researchers after the study has been completed. Although public access to depersonalized study data is a mandate now of most registered federally funded clinical studies (8), smaller studies that are funded through non-governmental sources may not be subject to these same public requirements. Therefore, investigators should carefully consider who may ultimately have access to the study database prior to designing it. If the database is going to be widely accessible to other researchers not familiar with the project, then the design, coding, functions, and presentation of the database should be universal and easy to access and use. Researchers may thus want to replicate an existing publicly available database or design their database around common themes and data storage procedures so as to encourage data sharing among investigators and minimize interpretation issues.

DISCUSSIONS AND CONCLUSIONS

This chapter has provided a structural framework for database design and maintenance as well as insights from the authors' own experience with database development and management in the STOMP study. Although the material provided cannot capture every aspect of data entry, management, and retrieval, it provides a comprehensive guideline for considerations and procedures critical to creating a study database that facilitates ease of data input and output. Readers are also encouraged to consult additional published resources for a more extensive review of the topic (12), and a list of helpful statistical and data management resources is included in Table 17-4.

In conclusion, there are several fundamental aspects of database design and management which the authors summarize as major points and take-home messages of the chapter. They are as follows:

- Database design should be initiated prior to or at the beginning of data collection. Following this procedure ensures that the flow of data from collection to storage occurs quickly, reducing the possibility of error and even loss in a dataset.
- Database design should be thoughtful, well-planned, and practical. It should directly answer the needs of the study by being structured around proposed hypotheses and associated statistical analyses as well as potential future uses of the dataset.

Table 17-4 Resources for Database Management and Statistical Analyses
Centers for Disease Control and Prevention website [Internet]. Data security and confidentiality. Atlanta (GA): Centers for Disease Control and Prevention; [cited 25 Sep 2013]. Available from: http://www.cdc.gov /nchhstp/programintegration/Data-Security.htm Cody RP, Smith JK. *Applied Statistics and the SAS Programming Language*. 5th ed. Upper Saddle River (NJ): Pearson Education; 2005.
Dawson B, Trapp RG. *Basic and Clinical Biostatistics*. 4th ed. New York (NY): McGraw-Hill; 2004.
dos Santos Silva I. Designing, planning and conducting epidemiological research. In: *Cancer Epidemiology: Principles and Methods*. France: International Agency for Research on Cancer; 2005. Available from: http:// w2.iarc.fr/en/publications/pdfs-online/epi/cancerepi/CancerEpi-18.pdf
Food and Drug Administration website [Internet]. Computerized systems used in clinical trials. Silver Spring (MD): Food and Drug Administration; [cited 20 Apr 2015]. Available from: http://www.fda.gov/regulatoryinformation /guidances/ucm126402.htm
Hulley SB, Cummings SR, Browner WS, Grady DG, Newman TB. *Designing Clinical Research*. 4th ed. Philadelphia (PA): Lippincott Williams & Wilkins; 2013.
O'Connell AA, McCoach DB, editors. *Multilevel Modeling of Educational Data*. Charlotte (NC): Information Age Publishing; 2008.
Singer JD, Willett JB. *Applied Longitudinal Data Analysis: Modeling Change and Event Occurrence*. New York (NY): Oxford University Press; 2003.

- Study investigators should fully account for the entirety of data collected and the manner in which it will be stored and analyzed when designing a database. It is far better to design a comprehensive database that is not used to its full capacity than to create a database that does not address the comprehensive needs of the data collected and omits certain variables or measurements.
- Procedures for data collection, entry, storage, maintenance, assessment, retrieval, and analysis should be thoroughly discussed and standardized among the research team. Management techniques associated with data accuracy and reliability should be instituted, and study staff should be cross-trained. Updates on data entry and database maintenance should be discussed at regular research meetings. The database should be considered as critical a piece of equipment to study efficacy and validity as any other equipment associated with data collection.
- The increasing use of electronic data collection will necessitate that investigators carefully consider how best to incorporate this methodology into database use, recognizing that the potential for efficiency and accuracy must be balanced with the need to maintain controls for security and storage (6).
- The myriad purposes of the database—for database storage, report generation, and collaboration between other sites and investigators—should be identified so as to build a database that is as universal and applicable as possible. A powerful database will inform future studies and allow for generation of pilot data and institutional collaborations that ultimately strengthen the science of the investigative team.

The STOMP study benefitted from the effective database built for the study, as it allowed investigators to transition between data collection and analysis with minimal delay. Moreover, although the main study results have been published (10,16), the authors continue to use the database for secondary analyses and to support the research and hypotheses of other investigators. Resultantly, the database has served as a powerful tool with which to address the original specific aims of the study, create new ones, and investigate important clinical data that may ultimately influence our understanding of the costs and benefits of statin therapy.

GLOSSARY

Cryptographic protocol: protection method used to encrypt protected health information on computers and accessory electronic storage drives

Data at rest: term referring to the physical storage of data

Data coding scheme: pre-selected identifiers assigned to quantitative and qualitative study data

Data in motion: term referring to the transmission of data

Outliers: extreme data points that arise from either measurement error or inherent physiologic variability

REDCap: research electronic data capture; a secure web application designed exclusively to support data capture for research studies

Relational database: database model allowing data (entered in tables in a tabular format) to be interlinked by a unique identifier such as a subject identification number, with relations existing between tables and within tables

Source document: a paper or electronic recording form developed for every measurement and participant contact in a study to ensure standardization of data collection

Standard operating procedure: manuals developed to standardize every aspect of data collection and patient contact for a study

Statins: HMG CoA reductase inhibitors or LDL-C–lowering drug

STOMP: the effect of statins on muscle performance study (RO1 HL081893)

REFERENCE

1. Atkinson G, Nevill AM. Statistical methods for assessing measurement error (reliability) in variables relevant to sports medicine. *Sports Med.* 1998;26:217–238.
2. Diffie W, Hellman M. Exhaustive cryptanalysis of the NBS data encryption standard. *Computer.* 1977;10:74–84.
3. Harris PA, Taylor R, Thielke R, Payne J, Gonzalez N, Conde JG. Research electronic data capture (REDCap)—a metadata-driven methodology and workflow process for providing translational research informatics support. *J Biomed Inform.* 2009;42:377–381.
4. Hopkins WG, Marshall SW, Batterham AM, Hanin J. Progressive statistics for studies in sports medicine and exercise science. *Med Sci Sports Exerc.* 2009;41(1):3–13.
5. Marks RG. Validating electronic source data in clinical trials. *Control Clin Trials.* 2004;25:437–446.
6. Marks RG, Conlon M, Ruberg SJ. Paradigm shifts in clinical trials enabled by information technology. *Statist Med.* 2001;20:2683–2696.
7. McPherson K. Statistics: the problem of examining accumulating data more than once. *N Engl J Med.* 1974;290:501–502.
8. National Institutes of Health Web site [Internet]. NIH Data Sharing Policy and Implementation. Bethesda (MD): National Institutes of Health; [cited 2003 Mar 5]. Available from: http://grants.nih.gov/grants/policy/data_sharing/data_sharing_guidance .htm#goals
9. Ott RL, Longnecker M. *An Introduction to Statistical Methods and Data Analysis.* 5th ed. Pacific Grove (CA): Duxbury; 2001.
10. Parker BA, Capizzi JA, Grimaldi AS, et al. Effect of statins on skeletal muscle function. *Circulation.* 2013;127:96–103.
11. Penny KI, Jolliffe IT. Multivariate outlier detection applied to multiply imputed laboratory data. *Stat Med.* 1999;18:1879–1895.
12. Ramakrishnan R, Gehrke J. *Database Management Systems.* 2nd ed. Boston (MA): McGraw-Hill; 2000.
13. Shoemaker JS, Painter IS, Weir BS. Bayesian statistics in genetics: a guide for the uninitiated. *Trends Genet.* 1999;15:354–358.
14. Staffa JA, Chang J, Green L. Cerivastatin and reports of fatal rhabdomyolysis. *N Engl J Med.* 2002;346:539–540.
15. Thompson PD, Clarkson P, Karas RH. Statin-associated myopathy. *JAMA.* 2003;289:1681–1690.
16. Thompson PD, Parker BA, Clarkson PM, et al. A randomized clinical trial to assess the effect of statins on skeletal muscle function and performance: rationale and study design. *Prev Cardiol.* 2010;13:104–111.
17. U.S. Department of Health & Human Services Web site [Internet]. Health Insurance Portability and Accountability Act of 1996. Washington (DC): U.S. Department of Health & Human Services; [cited 2015 May 25]. Available from: http://www.hhs .gov/ocr/privacy/hipaa/administrative/statute/

CHAPTER 18

Statistical Approaches to Data Analysis

Joseph P. Weir, PhD, FACSM

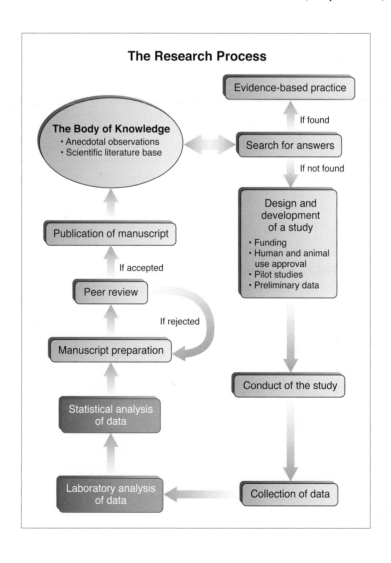

The Research Process

Evidence-based practice

If found

The Body of Knowledge
• Anecdotal observations
• Scientific literature base

Search for answers

If not found

Design and development of a study
• Funding
• Human and animal use approval
• Pilot studies
• Preliminary data

Publication of manuscript

Peer review

If accepted

If rejected

Manuscript preparation

Conduct of the study

Statistical analysis of data

Laboratory analysis of data

Collection of data

INTRODUCTION

Almost all research in the exercise sciences is quantitative in nature. That is, performance on a dependent variable is assessed by assigning a number to that performance. Typically, the magnitude of that number is reflective of the quality of that performance; for example, the greater the force output, the larger the amount of weight lifted. We use statistical methods to both describe the data and to make inferences from the data. This chapter provides a broad overview of the common statistical procedures employed.

A SIMPLE MODEL OF RESEARCH DESIGN

The process of designing research studies can be complex, and numerous graduate level textbooks have been written outlining the process of designing different types of research studies. However, from the perspective of a consumer of research studies, a simple and helpful model is to separate studies into two broad categories, which you have learned about in previous chapters: (a) observational studies and (b) experimental studies. All statistical approaches that will be addressed in this chapter center on quantifying the relationship between the independent variable(s) and the dependent variable(s). In an experimental study, the researcher manipulates the independent variable and examines the effect of that manipulation on the dependent variable. For example, say a researcher studies the effect of creatine monohydrate supplementation on anaerobic performance as quantified using the Wingate anaerobic power test. Subjects may be randomized to receive either creatine monohydrate or the placebo, and after an appropriate dosing period, subjects are tested on the Wingate test. Here, the researcher has manipulated the independent variable (subjects receive creatine monohydrate or the placebo) and examines the effect of that manipulation on the dependent variable (anaerobic power).

An observational study does not involve the manipulation of the independent variable; rather, the independent variable is quantified, and the degree of relationship between the independent variable and the dependent variable is determined. Most epidemiology studies are observational studies. For example, say an investigator studies the influence of television watching (independent variable) on physical activity (dependent variable). A survey instrument is developed to quantify the amount of time in hours of television watched per week, and the amount of physical activity is quantified using pedometer recordings. The investigator then quantifies the degree of relationship between hours watched and walking. Notice here that the researcher does not manipulate or control the independent variable. Instead, the score on the independent variable is simply quantified for each subject, as you have learned in previous chapters.

With respect to statistical analyses, the distinction between experimental and observational studies is not critical. As discussed in this chapter, the general procedures employed, such as analysis of variance and regression analysis, are in fact based on the same underlying statistical model (the general linear model) and distinctions between them are artificial. However, differences between observational and experimental research do affect the strength of the causal inferences one can make. In general, well-designed experimental research allows for stronger causal inferences than can be made with observational studies.

TYPES OF DATA

There are four broad classifications of data types, and these can influence the choice of statistical procedures employed. Recall from earlier chapters that these data types are called "nominal," "ordinal," "interval," and "ratio." Because of the different properties of these data types, the choice of statistical approach can be affected by the type of data, and so we will review them here.

- Nominal data are data where the number assigned reflects a specific category. For example, the researcher may wish to categorize whether subjects were successful or not in terms of smoking cessation. Subjects who did not cease smoking may be assigned a zero, whereas those who successfully stopped smoking would be assigned a one. Here, the use of the specific numbers of zero and one is completely arbitrary as long as the researcher is consistent when coding the data into the database. Similarly, the researcher may be interested in whether subjects were able to successfully lift a weight or not. Again we can assign arbitrary numbers to success and failure, and the numbers allow us to communicate that level of performance. Note that the numbers do not convey an amount of anything. They are simply used to categorize a performance.
- Ordinal data occur when the numbers assigned do indicate magnitude, but equal differences between numbers may convey a different amount of whatever is quantified. The 6–20 Borg scale of rating of perceived exertion (RPE) scale is an example of an ordinal scoring system. In the RPE scale, we know that a rating of 12 is greater than a rating of 11 (so that a person with an RPE of 12 is exercising harder than at an RPE of 11) and that a rating of 17 is greater than a rating of 16. However, we do not assume that the difference in effort between 12 and 11 is the same as the difference in effort between 17 and 16.
- Interval data are data where the differences between numbers do reflect equal amounts of what is being quantified; however, zero is an arbitrary value on the scale. The Celsius temperature scale is an example of interval data. Here, the difference between 10°C and 20°C is equal to the difference between 30°C and 40°C. However, because 0°C does not denote the absence of heat (rather it is the freezing point of water), it is inaccurate to say that 40° is twice as hot as 20°C.
- Ratio data have the properties of interval data, with the addition that zero on a ratio scale conveys absence of what is being measured. Range of motion at a joint is an example of ratio data because it is possible that a joint cannot move, in which case the score for range of motion would be 0 degrees. As the name suggests, with a meaningful zero point on the measurement scale, it is possible to create meaningful ratios. A range of motion of 90 degrees is twice the range of motion of 45 degrees. Many dependent variables in sports medicine and exercise science are measured on a ratio scale. However, the distinction can sometimes be tricky. For example, although range of motion at a joint is ratio data, joint angle is not. At the knee, we can define the knee at full extension to be 180 degrees. (We could also define full extension to be 0 degrees. Both reference systems

are acceptable.) If we move the knee 90 degrees starting from full extension (180 degrees), we have moved the knee through a range of motion of 90 degrees and we are now at a knee angle of 90 degrees (or 270 degrees depending on the frame of reference). But it is nonsensical to state that the knee at 90 degrees has half the joint angle of the knee at full extension because the reference point of 0 degree is arbitrary. From a statistical perspective, however, the distinction between interval and ratio data is unimportant as long as one does not try to analyze or interpret ratios created using interval data.

FREQUENCY DISTRIBUTIONS

When organizing data that have lots of scores, it is helpful to create a **frequency distribution** of the data. A frequency distribution is a distribution that notes the number of times a score (or scores within a specific range of values) occurs in a dataset. As it turns out, many phenomena in nature tend to exhibit what is referred to as a "normal (or Gaussian) distribution." This stems from the property that when one adds random numbers together and plots the frequency distribution of those sums, the frequency distribution is normal. Thus, randomness leads toward distributions that tend to be somewhat normal. Normal distributions have several properties, including that the distribution is symmetrical and the mean, median, and mode are the same value. We depend on the properties of the normal distribution in many of the inferential statistical processes described in this chapter.

DESCRIPTIVE STATISTICS

Researchers use statistics to describe their data and to make inferences about their data. As the term suggests, **descriptive statistics** simply describe the data in the study. We will focus on the two major types of descriptive statistics: (a) **central tendency** and (b) **variability**. Measures of central tendency are used to assess where scores tend to cluster. The most common measure of central tendency is the arithmetic **mean** or average. The mean is calculated by adding all the scores together and dividing this sum by the number of scores. In statistical shorthand:

$$\bar{X} = \frac{\Sigma x}{n}$$

where $\bar{X}$ (pronounced "X bar") is the symbol for the mean of the "x" scores, the symbol Σ is an operation that indicates summation, and n is the number of scores. Other indices of central tendency include the **mode** (most frequent score) and the **median** (half the scores are higher than the median, half are below).

The variability in a set of scores refers to how the scores tend to spread out or differ from each other. Two related indices are commonly used to quantify variability. These are the **variance** and **standard deviation**. In calculating the variance, it is important to note that if we simply calculated how each score deviated from the mean and then added up all the deviation scores, the sum of the deviation scores would always equal zero. Instead, we square the deviation scores and then add the squared values as a core part of the calculation—this is a "sums of squares" operation. We then divide the sums of squares by the number of scores if the scores are from a population, or we divide by n−1 if the scores are from a sample (which is typical). In equation form, the variance (V) calculation for a sample is:

$$V = \frac{\Sigma(x - \overline{X})^2}{n - 1}$$

Notice that the larger the difference between each "x" value from the $\overline{X}$, the larger will be the numerator and therefore the larger the variance, all else being equal. The standard deviation (SD) is simply the square root of the variance, such that:

$$SD = \sqrt{V} = \sqrt{\Sigma \frac{(x - \overline{X})^2}{n - 1}}$$

Table 18-1 is a simple illustration of the calculation of the variance and the SD. Each "x" score represents the one repetition maximum (1RM) bench press (kilogram). The mean of the five scores equals 85.8 kg. Because we recorded the bench press to the nearest kilogram, reporting the mean to a 10th of kilogram is not appropriate, but we will not round during the subsequent variance and SD calculations because that can exacerbate errors.

From Table 18-1, we see that the V = 1,356.8/4 = 339.2, and the resulting SD = $\sqrt{339.2}$ = 18.4 kg. Here it might make sense to round this to 18 kg because that is consistent with the level of precision of our bench press measurement. In practice, we rarely report the variance but should routinely report the SD. When the data are normally distributed, the SD can define specific areas of the normal distribution. As an approximation, about 68% of all scores fall between ±1 SD from the mean. Similarly, about 95% of all scores fall between ±2 SD from the mean, and about 99% of all scores fall between ±3 SD from the mean.

The concept of variance is central to our use of inferential statistics (described in the next section). Specifically, when we conduct research, we are interested in how scores differ. If all 1RM bench press values were equal between persons, then the one-repetition bench press would not be interesting. Instead, we want to understand the variance in the scores. Why are some people stronger than others? Why does blood pressure vary between individuals? Why do some people get cancer and others do not? It is therefore the understanding of the variance in the data that is central to our analysis of the research data, and as will be discussed in the following text, "analysis of variance" is a central method in our statistical toolkit.

Table 18-1 Calculation of Mean, Variance, and Standard Deviation		
x	$x - \overline{X}$	$x - (\overline{X})^2$
70	$70 - 85.8 = -15.8$	249.64
84	$84 - 85.8 = -1.8$	3.24
66	$66 - 85.8 = -19.8$	392.04
107	$107 - 85.8 = 21.2$	449.44
102	$102 - 85.8 = 16.2$	262.44
$\Sigma = 429$	$\Sigma = 0$	$\Sigma = 1,356.8$

INFERENTIAL STATISTICS

In contrast to descriptive statistics, in **inferential statistics**, we are trying to make generalizations specific to our sample population (called "inferences") about our data. More specifically, the process of statistical inference involves trying to infer population values from sample values. A sample is a subset of the population of interest, and we require that the sample be representative of the population.

When we calculate the mean from a sample, this serves as our best estimate of the population mean. We know, however, that the sample mean and population mean are unlikely to be exactly the same. The difference between our sample estimate and the population value is the **sampling error**. Because we don't know the population mean, we can't know the sampling error. However, we can make estimates of a range of values in which we estimate the population mean value to occur. We use a type of SD called a **standard error** to make these estimates. Imagine a computer simulation where millions of random numbers have been generated. The simulation then takes a sample of say 200 scores and calculates the mean of the sample. Those scores are placed back in the pool of numbers, and another sample of 200 is taken and the mean once again calculated. This mean will be somewhat different from the first mean, but they ought to be somewhat close to each other and somewhat close to the mean of the population of all scores. If we repeat this sampling process many times, we will get a distribution of the sample means which is called a **sampling distribution of the mean**. From the **central limit theorem**, we know that the sampling distribution of the mean is normally distributed and the mean of the sample means will equal the population mean. The SD of the sampling distribution of the mean is called the **standard error of the mean**.

From the point estimate (*e.g.*, sample mean), the standard error, and knowing the properties of the normal distribution, we can construct ranges of values where we are confident that the population value lies.

THE NULL HYPOTHESIS SIGNIFICANCE TEST

The typical way that inferential statistical analyses are conducted is to perform what is called the **null hypothesis significance test** (NHST). In this formulation, the data analyst generates two mutually exclusive and exhaustive statistical analyses called the **null hypothesis** (H_O) and the **alternate hypothesis** (H_A). The null hypothesis typically posits that there is no relationship between the independent variable and the dependent variable, whereas the alternate hypothesis is the logical alternative of the null hypothesis; in other words, there is a relationship between the independent variable and the dependent variable. To take a simple example, assume we want to study the effect of exercise on left ventricular mass in rats. Rats are randomized to either an exercise group or a control group, and after the training intervention, the rats are sacrificed, and the masses of the left ventricular quantified. We might then want to compare the mean mass of the exercised rats versus the mean mass of the control rats. We could set up the null and alternate hypotheses as:

$$H_O: \overline{X}_{exercise} = \overline{X}_{control}$$

$$H_A: \overline{X}_{exercise} \neq \overline{X}_{control}$$

Notice that H_O and H_A exhaust the possible outcomes as there is no possible third hypothesis and that only one hypothesis can be true. Further, note that H_A is typically consistent with the overall research hypothesis. The conceptual process of the NHST is to test the tenability of H_O given the data collected. In this example, if exercise (the independent variable) has no effect on left ventricular mass (the dependent variable), then our sample means from the exercise and control rats ought to be about the same. However, even if H_O were true due to sampling error, we would not expect the exercise and control means to be exactly the same, but they ought to be reasonably close to each other. When we statistically analyze the data in the NHST, we calculate a value (P) that quantifies the probability we could have gotten the data that we have, assuming H_O is true. If we calculate $P = .12$, then we are saying that if H_O is true, the probability of finding a difference as large or larger than what was found in this data is 12%. We evaluate that P value in the context of what is called **alpha (α)**. The α value is set by the researcher and defines what we described earlier as "reasonably close." As noted in Chapter 6, the typical α level is .05, although thoughtless adherence to this tradition is not recommended (5). The mechanics of the process is that if $P \leq \alpha$, we reject H_O and therefore accept H_A. When we reject H_O, we often state that the effect is **statistically significant**. So in the example with $P = .12$, if $\alpha = .05$, then we would not reject H_O. In contrast, if $P = .04$ and $\alpha = .05$, then we would reject H_O and by extension must accept H_A. Note that α is chosen by the investigator, whereas the P value is determined by the data.

When we perform an NHST, we are making a probabilistic statement about the tenability of H_O. If we reject H_O (*i.e.*, $P \leq \alpha$), we have either made a correct decision or we have committed what is called a **type I error**. A type I error occurs when H_O is rejected when in fact H_O is true. This is a false positive in that we are saying that there is a relationship between the independent variable and the dependent variable, when in fact there is no relationship. (The α value defines the risk of a type I error, assuming H_O is true.) In contrast, if we accept H_O (*i.e.*, $P > \alpha$), we have either made a correct decision or we have committed what is called a **type II error**. A type II error occurs when we accept H_O when H_O is false. This is a false negative in that we are saying that there is no relationship between the independent variable and the dependent variable when in fact there is a relationship.

A critical concept in the NHST test is the idea of statistical power. Statistical power is the ability of a test to detect an effect if the effect is present. The statistical power of a test is affected by factors such as the α level (all else being equal, decreasing α from say .05 to .01 also decreases statistical power) that is employed and the homogeneity of the scores. However, the primary influence on statistical power is the sample size. Holding all else constant, increasing sample size increases statistical power.

EFFECT SIZE

The evaluation of H_O is only one part of the inferential process and perhaps the least important part. When we state that an effect is statistically significant, the word "significant" should not be equated with important. Significant in this context means to signify or to signal. That is, we think an effect is not zero. An effect can be statistically significant but may be trivial in magnitude. In addition, because of low statistical power, an important effect may not be statistically significant. The magnitude of an effect can be quantified using a variety of metrics and fall under the concept of "effect size." It is important to note that "effect" sizes arose from psychologic data not physiologic data that it is often applied to. When comparing mean values, a common effect size metric is called **Cohen's *d*** (see also Hedges *g*) (7). The **effect size** (ES) here is calculated as:

$$ES = \frac{\overline{X}_1 - \overline{X}_2}{SD}$$

where the SD is often a pooled SD reflecting the variability in both groups, or if one mean is from a control group, the control group SD can be used (9). From the equation, we can see that ES is the mean difference normalized to SD units. For example, if ES = 0.25, we can interpret this as the mean difference = 0.25 SD. Cohen (2) has suggested the following guidelines for ES interpretation: 0.2 = small, 0.5 = medium, and >0.80 = large. However, these values are at best very general guidelines, and different ES values may be expected in the exercise sciences (8). Other ES include omega squared (ω^2) which quantifies the variance in the dependent variable that is shared with the independent variable and is often thought of as "variance accounted for" such that if $\omega^2 = 0.10$, we would say that the 10% of the variance in the dependent variable (*e.g.*, left ventricular mass) is accounted for the independent variable (*e.g.*, exercise training). In a subsequent section, we will address the Pearson r, an index of correlation. This is also an ES metric.

CONFIDENCE INTERVALS

A **confidence interval** (CI) is a range of values within which we are confident that the population value lies. As with choosing an α level, we choose a level of confidence when constructing a CI. A 95% CI is analogous to an α level of .05. We can construct a CI about a sample mean in the process of estimating the population mean. For example, assume that a sample of college offensive linemen in American football has a mean body mass index (BMI) of 25 kg/m^2 and that the resulting 95% CI is 22–28 kg/m^2. Our best estimate of the population BMI for offensive linemen is our sample estimate (*i.e.*, 25 kg/m^2). However, due to sampling error we would not expect the population mean to be exactly 25 kg/m^2. Instead, we can interpret the 95% CI such that we are 95% confident that the population of college offensive linemen has a mean BMI somewhere from 22 to 28 kg/m^2.

We can extend this idea to indices such as mean differences. Assume that the mean difference in left ventricular mass between exercise and control rats is +10 g (exercise minus the control) and the 95% CI = 6–14 g. We would interpret this such that we are 95% confident that the true difference in left ventricular mass is somewhere from 6 to 14 g.

CIs and *P* values from the NHST are calculated from the same underlying statistical models and indeed if the null hypothesis value is outside the CI for a chosen level of confidence, that is, tantamount to rejecting H$_O$ at the associated α level. For example, in the rat left ventricular mass, if H$_O$ is true (exercise has no effect on left ventricular mass), then we would expect a mean difference of about 0 g (the null value) to be within our CI. In our example, the fact that the 95% CI excludes zero also means that we would reject H$_O$ when α = .05. It should be noted that many argue that the use of the NHST should be discontinued and an approach based on estimating effects using CIs should be used instead (6).

ANALYSIS OF VARIANCE, REGRESSION ANALYSIS, AND THE GENEAL LINEAR MODEL

Most statistical analyses that are conducted are part of what is known as the **general linear model**. In general, the techniques known as **analysis of variance** (ANOVA) and **regression analysis** comprise the primary toolkit used to statistically analyze data. It should be noted that although a traditional overview will be presented, that is, ANOVA and regression as separate approaches, in fact, this is an artificial distinction. Both ANOVA and regression are the same underlying system of data analysis (3). Advanced statistical textbooks and courses tie these concepts together and show the homology of ANOVA and regression, but that is beyond the scope of this chapter. Furthermore, in practice, ANOVA and regression tend to be used in different contexts, and as such, the presentation of ANOVA and regression here will follow these contexts.

Comparing Means: ANOVA and the t Test

A common question posed of data is whether mean values differ between groups or time periods. In experimental studies, we typically ask whether the groups that received different treatments (*e.g.*, high- vs. low-intensity exercise training) differ on average on some measurement (*e.g.*, resting systolic blood pressure). Here, the independent variable is the type of exercise treatment (high or low intensity) and the dependent variable is resting systolic blood pressure. We could extend this to situations with more levels of the independent variable. For example, we could study three different exercise intensities instead of just two. Notice that the independent variable is a categorical variable (exercise intensity group) and comparing the means between the different categories (groups) should provide insight into the influence of exercise intensity on resting systolic blood pressure.

We can also compare means when assessing the same subjects on multiple occasions. For example, we may compare running time to exhaustion with caffeine versus placebo. Instead of randomizing subjects into two groups, one getting caffeine and the other placebo, subjects could be tested under both conditions (assume randomizing the order across subjects and blinding of caffeine vs. placebo). Here, we say the subjects serve as their own controls, and the design is a **repeated measures** design because the same subjects are tested on repeated occasions; this is also referred to as a **within-subjects** design. In contrast, a **between-subjects** design is employed when different subjects provide the scores from which the different means are calculated. You will recall these concepts from the chapters on research design.

When comparing means between groups, if there are just two means to compare, we typically perform what is called a **t test**. The two main types of t tests are the **independent t test** and the **dependent t test**. The independent t test is employed under conditions of a between-subjects design such that the scores that form the mean of group 1 come from different subjects than the scores that form the mean of group 2. That is, because subject 1 in group 1 is a different subject from subject 1 in group 2, the scores are independent of each other.

In a within-subjects design, we no longer have independent scores because score 1 that forms one mean value and score 1 that forms the second mean value come from the same subject. The computational differences between independent and dependent t tests are explained in statistical textbooks (9) and will not be addressed here. The interpretations, however, are similar. In an NHST, we compute a test statistic, called *t*, that is evaluated for statistical significance. The larger the t value, the less likely we could have gotten that value assuming the null hypothesis is true. If the t value is large enough, the *P* value will be less than the α level, and we reject the null hypothesis.

When there are more than three mean values to compare, we can employ ANOVA. Note that, in fact, the t test is a special case of ANOVA, and ANOVA is the more general system for making comparisons of mean differences, and we will get the same answer if we employ ANOVA under what might otherwise be considered a t test situation. As with the t test, we can use ANOVA with between-subjects or within-subjects (repeated measures) types of designs. (Reliability calculations [see Chapter 10] are derived from the variance components in a repeated measures ANOVA [10]). The computational details of ANOVA will not be discussed here. The mechanics of the process are similar to the t test, however. We compute a test statistic called "F." The larger the magnitude of F, the less likely it is that F could have been found under conditions of the null hypothesis being true. That is, from the calculated F value, we can determine the *P* value that reflects the probability that one could have gotten an F value of this size if the null hypothesis is true.

When the results of an ANOVA are such that the null hypothesis is rejected, if there are more than two mean values to compare, additional analyses are typically employed. Consider an example in which a researcher investigates the effects of three different exercise conditions (*e.g.*, high-intensity exercise, low-intensity exercise, and no exercise) on left ventricular mass in rats. The three groups of rats undergo eight weeks of training, then the animals are sacrificed, and the mass of the left ventricles is determined. Assuming the magnitude of the F statistic allowed rejection of the null hypothesis, all that has been determined is that somewhere among the three means there appear to be significant differences, but we do not know the specific pattern of the differences. Perhaps the high- and low-intensity groups had comparable left ventricular mass, but both exercise groups had greater mass than the no exercise group. Perhaps there was a dose-dependent response such that high intensity > low intensity > no exercise. The typical approach to gain greater detail from the data is to perform what are called **post-hoc comparisons**. Common post-hoc tests include the Tukey WSD, Scheffe, and Newman-Keuhls tests. These tests allow one to perform more specific comparisons within the context of the overall ANOVA.

As with the t test, ANOVA can be implemented under conditions of a between-subjects design (*e.g.*, the exercise intensity and rat left ventricular mass example from earlier) or a within-subjects design. As an example of a within-subjects design, say an investigator wishes to examine the effects of different caffeine doses on simulated cycling time trial performance. Subjects will randomly perform time trials under conditions of a high caffeine dose, a low caffeine dose, and placebo. Because the same subjects perform the time trials under all conditions, this is a repeated measures analysis. The interpretation of the results of the repeated measures ANOVA is comparable to that with a between-subjects design, but the computational details differ.

We often employ more complex designs that include more than one independent variable. Imagine we modified the caffeine study such that we included both highly trained and novice cyclists. We would now have a two-factor ANOVA. The two factors would be cycling group (highly trained vs. novice) and caffeine dose (high, low, and placebo). The dependent variable is still cycling time trial performance (time) as before. This two-factor design, which may also be referred to as a "two-way ANOVA" or perhaps a two-by-three ANOVA (because there are two levels of groups and three levels of caffeine dose), allows us to look at the effects of each independent variable separately as well as examine the interaction between the two. Note that there is one between-subjects factor (group) and one within-subjects factor (caffeine dose) in this example. We can perform multiple factor ANOVAs with only between-subjects factors, only within-subjects factors, or with a mixture of between- and within-subjects factors as in this example (hence, this is sometimes called a "mixed design"). When examining each factor, we refer to the effect of each factor as its "main effect" in which we examine the effect of each independent variable while collapsing across the effect of the other independent variable. For example, if there were 10 subjects in the highly trained group and another 10 subjects in the novice group, the main effect for caffeine dose would effectively be a repeated measures ANOVA with three levels of dose and a total of 20 subjects. That is, in the analysis of the main effect for caffeine dose, we would ignore the presence of the other factor (group).

The primary reason for use of a factorial ANOVA allows us to examine the interaction between two factors, which can be more interesting than the main effects of each factor separately. Consider the hypothetical data from our caffeine example in Figure 18-1. It appears that the highly trained cyclists respond to caffeine in a dose-dependent manner, whereas novice cyclists are unaffected by caffeine. This differential effect where the effect of one factor (caffeine) varies across levels of the other factor (group) is the essence of an interaction and can be tested statistically in a factorial ANOVA.

Correlation and Regression

In studies in which the independent variables are on an interval or ratio scale, the typical approach for data analysis is to employ what is referred to as "regression analysis," including indices of correlation between the independent and dependent variables. As noted

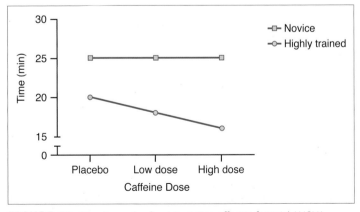

FIGURE 18-1: Example of an interaction effect in factorial ANOVA.

previously, ANOVA and regression are really the same underlying process, and both are part of what is referred to as the "general linear model." So the distinction between regression and ANOVA is quite artificial. Nonetheless, in practice, most data analysts employ ANOVA when the independent variables are nominal and employ regression when the independent variables are interval/ratio. Furthermore, in regression, we typically think of the independent variable as the "X" variable and the dependent variable as the "Y" variable.

A correlation coefficient is an index that quantifies the degree of relationship between two variables. The most common index is the Pearson product moment correlation coefficient, or the **Pearson r** for short. The Pearson r is a number that can vary between -1.0 and $+1.0$. A value of zero means that there is no relationship between the independent variable and the dependent variable. The closer the absolute value, that is, plus or minus, of r to 1.0, the stronger the relationship between the independent and dependent variable. The sign of the r value indicates the direction of the relationship. For example, we would expect the relationship between leg strength as quantified by the 1RM leg extension (X) and upper body strength as quantified by 1RM bench press (Y) to be positive. Example data from 10 subjects in this regard is presented in Figure 18-2. In fact, the r value for this data is $+0.83$, which indicates a strong positive linear relationship between upper and lower body strength. In contrast, as adults age, they tend to lose muscle mass, so we would expect a negative relationship between age and muscle mass and therefore a negative sign associated with the r value.

We can also test the statistical significance of the Pearson r, which is a test of whether we think the relationship is not zero. The statistical hypotheses are:

$$H_O: r = 0$$

$$H_A: r \neq 0$$

from which we can derive a *P* value to assess statistical significance. For the data in Figure 18-2, the *P* value is .003 which tells us that the probability we could have gotten

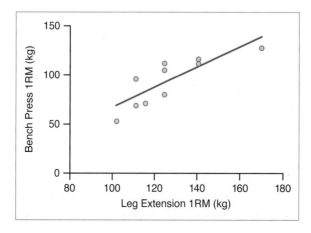

FIGURE 18-2: Example data showing a positive linear relationship between the independent variable (leg extension 1RM) and the dependent variable (bench press 1RM).

$r = 0.83$ with $n = 10$, if H_O is true ($r = 0.0$) is 3 in 1,000 or 0.3%. Assuming $\alpha = .05$, we would reject H_O and note that there is a statistically significant relationship between leg extension strength and bench press strength.

However, the test of statistical significance only assesses whether the correlation is not zero. As noted previously, the Pearson r is in fact an ES metric and the closer r to 1.0, the stronger the relationship. Cohen (2) has suggested that Pearson r values of 0.10, 0.30, and 0.50 reflect small, medium, and large ES, respectively. As with Cohen's *d*, these are simply guidelines and should not be strictly followed. Again, the Cohen's *d* values are derived from psychological data which differs from physiological data especially with measures of association. Another way of developing a sense of the magnitude of the relationship is to calculate what is called the **coefficient of determination**, which is simply the square of the r value (r^2). For reasons that go beyond the scope of this chapter, the r^2 value is analogous to ω^2 that was described in the context of ANOVA, and as such, it reflects the "variance accounted for" or shared variance between the independent and dependent variables. For the data in Figure 18-2, $r^2 = 0.69$, we can interpret this as saying that about 69% of the variance in bench press strength is accounted for by leg extension strength, or bench press and leg extension strength share about 69% common variance.

We can extend the idea of correlation to what is called **linear regression**. In linear regression, we develop an equation that best describes the linear relationship between the independent variable and dependent variable. This equation is sometimes called a "prediction equation" because it can be used to predict scores on the dependent variable based on scores on the independent variable. In linear regression, we use the following basic equation for a straight line:

$$Y = a + bX$$

where a is the y-intercept and b is the slope. The y-intercept (a) is the predicted score on the dependent variable (Y) when the score on the independent variable (X) equals zero. Visually, the y-intercept is where the line hits the y-axis. The slope (b) of the line reflects the change in Y associated with one unit change in X, which you may recall from junior high was rise over run, or mathematically $\Delta Y / \Delta X$. Extending the equation for a straight line to linear regression, we present the equation as:

$$\hat{Y} = a + bX$$

where $\hat{Y}$ is the predicted score for Y. Due to space constraints, we will not address the calculation of the slope and intercept. For the example data in Figure 18-2, the equation is:

predicted bench press 1RM $= -37.73 + 1.036$ (leg extension 1RM)

such that $b = +1.036$ and $a = -37.73$. It is important to note that the a and b terms have units. The units for a are the units of the dependent variable, which in this example is kilogram of bench press mass. The units for b are the y-axis units/x-axis units, which in this example is kilogram of bench press mass/kilogram of leg extension mass. For b, we can interpret this as for every 1-kg increase in leg extension 1RM performance, we should expect a 1.036-kg increase in bench press 1RM performance. Note that the intercept value is -37.73 kg which indicates that we would predict a person with zero 1RM in the leg extension would have a bench press of -37.73 kg which is nonsensical and illustrates that one must be careful when extrapolating beyond the actual range of the data. Employing the equation, we could predict 1RM bench press ($\hat{Y}$) for a person with a 1RM leg extension strength (X) of 120 kg:

$$\hat{Y} \text{ (kg bench press)} = -37.73 \text{kg bench press} + 1.036 \frac{\text{kg bench press}}{\text{kg leg extension}} (120 \text{ kg leg extension})$$

which equals 86.59 kg bench press. Thus, we would predict someone with a 120-kg leg extension 1RM to have a 1RM bench press of 86.59 kg. Note that the units of kilogram leg extension cancel in the equation such that we have kilogram bench press on both sides of the equation.

The test of significance of the regression equation is fundamentally a test of whether the slope (b) is significantly different from zero, such that:

$$H_O: b = 0$$

$$H_A: b \neq 0$$

It should be noted that the test of significance of r for these data will be completely redundant with the test of significance of b, and therefore the P value of .003 is identical to that found for the test of r. Furthermore, we can construct a CI about the slope coefficient. For the example earlier, the 95% CI for the slope is 0.469–1.604. Note that the CI excludes zero which is to be expected given the redundancy of the test of significance at a given α level with the construction of the CI at the associated level of confidence. Furthermore, the CI provides more information than just the determination of statistical significance. Here, we note that we are 95% confident that the population slope is somewhere from 0.469 to 1.604 kg bench press/kg leg extension. Although the CI excludes zero, it is rather wide, which stems from the relatively small sample size (n = 10). The precision of the estimate of the population slope (narrower confidence limits) could be improved with a larger sample size.

As with all statistical estimates, there is error in the prediction with regression. The regression line plotted in Figure 18-2 represents the predicted Y scores ($\hat{Y}$) for any X score in the data range. The vertical distance from each actual data point and the regression line is the error in prediction for that subject and is called the "residual." Similar to the calculation of the variance and SD, the sum of the residuals will always equal zero, so we need to square the residuals and then add them together to get a handle on the error in the prediction. The process of regression is sometimes called a "least squares" process because the regression line is the one straight line (among the infinite number of possible straight lines) that when fit to the data will have smallest sums of squares of the residuals. The SD of the residuals is called the "standard error of estimate" (SEE) and is a common metric for assessing the quality of the regression equation. The smaller the SEE, the less error in the prediction and the better is the prediction equation. The units of the SEE are the units of the dependent variable, which in this example is in kilogram of bench press 1RM.

As with ANOVA, we can extend regression models to include more than one independent variable. This process is called **multiple regression**. The generalized multiple regression equation is:

$$\hat{Y} = a + b_1X_1 + b_2X_2 + \cdots b_iX_1$$

where each b term is the slope coefficient for a particular independent variable. For example, we could extend the bench press example earlier to include other predictors such as body mass, arm length, years of weight training experience, etc. Of course, we would need to greatly expand our sample size to build such a model. Each of the additional variables listed would be separate independent variables in the model and have a separate slope coefficient. For example, if we were to add arm length (centimeter) to the model as X_2, we would have a slope with units of kilogram per centimeter. We might expect this slope to have a negative sign because longer arms tend to be a disadvantage in performing the bench press. If the slope were $b_2 = -1.5$ kg/cm, we would interpret this slope as indicating that for each 1 cm of additional arm length, bench press strength is on average 1.5 kg lower. As with simple linear regression, we can calculate a correlation that is typically denoted with a capital R and more commonly an R^2 value, which is an estimate of the variance in the dependent variable that is collectively accounted for by the independent variables in the model. In addition, the SEE from a multiple regression model is interpreted the same way except that it now incorporates information from multiple independent variables.

A common problem when building multiple regression models is that independent variables tend to be correlated with each other. In the example earlier, we might expect bodyweight to be not only correlated with our dependent variable (1RM bench press) but also our other independent variable (1RM leg extension). So our two independent variables have some redundancy. That is, if we know something about bodyweight, we also know something about 1RM leg extension. This problem is referred to as **multicollinearity** (or sometimes just collinearity) and can greatly affect the quality of the regression analysis. At a minimum, the ability to test the significance of the slope coefficients is compromised as the CIs widen. Ideally, the independent variables in the model are highly correlated with the dependent variable but only minimally correlated with the other independent variables.

SAMPLE SIZE DETERMINATION

It has been repeatedly noted that larger sample sizes increase statistical power and narrow CIs widths. How does one determine the right sample size? The general process is as follows. First, the researcher should determine the smallest effect that would be desired to detect. That is, the investigator should determine the smallest effect that is meaningful. For example, if one wishes to detect differences in systolic blood pressure of 2 mm Hg or larger and the SD of systolic blood pressure is expected to be 10 mm Hg, then one would like to detect an effect as small as a Cohen's $d = 0.20$. Given the minimal effect to detect, one needs to set α (typically .05) and the desired power (often 0.80 or 0.90). From these inputs, the necessary sample size for a particular statistical test can be calculated. Free software such as

G*Power (http://www.psycho.uni-duesseldorf.de/abteilungen/aap/gpower3/) will perform these calculations for most statistical tests used in the exercise sciences (1,4). These *a priori* sample size calculations are now a necessary component of most grant applications.

SUMMARY

Statistical analyses are used to help us understand quantitative data. Descriptive statistics are used to describe the data and typically focus on indices of central tendency and variability. Inferential statistics are used to make inferences about the data, specifically to estimate values in the population based on sample values. In the exercise sciences, common inferential approaches include tests of mean differences using t tests and ANOVA and analyses to quantify relationships between variables (*e.g.*, Pearson r) and to predict a variable using another variable(s) (*i.e.*, regression).

GLOSSARY

Alpha (α): a value set by the researcher which quantifies the risk being taken of committing a type I error if the null hypothesis is true

Alternate hypothesis: a statistical hypothesis that is the logical alternative to the null hypothesis; it typically states that there is a relationship between the independent variable and the dependent variable

Analysis of variance: a class of statistical procedures in which the variance in a set of data is decomposed into pieces associated with different factors (independent variables); typically employed in the context of comparing mean values

Between-subjects: different subjects provide the scores from which the different means are calculated

Central limit theorem: a theorem stating that repeated sample values (*e.g.*, sample means) taken from the population will be normally distributed even if the population from which the samples were drawn is not normally distributed and the mean of the sample means will equal the population mean

Central tendency: a description of where scores in a distribution tend to cluster

Coefficient of determination: an estimate of the amount of shared variance between an independent variable and a dependent variable; quantified by squaring the Pearson r

Cohen's *d*: a statistical calculation that provides an index of the strength of the relationship (association) between two variables; $d = 0.2$ is a small effect size, $d = 0.5$ represents a medium effect size; and $d = 0.8$ a large effect size

Confidence interval: a range of values within which the population value is believed to lie at a given level of statistical confidence (*e.g.*, 95%)

Dependent t test: a t test in which the scores come from correlated samples; typically, the scores being compared come from the same subjects tested on two occasions

Descriptive statistics: statistics that merely describe the sample data but do not provide inferences about population values

Effect size: an index of the magnitude of relationship between an independent variable and a dependent variable

Frequency distribution: a distribution that notes the number of times a score (or scores within a specific range values) occurs in a dataset

General linear model: a statistical model that forms the basis for many statistical procedures including analysis of variance and regression analysis

Independent t test: a t test in which the scores being compared come from different subjects

Inferential statistics: allows a scientist to draw conclusions about a population by using data from a subset (sample) of all individuals. The investigator attempts to reach conclusions that extend beyond the immediate limited data set

Linear regression: a mathematical model of the linear relationship between one or more independent variables and a dependent variable; uses a least squares criterion to fit the linear model

Mean: an index of central tendency calculated by dividing the sum of all the scores by the number of scores

Median: an index of central tendency that divides a distribution of scores in half such that 50% of the scores are larger than the median and 50% of the scores are smaller than the median

Mode: an index of central tendency consisting of the most frequent score on the distribution of scores

Multicollinearity: also known as collinearity; a state of strong interassociations among independent variables in a multiple regression analysis. The simplest solution is to reduce the number of collinear variables until only one remains

Multiple regression: a type of linear regression in which more than one independent variable is used to model the dependent variable

Null hypothesis: a statistical hypothesis which states that there is no relationship between the independent variable and the dependent variable

Null hypothesis significance test: a process of statistical inference in which, given the sample data, a decision is made to either reject or not reject the null hypothesis

Pearson r: a correlation coefficient quantifying the amount of linear association between two variables

Post-hoc comparisons: statistical comparisons of smaller pieces of a larger statistical analysis that are performed after an overall analysis of the larger statistical model

Regression analysis: a mathematical technique that determines the line that best represents the relationships between two variables (*i.e.,* the line of best fit), plotted as data points on a scatter graph

Repeated measures: same subjects are measured on multiple occasions

Sampling distribution of the mean: a theoretical distribution composed of mean values from repeated samples taken from a population

Sampling error: the difference between a sample estimate and the population value

Standard deviation: the square root of the variance; the typical index of variability when reporting the results of a research study

Standard error: the standard deviation of a sampling distribution

Standard error of the mean: the standard deviation of the sampling distribution of the mean

Statistically significant: a phrase that denotes that the null hypothesis has been rejected

t- test: a statistical analysis that determines if two sets of data are significantly different from each other

Type I error: a statistical error in which the null hypothesis is rejected when the null hypothesis is true

Type II error: a statistical error in which the null hypothesis is not rejected when the null hypothesis is false

Variability: a description of how scores in a distribution are spread out or different from each other

Variance: an index of variability in the data that is quantified by calculating the mean of the squared deviation scores about the mean

Within-subjects: same subjects are measured in multiple occasions (see repeated measures)

REFERENCES

1. Beck T. The importance of a priori sample size estimation in strength and conditioning research. *J Strength Cond Res.* 2013;27(8):2323–2337.
2. Cohen J. A power primer. *Psychol Bull.* 1992;112(1):155–159.
3. Cohen J. Multiple regression as a general data-analytic system. *Psychol Bull.* 1968;70:426–443.
4. Faul F, Erdfelder E, Lang A-G, & Buchner A. G*Power 3: a flexible statistical power analysis for the social, behavioral, and biomedical sciences. *Behav Res Methods.* 2007;39:175–191.
5. Franks BD, Huck SW. Why does everyone use the .05 significance level? *Res Q Exerc Sport.* 1986;57(3):245–249.
6. Hopkins WG, Marshall SW, Batterham AM, Hanin J. Progressive statistics for studies in sports medicine and exercise science. *Med Sci Sports Exerc.* 2009;41(1):3–12.
7. Nakagawa S, Cuthill IC. Effect size, confidence interval and statistical significance: a practical guide for biologists. *Biol Rev Camb Philos Soc.* 2007;82:591–605.
8. Rhea MR. Determining the magnitude of treatment effects in strength training research through the use of the effect size. *J Strength Cond Res.* 2004;18(4):918–920.
9. Vincent WJ, Weir JP. *Statistics in Kinesiology.* 4th ed. Champaign (IL): Human Kinetics; 2012.
10. Weir JP. Quantifying test-retest reliability using the intraclass correlation coefficient and the SEM. *J Strength Cond Res.* 2005;19(1):231–240.

Drawing Inferences, Logical Fallacies

*J. Larry Durstine, PhD, Raymond W. Thompson, PhD, and
Benjamin T. Gordon, PhD*

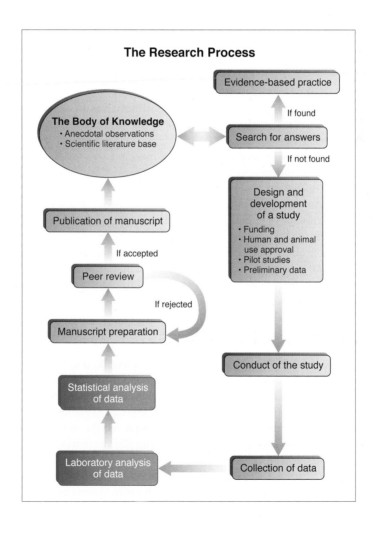

INTRODUCTION

Advances in technology have significantly changed every avenue of life in the past 50 years, resulting in faster and better communication. These changes have been helpful to all professions including those in science. For scientists, technology has enhanced the rate of information gathering, yet this change has not altered the importance of making strong inferences and logical conclusions. An **inference** is the process or act of deriving logical conclusions from premises or statements that are known, assumed true, or derived. Developing logical inferences is a crucial step in every aspect of the scientific process including developing questions, information gathering, making appropriate hypotheses, experimental design, data analysis, developing suitable conclusions, and, finally, communication of findings. Scientific information was once gathered by handwritten letters, telephone conversations, in-person meetings, and by searching through stacks of journals in the library. This painstakingly gathered information was used to construct appropriate inferences and make suitable hypotheses. Today, e-mails are directed to colleagues on other continents, and depending on the colleague, a reply may arrive within minutes. The telephone is still used but is now giving way to video conferences between colleagues in different countries. Library searches are still completed but from one's office and without the need to visit the actual library. Greater access to data in the information age has fostered the development of a greater number of hypotheses.

Clearly, today, the processes of information gathering in order to develop inferences and draw conclusions are the same, but the speed in obtaining this information to complete these processes is much faster. However, this increased speed does not always facilitate drawing proper inferences if appropriate caution is not taken. Developing a valid and sound inference is independent of the rate of information gathering and requires ample time, thought, and effort.

The purpose of this chapter is to introduce the theory and process for inference making, the development of sound and valid inferences, and to offer suggestions in order to avoid making invalid inferences. Logical inferences begin with valid premises and are the foundation of strong scientific investigations. Any misstep in drawing inferences may lead to conclusions that are not sound and logical fallacies. This chapter reviews the process of developing sound inferences based on available information while avoiding the pitfalls of logical fallacies.

INFERENCES AND THE SCIENTIFIC PROCESS

Today's universities place a strong emphasis on scientific inquiry in graduate education. This same emphasis now extends to undergraduate students as part of their academic preparation. As a result, students become acquainted with this process and begin to develop these skills earlier in their academic development. Regardless of academic training, a **scientific argument** is an application of logic, requiring the making of sound premises to draw valid inferences. Therefore, logical **reasoning** plays a central role in the generation and validation of all scientific understanding.

Errors in reasoning stem from inaccurate statements or invalid conclusions drawn from sound premises. These errors lead to invalid conclusions known as "logical fallacies."

Accordingly, fallacies are defined and categorized based on the error made. Logical fallacies are discussed in detail later in the chapter.

Throughout this chapter, examples of valid and invalid reasoning are presented to illustrate how reasoning affects reaching valid conclusions and provides the basis for better decision-making, research design, and appropriate data analysis to maintain or improve research quality. Presented here is an example from Ancel Keys's classic work regarding blood cholesterol concentrations and cardiovascular disease (CVD). In 1969, Dr. Keys presented Figure 19-1 which is a presentation of five cross-sectional studies from various countries representing blood cholesterol concentrations and aging. From this figure, one can observe that blood cholesterol concentrations in men rise with age. A second observation is that this rise appears to peak and then decrease after men reach the age of 65 years. Also noted is the relationship between CVD and blood cholesterol concentrations, which was well known at this time. These observations are rephrased in the following text as **logical constructs** with **premises** and **conclusions**.

- Logical construct 1:
  - Premise 1
    1. Blood cholesterol concentrations increase with age in men.
    2. As blood cholesterol concentrations increase, the risk of CVD also increases.
  - Conclusion 1: Therefore, as men age, their risk of CVD increases.
- Logical construct 2:
  - Premise 2: Blood cholesterol concentrations in men peak at the age of 65 years and then fall.
  - Conclusion 2: Therefore, CVD risk decreases after the age of 65 years in men.

In the next section, various types of inferences are discussed. As more information is gained regarding inference making and its applications, the determination of whether the conclusions drawn from the previous example were valid or invalid and why can be formed. But before going to the next section, consider the conclusion and practical implication reached using Figure 19-1. Once men reach the age of 65 years, blood cholesterol concentrations declined with further aging. Is the conclusion drawn from the premise sound? After other existing information is considered, is the conclusion as strong? With further examination, the data indicate that men with elevated blood cholesterol concentrations had died before the age of 65 years. Thus, the premise that once men reach the age of 65 years, blood cholesterol concentrations will become lower is false. But the conclusion is still true because men who survived past the age of 65 years had lower blood cholesterol concentrations during their lifespans than the men who did not survive. These men were at lower risk for developing CVD and were still alive after the age of 65 years. The invalid premise is that once men reach the age of 65 years, blood cholesterol concentrations will fall. Belief in this invalid premise leads to the belief that once the age of 65 years is reached, a reduction in blood cholesterol concentrations occur.

TYPES OF INFERENCES

Making an inference is the act of drawing conclusions from premises that are known or assumed to be true. Reasoning is simply the application of inference, and therefore throughout the rest of the chapter, the two are used interchangeably. Inference making is a natural process,

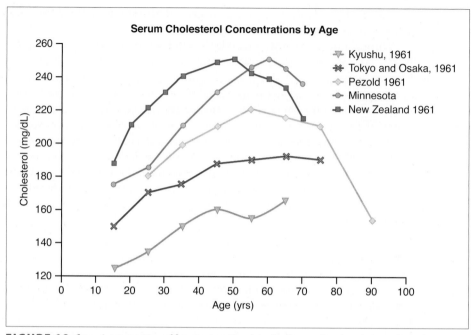

FIGURE 19-1:   A composition of five cross-sectional studies from various locations, representing cholesterol concentrations and aging. (From Keys A. Serum cholesterol and the question of "normal." In: Benson ES, Strandjord PE, editors. *Multiple Laboratory Screening*. New York (NY): Academic Press; 1969. p. 147–170.)

and regardless of the situation, the brain automatically tries to solve what is happening based on known or understood information from the past to predict what may happen in the future. Although inference making is natural, correctly inferring or drawing the proper conclusions within known confines is not always as innate. To determine whether a conclusion is valid, one must understand how a proper inference is made. To begin this understanding of inference, three groupings are generated to categorize different types of inference including deductive, inductive, and abductive (some consider abductive reasoning a mere subset of induction).

Deductive Reasoning

Deductive reasoning was introduced over 2,300 years ago when Aristotle released his ideas of reasoning in *Prior Analytics* (2). All other forms of reasoning were derived from Aristotle's work on deductive reasoning. In the broadest terms, deductive reasoning is defined as when general information is used to generate a premise, and from this process, a specific conclusion is drawn. Because the conclusion is built on a broad premise, deductive reasoning is also known as "top-down reasoning." This process uses one or more statements or premises that are linked to reach conclusions. When all terms used are clearly stated, the premises are true, and the rules of deductive logic are followed, the conclusion reached is valid. Like any other form of reasoning, deductive reasoning is evaluated on *validity* and *soundness*. A valid statement is obtained when it is impossible for the premise to be true while the conclusion is false (1). Conversely, an inference may be valid even while the premise is false. However, soundness is only awarded to inference if it is both valid and the premise is true. The following is a physiologic example of sound deductive reasoning.

- Premise
  1. Heart rate increases linearly with increasing exercise intensity.
  2. Running is a form of exercise.
- Conclusion: Therefore, heart rate linearly increases with increasing running intensity.

Several forms of deductive reasoning exist. The first form is the *law of detachment*, which describes the simplest form of deductive reasoning and is formed when a conditional statement is immediately followed by a hypothesis. The conclusion is drawn from the statements and hypothesis. The following is an example of the law of detachment:

- Premise
  3. All cells of the human body use adenosine triphosphate (ATP) as their energy source.
  4. The cells that make up the heart are cells of the body.
- Conclusion: Therefore, heart cells use ATP as their energy source.

The next form of deductive reasoning, the *law of syllogism*, is more complex and leaves a greater opportunity for causing a fallacy (untrue belief based on an unsound argument). With syllogisms, two conditional statements are used to derive a conclusion by combining the hypothesis of one statement with the conclusion of the other. Consider the following example:

- Premise
  1. Ben ran 5 mi everyday for four weeks and improved his performance in a time trial.
  2. Larry ran 5 mi everyday for four weeks and increased his maximal oxygen consumption ($\dot{V}O_2max$).
- Conclusion: Ben ran 5 mi everyday for four weeks and improved his performance *because he increased his $\dot{V}O_2max$.*

In the above example, the ultimate conclusion is deduced from the hypothesis of the first statement and the conclusion of the second statement. Unlike the law of detachment, with syllogism, the conclusion statement can be false. The logic considerations made in the previous statement are valid and the conclusion likely sound. However, because of the type of reasoning used, the possibilities of other sources of improved performance are not explored, leaving the possibility of a conclusion that is not sound.

The last form of deductive reasoning is known as the *law of contrapositives*. With contrapositive reasoning, a statement is proposed with a hypothesis and conclusion. If the conclusion is false, the hypothesis is then false as well.

- Premise
  1. During physical activity, blood flow to skeletal muscles is increased.
  2. Blood flow to skeletal muscle is not increased.
- Conclusion: Therefore, no physical activity is taking place.

The law of contrapositives is unique; if the conclusion is false, then the premise must be false. The converse is true; if the conclusion is true, the premise must be true. Remember, both the premise and conclusion are logically equal. Because both the premise and conclusion always have the same truth value in contrapositive deductive reasoning, they are popular for proving mathematic theorems.

When reviewing the previous examples, the following suggestions are helpful in evaluating a deductive argument. First, decide if the conclusion actually follows the premises. To accomplish this task, consider the question, "Is the argument valid?" If the argument is invalid, the premises do not support or establish the conclusion, and the conclusion is rejected. If the argument is valid, the next step is to determine the truth of the premises. If one premise is false, another reason is gained to support rejection of the conclusion. Thus, a conclusion is rejected if either the reasoning is invalid (regardless of whether the premises are true) or at least one premise is false (regardless of whether the reasoning valid).

Inductive Reasoning

Sir Francis Bacon formally introduced **inductive reasoning** as an alternative to deductive reasoning. Aristotle considered the concept of inductive reasoning nearly 1,500 years prior to Bacon but never formalized his theories. Bacon's inductive reasoning was later segued into the foundation of the scientific method (3). In the broadest sense, inductive reasoning is using evidence from particular instances to support more general ideas, which is basically the reverse of deductive reasoning. Inductive reasoning is closely associated with probability and the syllogism form of deductive reasoning. The main difference between inductive and deductive reasoning is that inductive reasoning leaves the possibility for a false conclusion even if all of the premises are true. Thus, inductive reasoning requires a substantial amount of supporting evidence that gives credence to the conclusion.

Inductive reasoning is the main foundation for what is collectively known as the "scientific method" which has been shaped, molded, and processed for thousands of years. As you've learned in the first portion of this text, the scientific method includes the formulation of a question, a prediction, testing the hypothesis for the question, and then analysis of the data collected to accept or reject the hypothesis. Although inference making in science is typically geared toward the analysis section, inferences are found throughout the scientific process. Flawed inferences are the result of incorrect assumptions. The following consideration is an example of inductive reasoning:

- Premise: All individuals measured in the study who did not exercise and were older than the age of 55 years had a heart attack within two years of completing the study.
- Conclusion: Individuals older than the age of 55 years who do not exercise will most likely have a heart attack.

In any situation using inductive reasoning, uncertainty can lead to false conclusions. For this reason, scientists primarily use derivations of inductive reasoning. **Abductive reasoning** is one such form of inductive reasoning and was developed by the American philosopher Charles Sanders Pierce (11). Like other forms of inductive reasoning, abductive reasoning is a form of logical inference in which moving from observation to a hypothesis accounts for the reliability of observations seeking to explain relevant evidence. Unlike deductive reasoning, when using abductive reasoning, the premise or evidence does not guarantee the conclusion. Abductive reasoning is also described as giving the best explanation.

Pierce himself referred to this form of reasoning as "guessing." Although abductive reasoning may be a guess, this form of reasoning has a place in forming a proper hypothesis when using the scientific method.

REASONING IN SCIENTIFIC RESEARCH

The scientific literature is replete with examples of deductive and inductive reasoning. The question is which type or types of inferences are used to reach a conclusion and where within a journal article do such statements appear. Inductive arguments are commonly found in the introduction and generally are used to provide support for the study's purpose by speculating a valid but uncertain conclusion in the form of a hypothesis (9). Deductive reasoning, however, is associated with the conclusions based specifically on the empirical findings reported in the results section and evaluated in the discussion section or occasionally in the methods section to justify a specific aspect of the methodology. The following section provides selected examples of how each type of reasoning is used in the scientific literature.

Deductive arguments are empirical and factual arguments that use premises taken from the current study and add facts from prior studies to form a conclusion. For example, a landmark physiology paper by Saltin and colleagues (14,15) reported the results from a longitudinal study that confined participants to bed rest for 20 consecutive days which was followed by 55 days of exercise endurance training. Several physiologic measurements including $\dot{V}O_2$max were made over multiple times during the course of the study. The authors employed *deductive* reasoning based on their data to infer what is now considered a basic and tested conclusion that patterns of physical activity (PA) and exercise partially determine $\dot{V}O_2$max.

Below are the premises stated from which a conclusion is drawn.

- Premises
  1. Twenty days of bed rest (detraining) decreased $\dot{V}O_2$max, stroke volume, and cardiac output.
  2. After 55 days of exercise training following the detraining period, subjects were able to improve $\dot{V}O_2$max above detraining levels.
- Conclusion: PA and exercise patterns affect $\dot{V}O_2$max.

Initially, what may not seem intuitive is how authors can use deductive reasoning to reach a valid logical conclusion or set of conclusions that are then used in an inductive argument to determine logical probability in support of a new study (13). For example, Blair and colleagues (7) attempted to establish and support the relationship between fitness and all-cause mortality. The researchers used inductive and deductive reasoning in different sections of this same article. They used inductive reasoning to support their assertion that their particular findings were a pertinent research question.

- Premises
  1. PA is inversely related to risk of morbidity and mortality.
  2. PA from hard work or leisure activities is protective and results in decreased risk of morbidity and mortality.

3. More PA is associated with increased longevity.

4. PA behavior does not necessarily improve physical fitness.

- Conclusion: Therefore, the health benefits of PA may not require improvements in physical fitness.

Note that the last statement is partially unstated by the authors although inserted here for completeness. At the time of their publication, the relationship between fitness and mortality was not clear. Therefore, the authors created an argument based on known information to draw a logical conclusion that was by no means certain or tested.

In the same article, the authors used deductive reasoning to support their conclusion that mortality is inversely associated with fitness in both men and women (7). The premises that support the argument and the conclusion drawn are as follows:

- Premise

  1. The least fit people have a greater risk of mortality than do the fitter.

  2. Greatest decreases in relative risk are between the least fit and next-to-least fit.

  3. Continued modest risk reductions are found with increasing fitness.

- Conclusion: The greater your fitness, the lower your mortality rate.

When reading a journal article, note the stated or underlying arguments in the introduction or discussion sections. Frequently, inductive arguments are found in the introduction stating what is currently known; this reasoning subsequently leads toward the purpose and research question(s) (12). Deductive reasoning is frequently found in the discussion section and uses the facts from the current study in combination with known facts to make a definitive conclusion.

Logical Disagreements: An Example of Factors Limiting Performance

The remainder of this section presents an example found in physiology literature in which different perspectives lead to logical disagreements in science. Although each perspective is different, the inference is still valid, showing that in science, two views can be upheld without either viewpoint being considered incorrect. Because all viewpoints are supported in the example, a better understanding for the physiologically limiting factors of $\dot{V}O_2$max is the result. Ultimately, science is about deriving the truth, whatever that truth is.

However, arriving at the truth may be an arduous process with opposing viewpoints and conflicting data. It is not unusual to find two (or more) entrenched ideologies regarding a particular controversial issue in science, politics, or just about any other field. Within the field of exercise physiology, one needs to look no further than the numerous discussions about physiologic factors limiting $\dot{V}O_2$max. A vigorous debate has raged here for many years, and for many scientists, this issue remains unsettled. The point to illustrate here is that the use of logic and the derivation of valid conclusions from factual premises is a legitimate part of the scientific process. However, different sets of premises can yield distinctly different conclusions. Bassett and Howley (5) published a commentary that discusses the history of $\dot{V}O_2$max and provides an overview of the different premises in support or to refute a particular conclusion. This paper is used to illustrate the use of premises and valid conclusions to reach different conclusions (5).

Logical Disagreement: Argument for the Pulmonary System as a Limiting Factor

The ability to oxygenate blood in the lungs is clearly an important issue and relates to the delivery and use of oxygen and thus is a potential key limiting physiologic site for $\dot{V}O_2max$. Some pulmonary diseases and genetic conditions are known to limit physical performance. However, the question here is whether or not the pulmonary system limits physical performance in otherwise healthy people.

- Premise
  1. Normal saturation of hemoglobin with oxygen occurs in the lungs and at sea level and is about 98%.
  2. During maximal exercise in recreational athletes, hemoglobin saturation decreases to approximately 95%.
  3. Maximal cardiac output in recreational athletes is around 25 L/min.
  4. In elite athletes, hemoglobin saturation may decrease to approximately 90% or less.
  5. Maximal cardiac output in elite athletes may reach 40 L/min.
  6. Addition of supplemental oxygen to elite athletes increases $\dot{V}O_2max$ from 71 to 74 mL/kg/min, whereas no change is observed in recreational athletes.

- Conclusion: The pulmonary system's ability to oxygenate hemoglobin is limiting $\dot{V}O_2max$ in elite athletes.

Logical Disagreement: Argument for Central Cardiovascular System or Heart as a Limiting Site

The argument for the central cardiovascular system as a limiting factor for $\dot{V}O_2max$ is based on the heart's ability to move blood to the lungs and peripheral tissues. A measure of central cardiovascular function is cardiac output. Clearly, this system is vital because of the transport of oxygen bound to hemoglobin from the lungs and delivery to the peripheral tissues where oxygen serves as the final electron acceptor for aerobic metabolism. A significant part of this argument relies on the principle of competing demands (*i.e.*, one has a fixed quantity of a resource that must be distributed for multiple purposes).

- Premise
  1. Human skeletal muscle can accommodate quite a large volume of blood flow.
  2. If all the muscles in the human body were maximally engaged in exercise, a cardiac output of greater than or equal to 50 L/min would be required, but such a value has not been reported previously in humans.
  3. Normal values for maximal cardiac output in nonelite athletes are 20–30 L/min.

- Conclusion: Heart function as measured by cardiac output sets the upper limit for oxygen delivery and thus $\dot{V}O_2max$.

Logical Disagreement: Argument for the Muscular System as a Limiting Site

Exercising skeletal muscle is the principal site for extraction of oxygen from blood and utilization of that oxygen. This argument centers on the number of mitochondria with their metabolic enzymes and the capillary density for blood flow in skeletal muscle.

- Premise
  1. Oxygen moves down a pressure gradient from the lungs to blood, then from the blood into the muscle cell, and finally into the mitochondria.
  2. Oxygen utilization by the mitochondria due to increased metabolic demand maintains this gradient.
  3. Endurance exercise training induces an increase in mitochondria and a twofold increase in mitochondrial enzyme levels, which increases the muscle's ability to use oxygen.
  4. Skeletal muscle capillary density increases approximately 20% after muscle is exercise-trained.
  5. Increased capillary density decreases diffusion distance for oxygen which enhances the delivery of oxygen to the muscle and the mitochondria.
  6. Increased capillary density also lengthens the transit time for red blood cells and enhances the unloading of oxygen to the tissues.
- Conclusion: Peripheral factors such as the number of mitochondria and capillary density determine the rate at which oxygen is used, and thus muscle is a site for limiting $\dot{V}O_2$max.

The discussion found in this section is not a debate regarding which of the above physiologic factors limits $\dot{V}O_2$max; rather, the point is to understand that premises are constructed with well-established facts, and conclusions are drawn from the premises. However, the inferences derived from different premises conflict even though the conclusions are all logically derived.

The arguments presented here are an attempt to illustrate various views taken by scientists to narrow the understanding for the physiologically limiting factors of $\dot{V}O_2$max. This discussion may seem esoteric to the casual reader, but these questions in the past have stimulated great debates among leading scientists (and still do) while having also stimulated an enormous amount of creativity in experimental research design that has resulted in novel findings leading to a better understanding of human physiology.

LOGICAL FALLACIES

In science, an inference is never infallible. In fact, the scientific method recognizes that inferences may be proven invalid. Nonetheless, inferences are supported by the available data. Properly performing scientific investigations necessitates that scientists do make inferences regarding what is found when completing the investigation. This process is completed through a combination of collecting evidence (known information and newly discovered data) and reasoning, whether this reasoning is deductive, inductive, or abductive (10). The driving aim of the investigator is to draw a sound conclusion—one that is supported by substantial evidence with valid and sound reasoning. This aim is not always reached, and when it is not, a **logical fallacy** is the result. Logical fallacies are errors in known information and reasoning. As is the case for reasoning, fallacies are divided categorically based on what type of error in reasoning is made.

Two broad categories of fallacies are formal and informal with classification based on the type of inference made. Formal fallacies are those originating from deductive reasoning. In the previous example from the law of detachment, the following statements were made:

- Premise
  1. All cells in the body use ATP.
  2. Heart cells are cells of the body.
- Conclusion: Therefore, heart cells use ATP.

Because all scientific evidence supports that cells of the body use ATP as their energy source and heart cells are cells of the body, the conclusion that heart cells use ATP is not refuted. Conversely, if heart cells were replaced with apical meristem cells from plants, then a formal fallacy would have been committed. Although the conclusion that apical meristems use ATP as their energy source is sound, the reasoning is not valid. Representations of formal fallacies in exploratory science are difficult to find because when using deductive reasoning, if the statement is valid, there is certainty in the statement. However, formal fallacies are not common.

Informal fallacies on the other hand are only committed when using inductive reasoning which commonly occurs during scientific investigations (8). Such fallacies occur when the stated premise of the study fails to support the proposed hypothesis. Inductive reasoning is typically judged in terms of the persuasiveness of argument, methodology used, and statistical evidence to support the argument. Informal fallacies or inductive fallacies are classified based on three characteristics which are *relevance*, *ambiguity*, and *presumption*.

Relevance fallacies originate when the inference is made on premises that are irrelevant to the conclusion. With any inference—whether in an argument or in scientific research—evidence must be provided to support that the premise is true. When relevance fallacies occur, evidence is provided that lends no evidential value to support the conclusion. The largest categorization of relevance fallacies is *irrelevant appeals*. Irrelevant appeals attempt to support a conclusion by providing powerful evidence even though the evidence is unconnected to the inference being made.

- John is a famous fitness trainer.
- John says walking on a motorized treadmill increases energy expenditure more than walking in the neighborhood.
- Walking on a motorized treadmill will expend more energy.

The premise "John is a famous fitness trainer" is irrelevant to the conclusion about energy expenditure. Although the statement that John is knowledgeable about energy expenditure during exercise may seem reasonable, the premise that John is a famous fitness trainer is not evidence for his knowledge regarding increased energy expenditure while using a motorized treadmill. Therefore, the argument is invalid.

Another form of a relevance fallacy is an *appeal to authority* and is an extremely common occurrence. With an appeal to authority, instead of relying on gathered evidence to support the conclusion, an attempt is made to support the conclusion by using the testimony of a person who is judged as an authority. The following is an example of an appeal to authority:

- Premise: A.V. Hill believed that caffeine had endurance performance-improving capabilities for exercise lasting over 60 minutes.
- Conclusion: Caffeine improves exercise endurance performance lasting over 60 minutes.

Dr. A.V. Hill was an astoundingly brilliant scientist and a Nobel Laureate who is responsible for coining many terms and concepts still used today in physiology. But his work never ventured into ergogenic aids and their effects on human performance (4). If the appeal to authority had relied on the testimony of Dr. David Costill, the inference and conclusion would have been more valid because some of Dr. Costill's most significant work was on the effect of caffeine on human performance.

An informal fallacy providing an inference that appears to support the conclusion merely because vague terminology is used within the inference is known as an "ambiguous fallacy." The most common ambiguous fallacy is the *equivocation fallacy*. These fallacies occur when a term is used that has two or more different meanings within a single argument. For example:

A theory is only an idea.
Evolution is a theory.
Evolution is only an idea.

Typically, equivocation fallacy will occur in debates and conversations but rarely occur in science. As in the previous example, a scientific term such as theory when used in social context may have more than one meaning.

Lastly, informal fallacies committed by using an unwarranted or unsupported inference to draw a conclusion are known as "presumptive fallacies." One of the most popular presumptive fallacies is the use of *circular logic* (12). The inference is circular if the conclusion is also part of the inference, leading to a logical construct that cannot support the conclusion. Some philosophers consider circular logic as needing a true question, which is why circular logic is also known as "begging the question." Consider the following example of circular reasoning:

- Premise: Question—Can an individual achieve any level of $\dot{V}O_2$max strictly through proper endurance exercise training?
- Conclusion: As long as an individual goes through endurance exercise training, attaining any level of $\dot{V}O_2$max is possible.

This example answers the question by restating the question, but there is no evidence that any level of $\dot{V}O_2$max can be attained with endurance exercise training. The text simply states that such an achievement is possible. Circular fallacies are accepted as sound inference by those who have already accepted the conclusion as true.

Methods for Reducing Logical Fallacies

Obviously, scientific research does not aim to create fallacies. However, fallacies do occur, and some are more difficult to avoid than others. Even when the guiding principles of the scientific process are closely followed, committing a formal fallacy is possible. For this reason, the process of peer review for manuscript publications was developed so as to reduce fallacies. The peer-review procedure is thought to be formally erected in the publication *Medical Essays and Observations* in 1731 (6). Although manuscripts are reviewed and inspected for potential fallacies, oral research presentations and defenses have no such filter. Because informal fallacies can happen when designing, implementing, defending, presenting, and writing a manuscript of scientific research, following simple guidelines can reduce their occurrence. By using such guidelines and by gaining experience with them, the occurrence of fallacies can be reduced.

The following section provides insights into avenues for developing and making logical inferences and arguments which make for better designed scientific studies. When properly formed premises are developed from known information, rather than assumed truths, stronger inferences and arguments are developed. Thus, well-built arguments are a result of appropriately composed premises that are arranged in a way to support the conclusion. Better inferences and conclusions are formed when:

1. Properly constructing premises are based on supported information that is both true and relevant to the issue.
2. Developed premises provide strong support for the intended conclusion and not another conclusion.
3. The most important or relevant aspects of the issue are addressed in making a premise.
4. The premise and conclusion focus on what is applicable to the issue.
5. Broad claims that are not supportable should be avoided.
6. All ideas are best presented in an orderly fashion so reviewers can easily follow the developed line of thought.

Fallacies do occur in scientific work, and their elimination makes for better oral presentations and greater likelihood for manuscript acceptance and publication. The following guidelines are useful in finding and eliminating fallacies. Working with a mentor is especially useful and will facilitate the use of these guidelines (16):

1. When developing inferences and conclusions, take an adversarial approach to explore various ways to disagree or find weaknesses with each inference or conclusion. This approach will facilitate evaluation and determination as to which inference or part of the argument is not supported or is weak. Once found, give special attention to strengthening these areas.
2. For each conclusion or argument, list main points. Once these points are identified, outline supporting and unsupported evidence for each. Following this process will allow for a precise review and evaluation of all points and will result in a clear understanding of whether the evidence for a particular claim is unsupportive, indifferent, or supportive. The overall goal is to complete a critical evaluation of the existing evidence.
3. Learn to understand your thinking and writing patterns by being introspective of your work. Early in a career, scientists are prone to making specific fallacies, and by knowing which types of fallacies are more likely to occur for any individual, a junior scientist can begin to find and reduce such fallacies. To accomplish this task, review earlier papers and determine which fallacies are more prominent. Compare this past writing to more current writing and see if the fallacies have been resolved.
4. Know that when developing a premise, broad claims need more supporting evidence than do narrow claims. The use of broad terms such as "all," "no," "none," "every," "always," "never," "no one," and "everyone" are usually red flags and are an indication that broad unfocused claims rather than a narrowly developed focus are presented. Focused premises require less proof and use words such as "some," "many," "few," "sometimes," and "usually."
5. When developing and making a presentation or writing and submitting a manuscript for publication, know the audience and background information pertaining to the audience. This guideline is broad and in the context of developing premises for designing a research project; giving this guideline consideration early in the development

process for a presentation or publication will provide an added dimension to making appropriate premises and inferences and therefore a better product.

SUMMARY

Developing a scientific argument is an application of reason. The intent of this chapter is to establish the importance for proper inference making, to give insight into the process for developing sound inferences in order to develop stronger scientific arguments, and to offer suggestions for ways to avoid making invalid inferences and logical fallacies. Improper reasoning (*i.e.*, invalid premises and unsound inferences) will lead to logical fallacies. Throughout this chapter, examples of valid and invalid reasoning are presented to illustrate the process for proper premise making necessary to reach valid conclusions. Improvements in logical constructs provide for enhanced decision making, better research design, and appropriate data analysis to maintain or improve research quality. Nonetheless, even with excellent reasoning skills, logical fallacies do happen in science when designing studies, implementing research protocols, and in manuscript writing. However, following a few simple guidelines can reduce their occurrence. Improved inference making results in stronger scientific arguments, and subsequently, the quality of science is enhanced.

GLOSSARY

Abductive reasoning: a form of reasoning which is sometimes considered a subset of inductive reasoning. In this form of reasoning, the premises do not guarantee the conclusions

Deductive reasoning: a form of reasoning in which a specific conclusion is derived from general statements

Inductive reasoning: a form of reasoning in which a general conclusion is derived from specific examples

Inference: the process of constructing logical conclusions from premises known or assumed to be true

Logical construct: a conceptual format that integrates thoughts in organized fashion to show the progression of reasoning

Logical construct conclusion: a propositional statement that is the final stage of inference. Often, these statements are indicated by phrases such as "therefore" and "it follows that"

Logical construct premise: a propositional statement that is stated explicitly and gives evidence for accepting the inference and conclusion that follows

Logical fallacy: an incorrect inference in a logical construct causing a lack of validity in the statement. Two general types of fallacies can be committed—informal and formal

Premise: an argument statement that will induce or justify a conclusion or a premise assumes that something is true

Reasoning: the action of thinking logically in a sensible way to support a conclusion

Scientific argument: the application of logic, making sound premises to draw valid inferences

REFERENCES

1. Aristotle. *Posterior Analytics*. Barnes J, trans-ed. New York (NY): Oxford University Press; 1994.
2. Aristotle. *Prior Analytics*. Smith R, trans-ed. Indianapolis (IN): Hackett; 1989.
3. Baronett S. *Logic*. Upper Saddle River (NJ): Pearson Prentice Hall; 2008. 321–325 p.
4. Bassett DR. Scientific contributions of A. V. Hill: exercise physiology pioneer. *J Appl Physiol*. 2002;93(5):1567–1582.
5. Bassett DR, Howley ET. Limiting factors for maximum oxygen uptake and determinants of endurance performance. *Med Sci Sports Exerc*. 2000;32(1):70–84.
6. Benos DJ, Bashari E, Chaves JM, et al. The ups and down of peer review. *Adv Physiol Educ*. 2007;31(2):145–152.
7. Blair SN, Kohl HW III, Paffenbarger RS Jr, Clark DG, Cooper KH, Gibbons LW. Physical fitness and all-cause mortality. A prospective study of healthy men and women. *JAMA*. 1989;262(17):2395–2401.
8. Engel SM. *With Good Reason: An Introduction to Informal Fallacies*. 3rd ed. New York (NY): St. Martin's Press; 1989.
9. Hacking I. *An Introduction to Probability and Inductive Logic*. Cambridge, United Kingdom: Cambridge University Press; 2011.
10. Kelly D. *The Art of Reasoning*. New York: W. W. Norton & Company, Inc.; 2011.
11. Magnani L. *Abduction, Reason, and Science: Process of Discovery and Explanation*. New York (NY): Springer Publishers; 2001.
12. Perkins R Jr. *Logic and Mr. Limbaugh: A Dittohead's Guide to Fallacious Reasoning*. 1st ed. Chicago (IL): Open Court Publishing; 1995.
13. Popper C. *Conjectures and Refutations: The Growth of Scientific Knowledge*. 2nd ed. London, United Kingdom: Routledge; 2004.
14. Saltin B. Hemodynamic adaptations to exercise. *Am J Cardiol*. 1985;55(10):42D–47D.
15. Saltin B, Blomqvist G, Mitchell JH, Johnson RL, Wildenthal K, Chapman CB. Response to exercise after bed rest and after training: a longitudinal study of adaptive changes in oxygen transport and body composition. *Circulation*. 1968;38(5 suppl):VII1–78.
16. UNC Writing Center Web site [Internet]. Fallacies. Chapel Hill (NC): UNC Writing Center; [cited 2013 August 1]. Available from: http://writingcenter.unc.edu/handouts/fallacies/

CHAPTER 20

Writing a Research Manuscript and Determining Authorship

Carl M. Maresh, PhD, FACSM, Jenna M. Bartley, PhD, and Colleen X. Muñoz, PhD

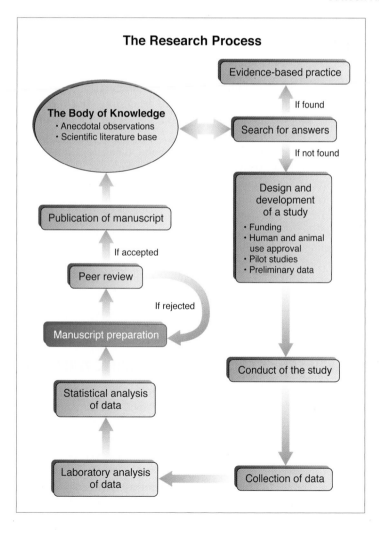

The Research Process

The Body of Knowledge
- Anecdotal observations
- Scientific literature base

Evidence-based practice

Search for answers

If found

If not found

Design and development of a study
- Funding
- Human and animal use approval
- Pilot studies
- Preliminary data

Publication of manuscript

If accepted

Peer review

If rejected

Manuscript preparation

Conduct of the study

Statistical analysis of data

Laboratory analysis of data

Collection of data

INTRODUCTION: NO SCIENTIFIC PUBLICATION, NO SCIENTIFIC PROGRESS

Manuscript publication permits researchers to share valuable information with other scientists, clinicians, practitioners, and the public. Without this avenue of communication, advancement of knowledge and scientifically based practice would cease. More important, this means of sharing scientific information incorporates the opportunity for peer review, which strengthens data quality and interpretation, and the author's ability to construct a quality manuscript prior to peer review is an inherent responsibility in scientific research.

Formal courses on scientific writing are not readily available, and learning to write in this way takes time; effective scientific writing techniques develop from practice more so than from verbal instruction. Nonetheless, basic principles, considerations, and tips provide the foundation for effective scientific writing. This chapter serves to relay the basic building blocks required for scientific writing, which will enhance the probability of publication success.

ALWAYS HAVE A PLAN

Adequate preparation prior to writing a manuscript always proves beneficial. Many researchers suggest that determining the specific manuscript objectives, authorship, and journal selection should occur prior to even beginning data collection (3,4,6). In fact, creating a clear plan that addresses these issues often prevents conflicts among peers and colleagues.

Initial preparations for both study design and manuscript construction include an extensive literature review (see Chapter 4), which will reveal the research rationale. Highly researched topics might present an abundance of published literature, which can greatly benefit from creating a summary table to synthesize the voluminous information. Once familiar with relevant literature, the researcher can develop the research question and hypotheses. Keeping the research question and hypotheses at the forefront during the study design and manuscript planning phases directs the researcher's efforts.

Another useful writing technique involves constructing an **outline** to organize and determine logical content flow. The specific guidelines of the anticipated scientific journal can dictate the outline's format. Furthermore, examining previously published articles in the anticipated journal provides formatting examples and commonly published topics to assure an appropriate fit for the manuscript.

DISTINCTIONS BETWEEN CREATIVE AND SCIENTIFIC WRITING

Most researchers began accruing their writing skills through a creative style. Although these rudimentary and descriptive writing courses provide fundamental knowledge of writing mechanics, grammar, and organization, obvious differences exist between creative and scientific writing styles. Most importantly, scientific writing demands clear and concise sentences that still incorporate ample detail. Therefore, expressive description and more relaxed organization (among other aspects) do not belong in scientific writing as they do in creative writing. Table 20-1 presents notable contrast between creative and scientific writing styles, which will assist in making the writing style transition.

Table 20-1 Notable Differences Between Creative and Scientific Writing

	Creative Writing	Scientific Writing
Purpose	Expression, narration	Clear communication
Details	Limited details and more generalized ideas	Highly detailed and specific, allowing for replication of methodology and clear logical progression
Content Characteristics	Subjective or objective, personal	Objective, impersonal, factual
Content Organization	Aesthetically shaped, integrated format	Structured by scientific purpose, guidelines dictate necessary headings and structure
Audience	General public	Scientific peers
Reader Interest	Designed to interest readers	Readers determine own interest based on content
Accuracy and Clarity	Not necessarily required	Required
Voice	Normally more active voice	More passive voice used to focus on subject matter
Sources	Personal knowledge and experience	Data and concepts from other peer-reviewed articles and scientific literature
Graphics	Embellished, illustration purposes	Structured, empirical demonstration of data or conceptual progression

Adapted from Goldbort R. *Writing for Science*. Binghamton (NY): Vail-Ballou Press; 2006. 110 p.

THE NAKED SCIENTIFIC MANUSCRIPT: JUST THE BARE BONES

A unifying, basic organizational skeleton of all scientific writing exists; this standardization permits ease in reading and collecting information from scientific publications. For the writer, one as opposed to numerous outline styles reduces the complexity of conveying information. As a student, laboratory-based courses often introduce this skeleton as the **title** followed by **introduction**, **methods**, **results**, **discussion**, and **references** sections. This same skeleton (with the addition of an **abstract**) applies for published scientific writing with only minor alterations depending on the research journal. Each section requires specific information, resulting in a logically progressing scientific story (Fig. 20-1 summarizes the components of a scientific manuscript).

Title

The title of a scientific manuscript successfully identifies the content in as few words as possible. Careful selection of title content proves imperative to the work's recognition, considering that search engine indexing in part relies on the title, and most individuals seeking scientific information triage articles by examining the title first to determine relevance (7). Title criticism often includes (a) too many words, (b) too general or insufficient information, and (c) incorporating unclear abbreviations. For example, the title *The Influence of a Long-Term Exercise Intervention on Skeletal Muscle* contains (a) non-descriptive

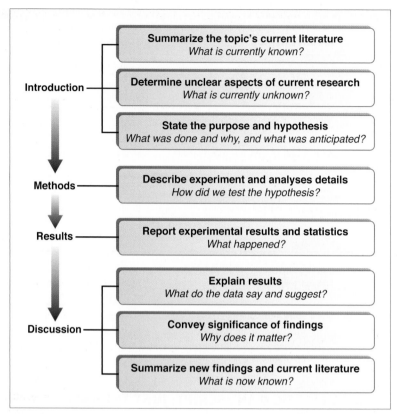

FIGURE 20-1:   The components of a scientific manuscript.

words (*e.g.,* "long-term" vs. an actual duration such as 18 weeks, "exercise intervention" vs. an exercise type such as run training, and "skeletal muscle" vs. a description of the variables examined such as skeletal muscle morphology) and (b) unnecessary words (*e.g.,* "The influence of a"). These changes create the more succinct and descriptive title: *Skeletal Muscle Morphology Following 18-Week Run Training.*

When should authors construct the manuscript title? Some argue that creating the title prior to writing the manuscript might not accurately capture the important aspects of the investigation, although others suggest that creating the title as the final step in the writing process might invite less care when selecting its words (5). However, most scientific writers agree that an initial working title helps them focus their thoughts, and the exact wording of the title can be altered throughout the writing process, which often occurs (3,6).

Abstract

As with the manuscript title, a successful abstract reports only the most critical information derived from each main section of the manuscript (excluding the references) in as few words as possible. Also similar to the manuscript title, many readers use this section to triage the manuscript for their purposes (6,7). This means that the abstract should stand alone as a brief yet encompassing representation of the manuscript. Careful word selection ensures that meaningful content will be identified during a web-based literature search. Abstracts do not require a full literature review or discussion but include research objectives and rationale, basic methods and results, and the most noteworthy conclusions; the author should continuously examine the necessity of the abstract content. Generally, acceptable abstract length ranges from 200 to 300 total words, depending on the journal requirements. Organization of the abstract content matches that of the manuscript, and many journals require headings within the abstract paragraph similar to those found in the manuscript (*i.e.*, methods, results, etc.). Abstract construction can commence at either the beginning or end of the writing process, dependent on personal preference.

Introduction

As the first primary section of the manuscript, the introduction attracts and tells the reader why the study was conducted. To do so, the writer includes background information on the topic, purpose of the study, and corresponding hypotheses.

Background information provides the reader with only the most critical knowledge of what currently does and does not exist among peer-reviewed sources (1,6). This requires authors to conduct a full literature search to present a comprehensive and objective view of the topic (see Chapter 4). To convey this information, writing begins with broader statements leading to more specific statements about the topic to acquaint the reader. All background information provided in this section necessitates appropriate citation in the text and inclusion in the references section at the end of the manuscript.

Following introduction of background information, the writer then conveys the importance of the investigation; this might include the environment, population, and other circumstances or details beneficial to data interpretation. This information leads the reader to assume the intentions of the study prior to any clear statement.

To this point, the introduction logically leads to a clear presentation of the purpose statement, which comprises one sentence precisely stating the aim of the investigation. For example, "The purpose of this study was to examine the influence of chronic creatine supplementation on body composition in recreational, female weight lifters." The subsequent sentence then presents the hypothesis statement, which describes the expected results. For example, "We anticipated that chronic creatine supplementation would improve lean body mass without influencing fat mass in recreational, female weight lifters." These critical statements express intention and direction of the manuscript and often dictate the success of publication within the scientific review process (3). Standing alone, these statements should convey the goals and educated expectations of the study.

In most cases, the introduction section extends approximately two to four paragraphs. Composition of the introduction section can occur either first or toward the end of the writing process. Like the title and abstract, some argue benefits for constructing a working introduction prior to writing the remainder of the manuscript and then adjusting its content throughout the writing process. Most importantly, the introduction must reflect the direction of the results and discussion sections, leaving some to argue that it might be best written later.

Methods

The methods section describes every detail involved in the data derivation. Extent of the detail provided should allow another researcher to replicate the investigation to determine the efficacy of the hypothesis being supported or to add to the replication of a study which strengthens the findings and can lead to the development of principles or theories (*e.g.*, size principle, sliding filament theory) (1,6,7). The methods provide information about the study population, research design, experimental protocol (including equipment, materials, and sample analyses), and statistical analyses; some of these titles often serve well as subheadings (3) (or variations of these depending on the journal).

Population

Humans, animals, or biological samples can define the study population, and generalizability of the research requires great detail of the examined population. Tips for describing study populations are available in Concept Box 20-1. Necessary details include the following:

1. Sample size (*e.g.*, number of human or animal participants)
2. Descriptive characteristics (*e.g.*, sex, animal model, cell line, etc.)
3. Group designations (*e.g.*, treatment, control, etc.)
4. Inclusion and exclusion criteria (*e.g.*, health status, habitual practices, genotype, cell strain, etc.)

Following the population details, research involving humans and animals requires a statement regarding ethical practice. For human research, authors need to include a statement acknowledging that participants provided informed consent, the study was approved through the local institutional review board (IRB), or the study complied with the Declaration of Helsinki. For animal research, authors need to include a statement affirming approval though the local Institutional Animal Care and Use Committee (IACUC) or a global equivalent. Refer to Chapters 11 and 12 for greater details regarding ethical practices.

Research Design

A statement pertaining to the research design not only provides details necessary for study replication but also supports the quality of the findings reported later in the manuscript. Details include definition of treatment and control groups, number of trials and experiments, order of trials and experiments, blinding, etc. (See Chapter 8 for research design classifications.)

CONCEPT BOX 20-1 Tips for Population Description

- Classify animals, plants, and microorganisms by genus, species, and strain (or appropriate identifying characteristics).
- Identify cell lines through reporting their sources and any specific biochemical, biologic, and/or immunologic traits. State any tests used for quality verification.
- Describe human participants' training status when necessary (type of exercise, years of participation, competition level, etc.).

CONCEPT BOX 20-2 **Tips for Methodologic Content and Grammar**

- Avoid including results in the methods section. Demographic data to describe a population sample are not results, as dependent variables are results.
- Seek related previous literature to serve as an example for variable collection details.
- Ask an uninvolved colleague to review the experimental protocol for sufficient details.

Experimental Protocol

The experimental protocol incorporates every process during data collection, from administering an intervention to analyzing samples. The information in this section should be in chronological order and as concise as possible, yet include enough detail for an experienced individual to replicate the entire experiment. Experimental protocol details include variables that were collected, how they were collected, when they were collected, and under what conditions.

Equipment manufacturer details, types and quantities of reagents, and exact experimental procedures must be noted. Tips for methodologic content and grammar are available in Concept Box 20-2.

Highly established protocols can simply be referenced with published research, whereas unpublished protocols require great detail within the manuscript's methods section. For example, when determining or estimating $\dot{V}O_2$max via an established protocol (*i.e.*, Bruce, YMCA, etc.), the author must reference the original publication validating the protocol. However, when determining $\dot{V}O_2$max through the modification of an established protocol, the author should describe the entire procedure including calibration of equipment where and when needed. Similarly, when using a commercially available enzyme-linked immunosorbent assay (ELISA), for example, the author simply references the manufacturer details. Conversely, newly developed or unpublished biochemical assays require the author to report every step and reagent used.

Statistical Analyses

The statistical analysis information typically comprises the final portion of the methods. Authors should report analyses in the same order in which they were conducted. Precisely *how* authors report this information is personal preference involving more or less statistical vocabulary. Although established statistical techniques require comment only, less established techniques necessitate an in-text reference of published work. Chapter 18 presents more information on statistical analyses, and Concept Box 20-3 provides tips for reporting statistical analyses.

Methods sections of scientific manuscripts can vary in length. A simple laboratory study might only require a few paragraphs, whereas a study introducing new methodology might require many pages. Furthermore, some manuscripts might benefit from including tables and figures (*i.e.*, equipment diagrams and protocol flow charts) for methodologic clarity.

CONCEPT BOX 20-3 Tips for Reporting Statistical Analyses

- Provide the statistical software package used, including the manufacturer's information.
- Report the *a priori* alpha level.
- Include any correction factors administered for multiple comparisons tests or assumption violations.
- Note the format of data central tendency and variability (*i.e.*, mean, median, standard deviation, standard error, interquartile range, etc.)

Authors should consult the journal guidelines to determine formatting specifics. Ultimately, a well-constructed methods section primes the reader to accept the results as valid and reproducible.

Results

The results section of the scientific manuscript contains findings from the previously described experiments with great clarity, brevity, and accuracy. Authors must present the experimentally derived data with statistical support while refraining from discussing its interpretations (6) unless this style is encouraged by the specific journal. This report includes text, tables, and/or figures without duplicating reports among these presentation formats (*i.e.*, values presented as text cannot also be presented in a table). When reporting numerical data, authors must report significant figures suitable for the variable (*i.e.*, reporting the same number of decimal places to resemble equipment accuracy) and include units of measurement according to International System of Units (SI) unless otherwise appropriate.

Results presented as tables or figures require in-text acknowledgment to guide the reader. For example, "$\dot{V}O_2$max decreased with age" (see Fig. 20-1). For uniformity and familiarity for the reader, authors should create the results section according to the format specified in the methods section (3) and in accordance with the journal requirements.

Tables and Figures

Some data become difficult to comprehend and evaluate when presented in text format. The use of tables and figures often puts data in a form more easily interpretable and aesthetically pleasing. However, this does not mean that authors should implement tables and figures overzealously. General rules dictate appropriate use of tables and figures.

Tables are useful when data may be too numerous or confusing as text or do not benefit from visual representation in the form of a figure. Tables allow the author to display large amounts of data in an organized and detailed form; however, tables can present too much data that leads to it being overlooked or misunderstood (3). Typically, in-text reporting suffices with less than 10 data points, yet a table format might highlight its importance. Trivial data do not necessitate table format.

Authors should organize tables as displayed most logically, but many scientists suggest an organizational rule of independent variables as the row headings and dependent variables as the column headings. Any abbreviations, further clarifications, or symbols indicating statistical significance reside in the footnotes, and table titles should be informative but concise. Authors must refer to journal formatting requirements for specific instructions and quantity limits.

Figures typically display data visually but can also support study methods to clarify procedures. In results, figures permit easy visual recognition of trends, patterns, and complex relationships, unlike text and tables. Figure elements include informative but concise titles and legends explaining pertinent details and statistical symbols. Ultimately, this information conveys the meaning of the figure without requiring clarification from the manuscript text.

Many figure variations exist, including photographs, diagrams, and graphs, and researchers select the type according to the nature of the data (or information type). Frequently, authors create figures before the writing process begins to aid in understanding the collected data. Journals generally call for specific figure formatting (color options, statistical symbols, etc.) and some have quantity limits. Authors must take great care in figure formatting because inappropriate formatting might create the appearance of artificial relationships and/or misleading conclusions. For tips on preparing figures and graphs, see Concept Box 20-4.

Discussion

The discussion section provides the opportunity to interpret the results and apply principles, associations, and generalizations that are within the scope of the data (3,6). Points of discussion must correspond with the results, such that the data statistically supports all elucidations. Nonetheless, theoretical explanations can provide value to data interpretation, but this text must be represented clearly with careful wording (*i.e.*, using words such as "potentially" or "might"). An effective discussion presents each main idea in a logical fashion, often beginning with the most critical findings in relation to the hypothesis to prepare the reader for the discussion's focus (3). Whenever possible, authors should compare their findings to previous literature (with in-text referencing) and offer explanations for similarities and discrepancies. With limitations in the number of references that can be used, often, authors will "cherry pick" only those references that they can handle and avoid ones that may

Concept Box 20-4 Tips for Figure and Graph Preparation

- The figure format type should accurately and comprehensively present the data.
- Photographs are appropriate formats for displaying unique equipment and protocols, microscopy, and other biochemical techniques.
- Suitable uses of diagrams include methodologic timelines and procedures as well as mechanistic, structural, and theoretical relationship paradigms.
- Graphs emphasize specific findings, magnitude differences, or relationships. Lines frequently depict temporal relationships, whereas bars clearly display group mean comparisons (however, their use pertains to the precise context). Pie charts (circle graphs) frequently illustrate proportions.

not support their data or be more difficult to explain in context with their findings. Such an approach to not take such matters head on can result in reviewers who are well aware of the literature and issues that exist and may turn in a more negative review. Many authors will also include directions for future research within their "Discussion" section (6). Responsible authorship incorporates unanticipated responses or relationships as well as study limitations (6), and this information left unreported might negatively affect future research and practical application; intentional failure to acknowledge these incidences is an ethical breach.

A final paragraph (or perhaps two) closes the discussion section by concisely presenting the most critical information gleaned from the investigation (3,6). This conclusion often includes practical applications and future directions for new research (3) (only if future directions are applicable and were not already included in previous "Discussion" paragraphs). A discussion section with concluding paragraph(s) greatly varies in length dependent on the data complexity and is often constructed in close proximity of the results section. For tips for a successful discussion section, see Concept Box 20-5.

References

All references cited in the text must reside in the reference list at the end of the manuscript; references not cited in the text do not belong in the reference list. Well-established and generally accepted concepts or processes do not need supporting references (*i.e.*, stating that the heart distributes blood does not require a reference). The author is obligated to review the content of manuscripts cited within his or her text and make sure one spans the life of the concept in the literature and not just the recent time frame or only five years back, as failure to do so could result in perpetual misinformation (5). Vast differences exist in the reference formatting styles demanded by scientific journals, and authors must familiarize themselves with these standards prior to the submission process. Fortunately, many software programs assist in reference formatting, and many journals collaborate with these programs to simplify the reference list construction.

Additional Sections

In many circumstances, author preference or journal requirements add supplementary sections at the end of the manuscript text. These often include statements of acknowledgment and conflicts of interest.

CONCEPT BOX 20-5 **Tips for a Successful Discussion**

- Variables and concepts must not first be introduced in the discussion; the reader should not feel that the discussion topics deviate from those in the introduction.
- Any questions and hypotheses raised in the introduction must be addressed in the discussion.
- Discussion points can reference and revolve around results figures. Authors can choose to include additional diagrams in the discussion section to argue theoretical framework.
- Discuss the impact of the data throughout the discussion section.

Acknowledgments

The optional acknowledgment section allows authors to recognize contributions of individuals who provided their time, materials, or a service but did not meet authorship criteria. Authors may also recognize funding sources such as grants and fellowships. Dependent on specific journal formatting, funding information might be represented as its own section separate from the acknowledgments.

Conflict of Interest

Although not all journals require a clear conflict of interest section, the authors should note potential conflicts to preserve ethical responsibilities. Potential conflicts of interest include receiving funding from a company that might benefit financially from the research findings or professional affiliations that could skew data interpretation. The official journal of the American College of Sports Medicine, *Medicine & Science in Sports & Exercise*, addresses conflicts of interest with the following statement:

> *Authors must state all possible conflicts of interest in the manuscript, including financial, consultant, institutional, and other relationships that might lead to bias or a conflict of interest. If there is no conflict of interest, this should also be explicitly stated as none declared. All sources of funding should be acknowledged in the manuscript. All relevant conflicts of interest and sources of funding should be included after the acknowledgments section of the manuscript with the heading "Conflicts of Interest and Source of Funding."*

For example: Conflicts of interest and source of funding: A has received honoraria from Company Z. B is currently receiving a grant (#12345) from Organization Y and is on the speaker's bureau for Organization X—the CME organizers for Company A. For the remaining authors none were declared.

BEGINNING TO WRITE CAN BE THE HARDEST PART

Many who exercise routinely can identify with the phrase "the hardest step for a runner is the first step out the door," and the same approach can be applied to writing. Authors frequently develop common excuses that prevent them from beginning to write, despite the actual truth of the matter (4). These include the following:

1. Feeling underqualified. In actuality, neither academic status nor experience necessarily dictates one's ability to write a quality scientific manuscript.
2. Assuming poor writing skills. In fact, good writing is largely good editing, and recognizing weaknesses predisposes improvement. Of course, seek assistance and practice, practice, practice.
3. Not worth the work. Particularly those new to research might feel this way, but publishing scientific work often opens doors for a successful future (*e.g.*, academic advancement, invitations to present data at conferences, collaboration or consulting offers, career opportunities, etc.).
4. Not enough time. Finding available time for writing challenges every researcher, but treating the writing process as a typical responsibility proves valuable. Concept Box 20-6 provides additional tips for finding time to write (4).

Concept Box 20-6 Tips for Finding Time to Write

- Break up sections within the writing process and set realistic and specific deadlines for their completion.
- Consider personal and professional commitments when setting deadlines.
- Arrive early or stay late at work or school to focus on writing.
- Schedule regular time blocks dedicated to writing only.
- Don't break scheduled writing appointments, as this often becomes a habit.

GOOD WRITING IS GOOD EDITING

Developing manuscript content comprises only one aspect of the writing process/battle, whereas the other aspects pertain to writing mechanics and grammar. Ultimately, good writing *is* good editing, supporting the practice of simply getting words on paper upon beginning the writing process. Little benefit results from attempting to create a finished product with a first draft, as this commonly hinders productivity (3).

Once the majority of the manuscript content has been written, first evaluate its organization. Paragraphs within each manuscript heading should clearly signify a single topic or theme, and the paragraph order should logically progress. The next step involves meticulous structural and grammatical editing by examining each sentence at a time. Although this practice might appear excessive, the end product improves clarity and reflects professionalism.

What components of the sentence require editing? Identify the sentence's verb. If the sentence contains a weak verb (*e.g.*, was, are, be), replace it with a strong verb. Weak verb substitution creates a more active as opposed to passive voice. For example, changing "body mass *was* made greater by the intervention" to "greater body mass *followed* the intervention" improves the sentence's impact. Although scientific writing commonly incorporates more passive voice than does creative writing, exclusive passive voice often results in wordiness and unclear communication. Replacing weak with strong verbs to create a more active voice will assist in concise, clear communication. Next, examine each sentence as a whole or for words that do not add meaning or clarity (3). Take them out! Unnecessary words potentially obstruct the message, and some people associate excessive words with carelessness or incompetence. For example, changing "the participants put on a heart rate monitor, they drank 500 mL of water, and then they walked into the environmental chamber" to "participants *donned* a heart rate monitor, *consumed* 500 mL of water, and then *entered* the environmental chamber" eliminates unnecessary words (underlined in the first example) and uses strong verbs. More tips for strong, concise writing are available in Concept Box 20-7.

GUIDELINES FOR DETERMINING AUTHORSHIP

Early in this chapter, we suggested determining manuscript authorship during the research planning process (as this early planning may reduce professional conflict). But who should

CONCEPT BOX 20-7 **Additional Tips for Improved Sentence Quality**

- Place words or ideas worth highlighting at the end of the sentence.
- Avoid fancy words (these might reduce clarity).
- Abstain from including excessive and unnecessary commas.

be an author on a scientific manuscript? Numerous scientific journals follow the recommendations put forth by the International Committee of Medical Journal Editors (ICMJE) (2), but each journal maintains the right to define authorship requirements. The ICMJE suggests authors meet *all* of the following four criteria:

1. "Substantial contributions to the concept or design of the work; or the acquisition, analysis, or interpretation of data for the work"
2. "Drafting the work or revising it critically for important intellectual content"
3. "Final approval of the version to be published"
4. "Agreement to be accountable for all aspects of the work ensuring that questions related to the accuracy or integrity of any part of the work are appropriately investigated and resolved"

If considered carefully and taken seriously, these criteria pose important responsibilities. Any individual who contributed to the research but failed to meet all four above criteria might best receive recognition in the acknowledgment section of the manuscript. Additionally, some scientific journals limit the number of authors deemed acceptable for manuscript publication; although some journals do accept requests for author justification when limits are exceeded, these requests can be denied. Knowing the specific journal requirements for authorship at the early stages of the research planning process prevents complications pertaining to the number of authors.

Once authors have been identified, decisions follow as to the order by which the authors' names appear on the manuscript. Generally, the first author of a manuscript is the individual who contributed the majority of the work leading to the research and manuscript writing as measured through the previously described authorship criteria categories. Following the first author, the rationale for the order of subsequent authors is less clear. Some might suggest that subsequently listed authors should be presented in the order in which they contributed (from more to less) to the research project, but this can be an extremely difficult and subjective practice. Others might choose to list subsequent authors in alphabetical order, a practice that is no more objective and possibly less fair to those involved. Regardless of the process used for determining the order of authorship, there is no universally accepted practice for this process. Finally, it is often typical practice to place the research's director (principal investigator or laboratory director) as the last author listed. This individual should, of course, meet all of the authorship criteria but is placed last among authors for the purpose of authoritative distinction.

IN A NUT SHELL

Scientific authorship permits the dispersal of facts and ideas while marking a point in scientific history. Writing scientifically takes practice, but every good scientific writer, too, began as a novice. Successful authors employ detailed plans to promote smooth and conflict-free publication processes and follow commonly used manuscript section headings to develop logical content flow. Although many circumstances make scientific writing challenging, authors are encouraged to begin rough drafts without focusing on initial quality and to follow disciplined time management strategies to ensure timely manuscript construction. Great responsibility exists in determining authorship, and many journals and organizations put forth authorship guidelines to assist researchers. Taken together, scientific writing and publication presents many challenges, but the individual and population benefits prove critical.

GLOSSARY

Abstract: a summary of the entire manuscript that identifies the key aims, methods, and findings in an easy-to-read format

Discussion: a manuscript section that provides interpretation, impact, and future directions of the research

Introduction: a manuscript section that presents background knowledge and the purpose of the presented research

Manuscript publication: the distribution of original work that follows a rigorous peer review process and allows the communication of experimental findings to the scientific community

Methods: a manuscript section that describes details of the research participants, experimental protocol, reagents, equipment, and statistical approach

Outline: a general, truncated content guide for a scientific manuscript

Reference: a record of previous literature used to support the claims, theories, and methodology used to develop the research

Results: a manuscript section that presents the research findings supported by the statistical analyses

Title: a succinct phrase that identifies the manuscript topic

REFERENCES

1. Cetin S, Hackam DJ. An approach to the writing of a scientific manuscript. *J Surg Res.* 2005;128(2):165–167.
2. International Committee of Medical Journal Editors Web site [Internet]. Vancouver (Canada): International Committee of Medical Journal Editors. Available from: http://www.icmje.org/
3. Kliewer MA. Writing it up: a step-by-step guide to publication for beginning investigators. *AJR Am J Roentgenol.* 2006;34(1): 53–59.
4. Morton PG. Publishing in professional journals, part I: getting started. *AACN Adv Crit Care.* 2013;24(2):162–168.
5. Roberts WC. How I prepare a manuscript for publication in a medical journal. *Methodist DeBakey Cardiovasc J.* 2012;8(4): 53–54.
6. Roederer M, Marciniak MW, O'Connor SK, Eckel SF. An integrated approach to research and manuscript development. *Am J Health Syst Pharm.* 2013;70(14):1211–1218.
7. Veness M. Strategies to successfully publish your first manuscript. *J Med Imaging Radiat Oncol.* 2010;54(4):395–400.

Submitting a Manuscript for Publication: Finding the Publication Outlet

*William J. Kraemer, PhD, FACSM, David P. Looney, MS, CSCS,
David R. Hooper, MA, Tunde K. Szivak, MA, and Shawn D. Flanagan, MA, MHA*

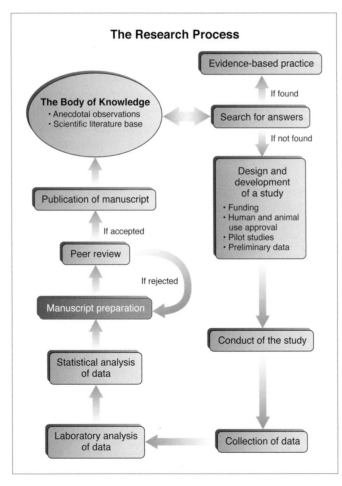

The Research Process

- The Body of Knowledge
  - Anecdotal observations
  - Scientific literature base
- Evidence-based practice
- Search for answers (If found → Evidence-based practice; If not found →)
- Design and development of a study
  - Funding
  - Human and animal use approval
  - Pilot studies
  - Preliminary data
- Conduct of the study
- Collection of data
- Laboratory analysis of data
- Statistical analysis of data
- Manuscript preparation (If rejected)
- Peer review (If accepted →)
- Publication of manuscript

INTRODUCTION

The purpose of this chapter is to provide an overview of the process of successfully submitting a manuscript for publication in an academic journal. Topics include the importance of publishing research, how to critically evaluate your manuscript, choosing a relevant journal for your manuscript, formatting your manuscript according to a journal's specifications, and finalizing the submission process. Ultimately, the primary objective of this chapter is to prepare the reader to successfully submit a manuscript for publication. It is the peer reviewed scientific journal that is the "gold standard" for scientific information coming out of laboratories around the world. A scientist's contribution and work in research are validated by such journal contributions. Universities, research institutes, and a host of other scientific entities including the lay public view peer reviewed journal contributions as the "coin of the realm" for efficacy of scientific/medical findings.

Websites, blogs, and social networks have made information immediately available to people across the globe. Although anyone can post his or her work to a blog or personal website, a manuscript is not considered "peer reviewed" unless it is submitted to a journal that uses a peer review process. It is important to note that journals will not accept papers that have already been published in such a manner as they are considered to already be in the public domain. Therefore, the only way to make your research publicly available without compromising its eligibility for inclusion in a peer reviewed scientific journal is to present the research as an abstract in a scientific meeting or in a university index service (for theses or dissertations). Although thesis indexing may be a requirement for graduation, the indexing process should be contemplated with care, especially as it pertains to information that may have proprietary value. Many universities offer a grace period, which can be used to protect ideas, discoveries, potential patents, and/or technologies until they can be published in an appropriate **peer reviewed scientific journal** where findings are formally attributed to the investigator.

Peer reviewed journals are essential for the advancement of human knowledge. Interestingly, manuscripts written long ago were not peer reviewed, but they still served as the primary avenue of communication for the sharing of ideas, methods, and experimental results (6). As described later in this textbook, the peer review process mandates that a manuscript meet a number of demands, including evaluation by at least one scientific expert on the manuscript topic. This requirement is designed to assure that manuscripts are of acceptable scientific quality and importance. Although imperfect, the peer review process attempts to screen for papers with "fatal" flaws in experimental design or scientific methods. Before submitting a manuscript for peer review, the first step is to identify the most appropriate journal for your research. The overall general process of manuscript submission is shown in Figure 21-1.

DETERMINING WHERE TO SUBMIT YOUR MANUSCRIPT

Once your study has been completed, you must carefully reflect whether the data is important and novel enough to contribute to the body of knowledge and merit publication.

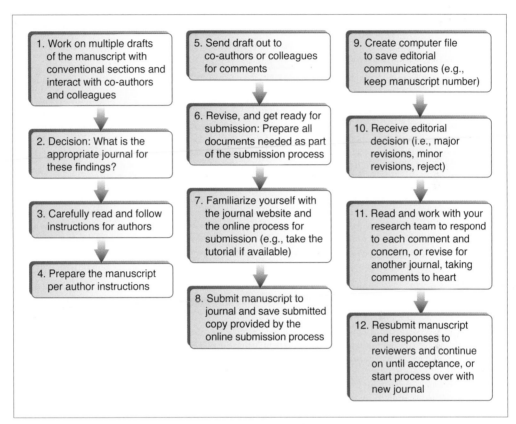

FIGURE 21-1: Steps in the process of submitting a manuscript for publication.

This is a very important first step. For example, you complete a training program and nothing happens with your treatment group, is this important or was it that there were issues with study design? What is the context, what does it mean, is more research needed to make a statement about a particular topic? Not all research done is worthy of publication, as it does not impact the field even if there are no fatal flaws. This is a hard decision to make but is important to do so. After you have determined that your study has merit, the next step is to publish your findings, but now you must decide the most appropriate journal for publication. As a student, consultation with your major advisor or a faculty mentor is important to help guide you through the process. When submitted for publication, other scientists will expect the insights of investigators with extensive experience, who understand the intricacies of issues in the current literature and can make critical evaluations. The types of articles that journals publish are overviewed in Table 21-1.

Before you can determine whether a journal is a viable option for your manuscript, it is important to decide the type of article you will be submitting, the extent of its area of study, and the overall impact of its findings on the scientific community. Being able to accurately

Table 21-1 Types of Manuscripts

There are various types of manuscripts that can be submitted to scientific journals, and authors must carefully review the types that a specific journal will consider.

Original investigation: a manuscript that presents novel data that have not been previously published and have been derived from experimental and analytical research processes

Case study: Different from an original investigation in that it is a report on a single unique individual profile or unexpected situation that could not be typically replicated in an experimental design with an adequate size due to the novel nature of profile or situation. Case studies can be used to inform scientists about previously unforeseen effects of a particular intervention and open up new topics that can be more intensely examined in future research. The conclusions derived from the case study stem from a highly unusual event or individual profile and may not apply in every related set of circumstances.

Review: A review article is unique in that it does not contain original research but is a critical examination of previously published articles whose contents share a particular topic or component. The results of the studies contained within the review article can be combined together to generate a larger scale perspective on the topic. Certain restrictions may apply to authorship of a review article. For example, *Medicine & Science in Sports & Exercise* requires that the author of a review article be a recognized expert in a particular field, which is determined by the editor-in-chief. Each journal has its own demands for a review manuscript, and this needs to be carefully evaluated. Review types include opinion reviews, systematic reviews, and meta-analyses, and each is an attempt to evaluate the current state of the literature.

Technical report: Technical reports are valuable in that they can explain the procedure and/or outcomes of a specific scientific experiment or summarize the current conditions revolving around a topic of debate. Often, technical reports are written to provide further detail to a particular scientific method.

Research note/brief report/hot topics: These articles vary in nature but constitute brief summaries of experimental findings that may give important and impactful new findings from which other scientists, field professionals, or the medical field may benefit immediately. It may also represent research data that sets the stage for more extensive research studies now given important new directions from this preliminary discovery not currently known. Such articles provide a means of expediting the process and sharing the results.

Letter to the editor: A letter to the editor or similar article type is typically a short submission that is written in critique of a previous publication, usually that appeared recently. The intent is to have the author(s) respond to the criticisms or in a worst-case situation create a debate to gain attention. Many journals have a pre-determined time frame for how long a letter to the editor can be written about a publication. For example, letters to the editor in *Medicine & Science in Sports & Exercise* must be in reference to a paper published in the previous 12 months. A letter to the editor is a great example of how peer review does not end on publication. In fact, once a paper is published, the work will continue to be critiqued in textbooks, publications, during conference presentations, and in classrooms. Care is taken by journal editors to make sure it is not just an attempt by antagonists to gain publicity and notoriety from criticism but to provide an opportunity for the author to provide new insight into their study. This article mechanism is often abused for the above reason, and readers must be carefully attentive to the history and nature of such complaints.

Symposium: A symposium generally refers to a meeting of experts to discuss a particular subject. The transcript recorded from a particular symposium can be published as symposium proceedings. Depending on the location and nature of the meeting, certain laws and regulations of the organization that held the symposium may dictate whether and to what extent the symposium proceedings can be published. A symposium can also refer to a selection of articles written by different authors that address a particular, singular topic from various perspectives.

Invited commentary: Invited commentaries are short, self-contained presentations on the significance of a particular manuscript from an overall perspective. Emphasis is placed on condensing the length of the piece as much as possible and only using references that are absolutely necessary for documentation or enrichment. Viewing the invited commentary as a place for extensive discussion of the author's opinions on the subject at hand is generally highly discouraged.

categorize and critically evaluate your manuscript will greatly assist in the process of choosing an appropriate journal. Several steps to help assess your manuscript are described in the following sections.

Identify Your Target Audience

Once you have chosen the type of manuscript you will write, it is important to identify your **target audience**, which should be the audience most interested in your research. This is where research on the journal, its scope, current and past publications, and the organization(s) that sponsor it becomes important. You may be a member of the organization that owns a journal of interest and have exposure to the type of research and professionals that the journal targets. However, even if you are not a member of the organization that publishes the journal, it is a good idea to examine the journal's mission and the types of manuscripts the journal publishes. As an example, some journals only publish reviews, whereas others rely heavily on short communications, and most still on full original research articles.

Carefully Read the Instructions to Authors

A common complaint of journal editorial staff and reviewers is that authors do not carefully read and conform to the author instructions of the journal. This may occur as a result of a hurried submission of thesis or dissertation or a manuscript prepared for a different journal that uses a markedly different formatting structure. Accordingly, many journals will automatically "unsubmit" and return your manuscript if not properly formatted. Although comprehensive and at times exhausting, adherence to author instructions is thus vital to successful manuscript submission.

A journal's instructions to authors will cover important areas, which include the following:

- General requirements
- Authorship requirements
- Open-access options
- Copyright assignments
- Conflicts of interest
- Misconduct
- Reproduction of text and figures
- Publication and page charges
- Submission requirements
- Type of review process
- Human and animal use requirements
- Submission article types
- Manuscript formatting and submission details
- Online submission processes
- Manuscript format and order of sections
- Reference formatting

- Technical guidelines
- Other content submission types

Match Your Research to the Journal's Mission

What type of research did you conduct, and how does it match the mission, scope, readership, and types of papers published by the journal? A strong and impactful study that does not fit with the editorial mission of a journal has little chance of acceptance. For example, you might have examined the effects of different training programs on maximal oxygen consumption and other performance outcomes, including a control group, but you have no data to explain possible mechanisms for these effects. Some journals will consider this work impressive, interesting, and worthy of publication. Other journals interested in basic science or the physiologic mechanisms behind such results may not feel that your research contributes substantively to their mission or the interests of their intended readership. Careful consideration of the nature of your research and its relationship to a journal's mission is of vital importance. Many journals publish their aims and scope in each printed issue, but the official journal website is the most reliable place to find this information. Along the same lines, reading recent publications can clarify the appropriateness of your manuscript and provide an idea of the topics that are currently considered noteworthy and groundbreaking.

In the contemporary publication environment, an important issue to consider is the importance of the research question. Does it have an impact on the specific field of science, and does it move the field forward from either a basic or applied perspective? Technology is now at the forefront of science more than ever, but technology should not obviate the importance of a study's experimental design and rationale. Each element of a study should be solid going from the importance of the question to the hypothesis-driven introduction and rationale to a strong experimental approach to the problem to a design with appropriate independent and dependent variables to the use of cutting edge technology to appropriate statistical analyses to impactful. The technology must be appropriate for the purpose or question to be addressed. Still, technology should not be what "carries the day" alone in a research study.

Although technology and scientific innovation go hand in hand, a research study with advanced technologies but a substantially flawed design may still be published due to reviewers being too impressed or focused on the technologic aspects of the study, a fault of the review process. On the other hand, clever and meaningful research that used older techniques may face a more difficult path to publication. Reviewers may fail to fully understand the limitations and disadvantages of new technologies or overlook otherwise fatal flaws because of it. Moreover, scientific journals prefer increasingly direct measurements of primary dependent variables so that the highest degree of accuracy and sensitivity are achieved (*e.g.*, electronic timing of sprints compared to using a handheld stop watch). Therefore, it is important to carefully review your methods and persuasively speak to the unique aspects of your research approach. The sustainability of a journal depends on continued support from its readership. Therefore, it is in your best interest to identify journals with target audiences that find your research interesting. Editors, reviewers, and readers will also appreciate your manuscript if it provides new information or builds on existing concepts relevant to their field of study.

Evaluate the Impact of Your Findings

Although it is difficult, developing the ability to critically evaluate your research is a vital component of journal selection. This can be done in concert with your major advisor and research team. Getting input on potential journal outlets can be very helpful, especially when the input comes from advisors with extensive publication experience. Although any source of new information adds to the body of knowledge, the magnitude of change varies substantially. Before you select a journal, make sure you understand the question your experiment answered and to what extent. This evaluation is important, as journals commonly require reviewers to rate the overall impact of the paper, and manuscripts that are not rated in the top 25% are often automatically rejected. Statements such as "this is the first time such a study has ever been done" do not sufficiently indicate or justify the importance of the work. Furthermore, a study on the lactate response to maximal exercise may be outstanding and without experimental flaw. Nevertheless, the impact may be considered low because this information has been repeatedly demonstrated for over 50 years. Thus, without a compelling rationale or new insight, rejection of the manuscript is likely to occur before peer review. This is called "administrative rejection," which is a decision made by the editor who initially receives the manuscript.

THE BEGINNING OF THE PUBLICATION PROCESS

From the point of submission, completion of the publication process with a paper published in a journal with volume and page numbers, it can take up to a year or longer. Most higher-end journals attempt to make a decision on an initial review within three to six weeks. Revision is almost always required and is a solid outcome to a first review. It is typical for most papers to have one or two revisions prior to acceptance which can take three to six months. The majority of rejections will occur upon initial review with the rest occurring after the first revision when the authors do not meet the demands of the reviewers and/or editor. Most journals today have rejection rates that are over 70%.

Valuable time can be wasted if you select a journal for submission and go through the publication progress only to be rejected. Many times, this involves a simple mismatch with a journal's mission. For example, you have a great study on the effects of swimming training tapering programs on swim performances in a meet but send it to a journal that is interested in the underlying physiologic mechanisms of an end point variable, or what mechanisms explain how this adaptation occurred, and not just the performance adaptation. Although this happens to even the best scientists, it is important to take the time to carefully select the most appropriate journal for your data. Consequently, your ability to navigate through the assortment of available scientific journals and select the right one is imperative in order to be successful in the publication process. The top five reasons for manuscript rejection can be summarized as follows:

- Poor fit for the mission of the journal, usually resulting in administrative rejection
- Fatal design flaws
- Gross methodologic flaws
- Poor presentation, writing, or clarity
- Lack of impact

It is important to note that all legitimate scientific journals have policies against **duplicate submission** or submitting your manuscript to multiple journals at the same time. The practice involves submitting a manuscript to two or more journals, intending to pick the journal that accepts the research first or the journal with higher perceived impact, and then withdrawing the submission from the other journal(s). This is clearly a highly unethical practice that amounts to a waste of valuable reviewer and editor time; when discovered, the paper will not be reviewed, and in some cases, the authors may be banned from publishing in that journal.

The lack of professional credit given to reviewers and editors in today's academic world has made it increasingly harder to find experts who are willing to contribute their time as a "service" to the profession, and the practice of double submission further exacerbates this issue.

Accepted Papers

Once accepted, the authors must wait for the paper to receive page numbers in an upcoming journal edition, which may take from three months to over a year. During this period, the paper will be reviewed in additional detail for formatting; grammar; and in higher-end journals, technical descriptions and term usage. The process yields a galley proof, which is revised by the authors to form a final manuscript. However, with today's technology, many papers are made available immediately upon acceptance, which is referred to as being published "ahead of press." This makes the paper publicly available and citable by a **digital object identifier** or DOI. This is up to the publisher and the editor-in-chief as to what status the paper is when it goes online. Some print the paper as it was accepted, but others wait until it makes it through the first round of galley proofs.

Finding Journals

There are countless peer reviewed academic journals in circulation throughout the world, covering a multitude of topics. Although it may seem daunting, there are many different tactics you can use to narrow the list of potential journals to a select few. One of the first places to look is in the reference articles used for your experiment. This will help direct you toward journals that have placed importance on articles with similar contents to your own. In this process, it is important to focus on papers cited in the introduction and discussion sections of the paper, as these references will share important elements of the theoretical paradigms of your topic.

As you learned in Chapter 4, numerous online databases also provide you with the ability to scour through countless articles and journals. One of the best services you can use to find journals and articles is PubMed, which is provided by the U.S. National Library of Medicine (4). PubMed indexes the online database MEDLINE, allowing you to search through millions of citations; abstracts; and articles from life science, health, and biomedical journals. ScienceDirect is another scientific database that offers thousands of full-text online book chapters and peer reviewed journal articles. One of the key advantages of ScienceDirect is that it provides access to its content before they are published on both computers and mobile devices. A third scientific database is Scopus, which is designed for allowing rapid, thorough searches for abstracts and citations from peer reviewed publications. Searches can be made even easier with Hub, which allows simultaneous cataloguing of full-text journals through both ScienceDirect and Scopus while eliminating duplicate results. Although the contents of your journal may fit within the scope of a multitude of journals, they may resonate with the readership of a journal that predominantly focuses on topics related to the field of exercise science. Therefore, it is in your best interest to become familiar with the journals that best represent your field of study. Some of the most prominent academic journals related to exercise science are described in Table 21-2.

Evaluating the Reputation of a Journal

Impact Factor

The most commonly used reputational measure for an academic journal is its **impact factor (IF)**, or the average number of times a journal's articles are cited over the past two years (2). A higher impact factor indicates that articles in the journal have been cited a greater number of times. Impact factors are calculated from the Web of Science database, maintained by Thomson Reuters. However, IF is now a point of controversy, as it started out as a simple matrix for budgetary priorities in libraries in the 1970s and has now escalated to the point of being used to evaluate the work of scientists, the journals in which they publish, and even tenure decisions. This concern about IF-based evaluations of journals or scientists is highlighted in an editorial on the San Francisco Declaration on Research Assessment (DORA) by the editor of *Science*, considered one of the top two journals in science today:

> *To correct distortions in the evaluation of scientific research, DORA aims to stop the use of the "journal impact factor" in judging an individual scientist's work. The Declaration states that the impact factor must not be used as "a surrogate measure of the quality of individual research articles, to assess an individual scientist's contributions, or in hiring, promotion, or funding decisions . . . " These recommendations have thus far been endorsed by more than 150 leading scientists and 75 scientific organizations, including the American Association for the Advancement of Science (the publisher of* Science*). (1)*

In essence, use of the IF has far exceeded its intended purpose, and this "mission creep" has led to ridiculous IF matrix gaming, the senseless destruction of careers, and misinterpretation of the roles of various journals' importance to an organization's readership and the field in which it resides. This is especially true for many exercise and sport science journals, where the number of laboratories doing certain types of research is limited, thereby limiting how many other scientists will cite it in other journals, which results in lower IF for the journal(s) that publish the manuscript. As noted earlier, this in turn can also lead to an inappropriate evaluation of the investigator.

As the number of citations a published article receives is highly dependent on the generalizability of its findings, it is important when making comparisons between journals to take the subject discipline into consideration. The findings of an academic publication may be of great relevance in its individual field but may be considered too specific to attract the attention necessary to elicit a greater number of citations. Moreover, the types of articles published

Table 21-2 Common Exercise Science Journals

For selected journals, full descriptions are provided to illustrate information commonly found on journal websites.

Medicine & Science in Sports & Exercise

Medicine & Science in Sports & Exercise (*MSSE*) is the flagship journal of the American College of Sports Medicine (ACSM). The goal of *MSSE* is to provide monthly information on current topics in biodynamics, epidemiology, physiology, physical fitness, and performance as well as sports medicine practice. It is important to note that *MSSE* is not interested in simply analyzing outcomes of a particular intervention but the physiologic mechanisms that were responsible. In addition to both original and clinical investigations, *MSSE* publishes brief and comprehensive reviews, case studies, letters to the editor-in-chief, methodologic advances, plus symposium proceedings. Although *MSSE* accepts submissions from authors unaffiliated with ACSM, its readership consists of predominantly ACSM members as well as athletic trainers, exercise physiologists, physiatrists, physical therapists, and team physicians. More information can be found at the official website of *MSSE* at http://www.acsm-MSSE.org/.

Exercise and Sport Sciences Reviews

Exercise and Sport Sciences Reviews (*ESSR*) is another official publication of ACSM. *ESSR* publishes a collection of review articles and invites commentaries every three months that touch upon emerging issues in exercise science and sports medicine. Typically including only invited reviews, *ESSR* makes exceptions for manuscripts that examine a topic of interest in a thoroughly innovative fashion and are supported by original published research. The articles found in *ESSR* are written in a clear and concise manner to allow for the sharing of information with those who may not be experts in the field without sacrificing accuracy and scientific merit. Subsequently, the readership of *ESSR* is highly diverse, ranging from students and professors to clinicians, scientists, and health and fitness professionals. More information can be found at the official website of *ESSR* at http://www.acsm-essr.org/.

Current Sports Medicine Reports

Similar to *ESSR*, *Current Sports Medicine Reports* (*CSMR*) is another publication affiliated with ACSM that publishes review articles. However, the review articles found in *CSMR* address the latest trends, developments, or debates in sports medicine in a manner specific to practicing clinicians. Therefore, the readership of *CSMR* is predominantly composed of experts in the field of sports medicine. Accordingly, authors are encouraged to share their own personal experiences and methods. Uninvited submissions are uncommon but are allowed if they present recent developments, findings, or trends considered especially relevant to sports medicine clinicians. More information can be found at the official website of *CSMR* at http://www.acsm-csmr.org/.

ACSM's Health & Fitness Journal

ACSM's Health & Fitness Journal aims to provide current information on exercise and nutrition that members of the health and fitness community can readily apply to their work. Topics include recent trends in general health and fitness, injuries, professional development, psychology, special populations, as well as sports law. The target audience of the journal stretches from exercise enthusiasts, personal trainers, and rehabilitation specialists to health/fitness directors and instructors. As such, articles are written informally, kept relatively brief (2,200–2,600 words), make ample use of figures and illustrations, and refrain from reporting on individual studies and their results. The journal also includes information on ACSM certification workshops and other opportunities for continuing education credits, making it an ideal choice for articles geared toward current practicing members of ACSM. More information can be found at the official website of *ACSM's Health & Fitness Journal* at http://www.acsm-healthfitness.org/.

Table 21-2 Common Exercise Science Journals *(Continued)*

Journal of Strength and Conditioning Research

Published monthly, the *Journal of Strength and Conditioning Research* (*JSCR*) aims to advance the understanding of strength and conditioning through applied exercise science in order to provide an ever-improving scientific basis for sports performance and training practices. Each edition of the *JSCR* includes a variety of articles, including original investigations, symposium proceedings, brief reviews, technical reports, and research notes. The primary focus of the articles found in the *JSCR* is on the effects of training techniques, nutrition, and technologic advancements on topics such as athletic performance, biomechanics, exercise physiology, motor learning, and sports psychology. In addition to the presentation of their research, authors offer recommendations for practical applications of their findings. Although it is the official research journal of the National Strength and Conditioning Association (NSCA), authors are not required to be official members in order for their work to be published in the *JSCR*. However, in order to lend credibility to their manuscripts' contents, authors are expected to have demonstrated significant research experience in the manuscript's area of study. Due to its emphasis on both research and practical applications of its articles, the *JSCR* remains a popular journal among exercise scientists, strength and conditioning coaches, fitness professionals, and general members of the NSCA. More information can be found at the official website of the *JSCR* at http://journals.lww.com/nsca-jscr/.

Strength and Conditioning Journal

The *Strength and Conditioning Journal* (*SCJ*) is a bimonthly publication that is also affiliated with the NSCA. The *SCJ* places less emphasis on analysis of research pertaining to the field of strength and conditioning and more on the practical applications of research findings. Accordingly, the readership of the *SCJ* consists of strength and conditioning coaches, athletic trainers, health professionals, personal trainers, and physical therapists. Each issue is composed of brief but concise articles, reviews, columns, and letters to the editor-in-chief focused on specific topics and their applicability in the practical setting. More information can be found at the official website of the *SCJ* at http://journals.lww.com/nsca-scj/.

Journal of Applied Physiology

The *Journal of Applied Physiology* (*JAP*) is an official journal of the American Physiological Society and publishes a wide variety of original research within the scope of the biochemical, biologic, pharmacologic, and physiologic sciences. Articles found in the *JAP* can be focused at the molecular level all the way up to the entire organism. However, the majority of these articles concentrate on the physiologic mechanisms fundamental to how the human body adapts and responds to different stimuli including aging, development, environmental factors, and pathophysiologic conditions. Notably, the *JAP* prefers research using state-of-the-art technology and procedures. Therefore, the target audience for the *JAP* consists primarily of active or future members in the field of applied physiology. More information can be found at the official website of the *JAP* at http://jap.physiology.org/.

Additional Exercise Science Journals

- *American Journal of Physical Medicine and Rehabilitation*
- *American Journal of Physiology*
- *American Journal of Sports Medicine*
- *Applied Ergonomics*
- *Applied Physiology, Nutrition, & Metabolism*
- *Applied Psychology—International Review*
- *Archives of Physical Medicine and Rehabilitation*
- *Australian Journal of Physiotherapy*
- *Australian Journal of Science and Medicine in Sport*
- *Aviation Space and Environmental Medicine*
- *Behavior Research Methods*

- *Biology of Sport*
- *British Journal of Sports Medicine*
- *Clinical Biomechanics*
- *Clinical Journal of Sport Medicine*
- *Clinical Nutrition*
- *Clinics in Sports Medicine*
- *Ergonomics*
- *European Journal of Applied Physiology*
- *European Journal of Clinical Nutrition*
- *European Journal of Sport Science*
- *Exercise and Immunology Reviews*

(Continued)

Table 21-2 Common Exercise Science Journals *(Continued)*

- *Gait and Posture*
- *High Altitude Medicine and Biology*
- *Human Movement Science*
- *International Journal of Sport Nutrition and Exercise Metabolism*
- *International Journal of Sport Psychology*
- *International Journal of Sports Medicine*
- *Journal of Aging and Physical Activity*
- *Journal of Applied Biomechanics*
- *Journal of Applied Sport Psychology*
- *Journal of Athletic Training*
- *Journal of Biomechanics*
- *Journal of Clinical Psychology*
- *Journal of Electromyography and Kinesiology*
- *Journal of Epidemiology and Community Health*
- *Journal of Human Kinetics*
- *Journal of Motor Behavior*
- *Journal of Nutrition*
- *Journal of Occupational and Environmental Medicine*
- *Journal of Orthopaedic and Sports Physical Therapy*
- *Journal of Physiology*
- *Journal of Science and Medicine in Sport*
- *Journal of Social and Clinical Psychology*
- *Journal of Sport and Exercise Psychology*
- *Journal of Sport Management*
- *Journal of Sports Science and Medicine*
- *Journal of Sports Sciences*
- *Motor Control*
- *Nutrition and Dietetics*
- *Pediatric Exercise Science*
- *Physical Therapy*
- *Physical Therapy in Sport*
- *Psychology of Sport and Exercise*
- *Research Quarterly for Exercise and Sport*
- *Scandinavian Journal of Medicine and Science in Sports*
- *Sociology of Sport Journal*
- *Sport, Education, and Society*
- *Sports Biomechanics*
- *Sports Medicine*
- *Sports Medicine and Arthroscopy Review*
- *The Sport Psychologist*

by a journal can skew its impact factor. For example, journals that primarily or solely publish review articles will typically receive more citations due to limitations in the number of references that can be used in a manuscript and the ability of a review paper to cover more concepts than an original research article. Ultimately, you should publish your study in journals that have the scientists and readership most interested in your topic of study.

Source-Normalized Impact per Paper

Direct comparison of academic journals in different subject areas can be better made with the **source normalized impact per paper (SNIP)** (3). A journal's SNIP is the ratio of the average number citations for each of its published articles and the citation potential of the journal's subject field over the previous year. The SNIP is advantageous in that it considers field-specific properties such as the number of citations per article, the amount of indexed literature, and the rate of publication. The normalization factor results in an average SNIP score across all journals approximately equal to one.

SCIMago Journal Rank

Although calculations based on the raw number of citations across all journals may provide insight into how many times an article is cited, they do not provide any information on the quality of the citing articles. The **SCIMago Journal Rank (SJR)** provides a means of assessing both the number of citations received by a journal and the perceived prestige of the journals from which the citations were made (5). The average prestige per journal article is calculated based on its subject field, quality, and reputation (similar to the SNIP), where the average of all SJR values is equal to one.

FORMATTING YOUR MANUSCRIPT

Although a topic such as manuscript formatting might seem elementary, it is actually a stage of the submission process that is often performed incorrectly. Improper formatting can cost an author valuable time for a number of reasons. First, after submission, the initial correspondence received from the journal could be an administrator notifying you of the formatting that must be corrected before the article will even be considered for review. Second, errors could be noticed by the reviewers and will need to be corrected before the paper can be published.

As previously mentioned, the length of time from initial paper submission to public appearance can, in some cases, exceed 12 months. Therefore, if there is any way that authors can expedite the process, especially by completing a task as simple as following the author instructions, it is certainly in their best interest to do so. Not only can failing to follow author instructions cause unnecessary delays in the process, but it is also not looked upon favorably by reviewers for the journal, particularly if the article has been formatted for a different publication. In this case, reviewers may be savvy to the fact that the paper was rejected from a prior journal and has since been resubmitted to the current journal as is. Thus, correct formatting is requisite when submitting a manuscript for the purpose of saving time as well as showing a level of courtesy and respect to the journal.

Manuscript Specifications

Each individual journal will have its own specifications, and the importance of reading the specific author instructions cannot be understated. File formats, font style and size, page margins, spacing, word limits, and even section headings will vary depending on the journal. Other requests, such as numbering paragraphs or providing line numbers in the text file, are also common. Again, the authors will find the specific requirements for the journal to which they are submitting in an author instructions section or file provided by the journal.

Language

One of the first things you will need to consider is the language of the journal. Even assuming the language is English, you will still need to be sure you are using the correct version of English (*i.e.*, British, Canadian, Australian, or U.S. English). The differences in the languages are subtle, but reviewers will correct you if you have made an error. A simple way to correct yourself when writing the manuscript is to set the spellcheck in your word processor to the correct version of English.

An important terminology to learn when you are referring to your subjects is the difference between "gender" and "sex." *Medicine & Science in Sports & Exercise* (*MSSE*) uses the terms as defined by the World Health Organization. "Sex" refers to the biologic characteristics of the individual that define men and women (7). "Gender," however, refers to the behaviors, activities, and attributes that a specific society considers appropriate for men and women. Other language issues to consider are that non-sexist language should be used. Only standardized acronyms should be used, and when they are, they should appear in full the first time they are used in the text.

Manuscript Sections

Most exercise science journals follow a similar layout, but the terminologies used may change. For example, introduction or literature review may be used. As another example, some journals combine the results and discussion sections or give authors the option of doing so. Some journals place the methods section last, and others encourage or require the submission of datasets and other supplementary information or figures. But a more distinct difference may be the inclusion of a unique section, such as the "practical applications" section of the *Journal of Strength and Conditioning Research* (*JSCR*), for which all authors are required to explain how their article will impact the practice of strength and conditioning coaches. If these types of sections are not clearly included (*i.e.*, the information is written, but in the discussion section), it will not be looked upon favorably by reviewers. Concept Box 21-1 provides a review of the basic sections of a manuscript, which you learned about first in Chapter 20.

Letter of Intent

The **letter of intent**, also referred to as "cover letter," addresses the editor or editorial office of the journal and is designed to convey a number of important pieces of information to the journal. First, the letter of intent confirms that the data are original and have

---

CONCEPT BOX 21-1   Typical Sections of a Manuscript

An Introduction or Literature Review
As you learned in Chapter 20, this section provides the reader with the important background information that is required to understand the context of the research and justify the need for it to be conducted.

Methods
This section should be written in enough detail that it can be exactly reproduced by another investigator as it is written here.

Results
This section should only include raw data with no interpretation of the results.

Discussion
The discussion section should describe the meaning of the results and also make comparisons with prior work.

not been published nor will be submitted elsewhere until the editor of the journal makes a decision. The letter may also speak to issues related to their institutional review board (IRB) stipulations (*e.g.*, exempt research so no informed consent was needed), authorships, and other conflicts that might need to be understood by the editors. The letter may also highlight the importance and impact of the manuscript, but this should not be longer than a sentence or two. Finally, requests for exceptions to common rules can be made. The most common example is the request that authorship limits be waived because many journals limit the number of authors that may be listed, when in reality, more made substantive contributions to the manuscript. Requests for the allowance of additional references are also commonly made.

Reference Style

All journals will have their own specific reference style, which will be found in the author instructions. The way that references appear in the body of the text will typically be in parentheses either by name and year or by a number that corresponds to the listing of references at the end of the manuscript. The number will be in regular form in parentheses or superscript form without parentheses. There are pros and cons to either system; for instance, names and years appearing in the text quickly provide the reader with the age of the article but can interfere with the flow of the paper, especially when there are many citations in quick succession. However, as mentioned, this is not a decision for the author but one that has been made by the journal.

The major concerns of the author regarding reference style is first getting it right (so as to not be delayed with administrative tasks) and perhaps more important, time. Setting up a reference list can take a substantial amount of time, particularly, for example, if a numbered system is used and an edit is made to include a reference at the beginning of the manuscript. Now, all future references will have to be edited to accommodate the new order. This is where programs such as RefWorks or EndNote can be invaluable because they will automatically format your reference list to whatever the journal guidelines are. Many journal styles are already included in the software, and journals often provide reference files on their website. In a worst-case scenario, a style can be quickly made and saved for future use. As a result, these software packages are a must-have for authors who frequently submit manuscripts.

Tables and Figures

A common mistake that is highlighted during the peer review process is incorrect formatting of tables and figures. A good rule to follow is that tables and figures should stand alone from the text in the manuscript. This way, a table or figure along with its legend could be used in a scientific presentation and be quickly and easily understood by the audience. The legend, therefore, which is a strand of text that appears in conjunction with the figure, should provide a detailed description of all the information that is pertinent to understanding the figure. For example, these may include an explanation of symbols (*e.g.*, $* = P \leq .05$) or spelling out any acronyms or abbreviations that appear in the figure as label axes.

Depending on the style they are using, journals will often ask that tables and figures be submitted in a file separate from the text document. As a result, the author is typically required to specify where in the text document each individual table or figure is supposed to appear. This is not part of an American Psychological Association (APA) style for formatting which emphasizes the importance of reading and following author instructions for each individual journal. This is especially important when getting ready to send your paper off to another journal after it was rejected by another one. This is accomplished by writing "Table X about here" or "Figure Y about here" in between the paragraphs at the desired position.

Authorship

As you learned in Chapter 20, an important decision to make before submitting a manuscript is the **author list**. Deciding which names to be included on the author list has important academic as well as financial implications. In the author guidelines for *MSSE*, each author listed on a publication is required to have contributed to two of the following areas: significant manuscript writer, significant manuscript reviewer/reviser, concept and design, data acquisition, data analysis and interpretation, and statistical expertise. Among the author list, an important designation is assigned to one author as the **corresponding author**. This person has an important responsibility to handle all communication with the journal during submission of the manuscript as well as throughout the peer review and publication process. In addition, the corresponding author should be available after publication to respond to questions or criticisms of the article.

The order in which the authors are listed is also important. The first author listed will be the name used in future citations of the article, and this is prestigious in the academic community. The last author listed is also a notable position (and often referenced when the manuscript is discussed) and is often reserved for the corresponding author in the case that the corresponding author is not the first author. This can be the case if a student investigator is the first author and the last author is the student's academic advisor.

Conflict of Interest

To review Chapter 20, a **conflict of interest** occurs when one or more contributors has motivations that clash with the ethical, moral, or scientific objectives of the manuscript. Examples of such conflicts of interest include financial, consultancy, institutional, or any other relationships that could lead to a bias or a conflict of interest. If the author believes that this does not apply, it must be explicitly written in the manuscript that there are no perceived conflicts of interest. Failure to address any potential conflicts of interest, regardless of the extent to which they are real or meaningful, may result in rejection of the manuscript or cause the findings and conclusions of the piece to be undermined.

SUBMITTING YOUR MANUSCRIPT

After you have reviewed your manuscript to ensure that it is properly formatted for the journal you have selected, the next step is to officially submit your manuscript. The submission process for journals now occurs online, drastically speeding up the process from the previous paper-based systems. In the case of *MSSE*, Editorial Manager is used and can be accessed at www.editorialmanager.com/MSSE. Other very commonly used processing systems are Manuscript Central and Scholar One. Along with the manuscript itself, accompanying documents are typically required such as a completed mandatory submission form, a copyright transfer agreement, a submission fee, and a letter of permission to reprint figures or tables.

Submission Form

Many publications require a specific **submission form** to be filed along with all other necessary materials. Although there is some variety in their composition, most submission forms contain the same basic components. Often, a checklist of items and steps necessary for the submission of a manuscript is included to remind the author to follow every step according to journal's directions. Authors are also asked to indicate that they have read through the author instructions and agree to pay all fees associated with publication. The submission form generally has to contain the signature of the corresponding author in order to confirm the authenticity of the document.

Copyright Transfer Agreement

Depending on the journal, all authors may be required to sign a **copyright transfer agreement**, which will need to be submitted along with the manuscript. In the case of *MSSE*, a link is provided in the author instructions. It is important to understand the rights you retain as an author if your manuscript is accepted by the journal. Depending on your agreement with the journal, there may be limitations placed on the form, extent, and situations by which you are able to reproduce or share the contents of your manuscript. Additionally, you should be aware of what protective measures the journal will enforce to safeguard against the misuse, plagiarism, or replication of your work by outside parties.

Submission Fee

Although a number of academic journals will allow for the submission of manuscripts free of charge, others will charge the authors a certain amount of money known as a **submission fee**. This not only helps the journal offset costs of the submission process but also deter authors without a strong commitment to their manuscript. Some journals such as *MSSE* have higher submission fees for authors who aren't members of their affiliated organization. This can help encourage those belonging to an organization to submit their manuscripts to their associated journals while encouraging non-members to become involved with the organization.

Letter of Permission

A **letter of permission** is a necessary inclusion during submission when figures or tables incorporated within the manuscript have already been published in previous literature. In order for it to be valid, each letter of permission must contain the written consent and signature of the copyright holder, which is often the publisher. The letter of permission authorizes the authors of the manuscript to reproduce the figure or table in question. Failure to secure a letter of permission can have significant financial and legal consequences, so it is best to make absolute certain you have permission to include all of your figures and tables.

Open Access

When submitting a manuscript, there may be an opportunity to designate the article as an **open-access article**. Making an article open-access allows it to be available for unrestricted online access as soon as it is accepted for publication rather than only available for those who have a subscription for that particular journal. Although there can be a significant cost involved (for *MSSE* it is $3,000), an open-access article has the opportunity to be read by a much larger audience while still allowing authors to retain all copyright privileges.

CONCLUSION

As is evident throughout this chapter, following through each step of the submission process can be a long and arduous process. However, you should now have a greater appreciation of why each step is necessary for the development of the body of knowledge and the preservation of its integrity. Authors who are familiar with the concepts and procedures previously discussed can avoid many of the unnecessary complications caused by simple ignorance. In summary, understanding how to submit a manuscript is an essential part of becoming a successful scientist and will continue to be instrumental throughout the entirety of your career.

GLOSSARY

Author list: the list of the primary contributors to a manuscript whose order is typically reflective of their level of contribution

Conflict of interest: when one or more contributors of a manuscript have financial, institutional, or other biased motivations that clash with the ethical, moral, or scientific objectives of the manuscript

Copyright transfer agreement: document signed by authors which confirms their agreement to terms set by the journal concerning the use and reproduction of their submitted work

Corresponding author: the author responsible for communication with the journal during the submission and publication process

Digital object identifier (DOI): unique combination of characters assigned to an original electronic publication for identification purposes

Duplicate submission: the submission of the same manuscript to multiple journals simultaneously

Impact factor (IF): qualitative measure of an academic journal which represents the average number of times the journal's articles have been cited over the previous two years

Letter of intent: document addressed to the editorial office of a journal which confirms the originality of the manuscript, highlights its importance, and contains any requests for exceptions to journal guidelines

Letter of permission: document signed by the copyright holder of the manuscript permitting the authors to reproduce content found in the manuscript

Open-access article: article which can be freely accessed without requiring subscription to the publishing journal

Peer reviewed scientific journal: journal containing manuscripts that have been screened and evaluated by a group of reviewers and the editorial office to ensure their originality, authenticity, impact, and quality

SCIMago Journal Rank (SJR): qualitative measure of an academic journal based on both the number of citations and the perceived prestige of the journals from which the citations were made

Source normalized impact per paper (SNIP): qualitative measure of an academic journal based on the ratio of the average number citations for each of its published articles and the citation potential of the journal's subject field over the previous year

Submission fee: cost that must be paid by authors in order to submit their manuscript to a particular journal

Submission form: document signed by the corresponding author of a manuscript, which generally consists of a list of submission requirements, acknowledgment that all proper steps have been followed, and confirms agreement to pay all necessary publication fees

Target audience: the population of readers for which your manuscript has been written

REFERENCES

1. Alberts B. Impact factor distortions. *Science*. 2013;340(6134):787.
2. Garfield E. The history and meaning of the journal impact factor. *JAMA*. 2006;295(1):90–93.
3. Journal Metrics Web site. SNIP & SJR: new perspectives in journal metrics. Atlanta (GA): Elsevier; [cited 2013 Sep 27]. Available from: http://www.journalmetrics.com/documents/Journal_Metrics_Factsheet.pdf
4. PubMed.gov Web site [Internet]. Bethesda (MD): U.S. National Library of Medicine, National Institutes of Health; [cited 2013 Sep 15]. Available from: http://www.ncbi.nlm.nih.gov/pubmed
5. SCImago Journal & Country Rank Web site [Internet]. SCImago Journal & Country Rank; [cited 2013 Sep 12]. Available from: http://www.scimagojr.com
6. Spier R. The history of the peer-review process. *Trends Biotechnol*. 2002;20(8):357–358.
7. World Health Organization Web site [Internet]. What do we mean by "sex" and "gender"? Geneva (Switzerland): World Health Organization; [cited 2013 Sep 29]. Available from: http://www.who.int/gender/whatisgender/en/

CHAPTER 22

Demands of the Peer Review Process

Bradley C. Nindl, PhD, FACSM, Andrew J. Young, PhD, FACSM, and
Kent B. Pandolf, PhD, MPH, FACSM

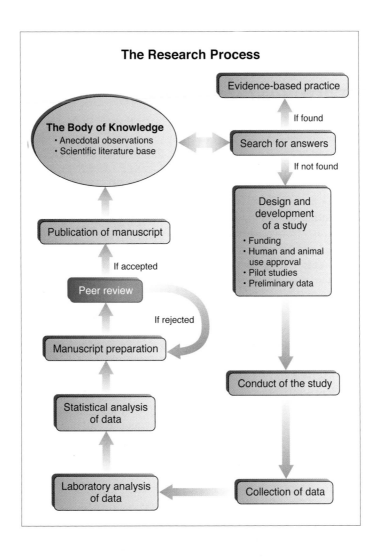

The Research Process

Evidence-based practice

If found

The Body of Knowledge
• Anecdotal observations
• Scientific literature base

Search for answers

If not found

Design and development of a study
• Funding
• Human and animal use approval
• Pilot studies
• Preliminary data

Publication of manuscript

If accepted

Peer review

If rejected

Manuscript preparation

Conduct of the study

Statistical analysis of data

Laboratory analysis of data

Collection of data

INTRODUCTION

The peer review process is in an important and essential step in science and one that helps ensure the quality of published research. Peer review assists journal editors and publishers in determining whether scientific work is credible and valid and meets a threshold of merit that warrants publication (3,5,6,10). Peer review can be operationally defined as a systematic and unbiased evaluation of scholarly scientific work by one's peers that lead to a decision about whether the work gets accepted or rejected for journal publication (10). In essence, peer review is a critical and fundamental quality control step in the scientific method.

This chapter introduces the reader to the demands of the peer review process and serves as a primer for the apprentice scientist/researcher in kinesiology, exercise science, and sports medicine. Here, we will help the reader navigate the peer review process to help facilitate the likelihood of a successful experience. As a representative example, this chapter provides particular guidance on the peer review process for *Medicine & Science in Sports & Exercise* (MSSE), the flagship journal for the American College of Sports Medicine (ACSM).

WHY IS PEER REVIEW IMPORTANT TO SCIENCE?

Of the steps of the scientific method that you learned about at the beginning of this text, the last step before publication involves the peer review process. It is imperative for apprentice researchers to fully understand and embrace that research unpublished is research that has not completed the scientific method and is therefore not yet complete (3,7). As you have learned in Chapters 20 and 21, for the body of knowledge to advance, a sharing of research findings with other scientists is necessary, and this is accomplished by publishing in a peer reviewed scientific journal (3,6,7). Peer reviewed, published research in reputable scientific journals contrasts from scientific claims reported in magazines, newspapers, infomercials, websites, blogs, radio, television, etc., in that it has been vetted by scientific subject matter experts (10). This vetting process helps ensure that the manuscript has a clear research question, has an appropriate and sound experimental design, is innovative and original, adds to the existing body of knowledge, is described in sufficient detail to be replicable, uses sound statistical analyses, and was ethically performed (10). The peer review process assists in preventing unsupported, invalid, significantly flawed, unethical, or fraudulent scientific claims from becoming accessible to the public and the scientific community at large. Although the peer review process is not perfect, it is an accepted part of the scientific culture and has been integral to ensuring quality science since the 18th century (7).

The hallmark of success or the "coin of the realm" in research is the peer reviewed publication (3,6,10). A scholar's peer reviewed publication will also influence one's career in terms of promotion, recognition, grant success, tenure, and more. Peer reviewed journals have survived the test of time due to the fact that they are useful vehicles for disseminating research results, are important for archiving knowledge, shape thought and knowledge, provide a stamp of quality and authority to work, provide recognition to the person who carried out the research, keep other researchers and practitioners up to date, advance the knowledge base of the discipline, help researchers advance their own careers, and provide a conclusion for a study.

HOW DOES THE PEER REVIEW PROCESS WORK?

Selecting a Journal

The peer review process starts after an author has concluded an experiment, conducted adequate analyses, interpreted the data, drawn conclusions, and finally drafted a manuscript for submission. After an author has a manuscript draft, the first decision point is to decide to which journal to submit. Two major criteria when selecting a journal are (a) the appropriateness or "fit" of the data for a particular journal and (b) the selectiveness of the journal based on the quality of the study findings. Students and apprentice scholars are encouraged to be familiar with journals within their field. Journals will typically have websites that include information about the type of research that is featured in the journal. For example, on the *MSSE* website, the following statement appears:

> **Medicine & Science in Sports & Exercise** *features original investigations, clinical studies, and comprehensive reviews on current topics in sports medicine and exercise science. With this leading multidisciplinary journal, exercise physiologists, physiatrists, physical therapists, team physicians, and athletic trainers get a vital exchange of information from basic and applied science, medicine, education, and allied health fields.* (11)

If a manuscript is submitted to a journal that the editor does not deem a good "fit" for the scope of a journal, the editor could choose to administratively reject the manuscript and not send it out for peer review. An administrative rejection does not necessarily mean that a manuscript does not have merit but rather that another journal may be a better match between the study results and journal scope. Authors are often encouraged to contact a journal's editors directly with an abstract before submitting manuscript in order to determine if the manuscript will be a good fit for the journal. For students in kinesiology, exercise science, and sports medicine, Table 22-1 lists 60 different reputable peer reviewed journals for consideration.

When submitting to a journal, potential authors are also encouraged to carefully read the instructions to authors; as you learned in Chapter 21, these offer specific information on manuscript requirements. General information, manuscript submission requirements and preparation, technical guidelines, and human and animal experimentation policy statements are all provided on the *MSSE* website. Table 22-2 lists some excellent reference material and resources for beginning writers.

Once an author has decided which journals are most appropriate for the manuscript, the goal should be to submit and publish in the most well-respected and reputable journal possible. An index that is used in an attempt to quantify the quality of scientific journals is the **impact factor**. The Institute for Scientific Information (ISI, a subsidiary of Thomson Reuters) compiles impact factors on a yearly basis. These journal citation reports can be accessed through the ISI Web of Knowledge which requires institutional subscriptions (4). Students are encouraged to seek assistance from a reference librarian if not familiar with how to access impact factors from the ISI Web of Science.

Impact factors are calculated by determining the average number of citations per published manuscript in a given journal during the previous two years. Impact factors have been calculated since 1975. For example, the impact for *MSSE* in 2013 was 4.5, which means

Table 22-1 Impact Factors for Exercise and Sports Medicine Journals with Impact Factors ≥1

Impact Factor	Journal	Impact Factor	Journal
7.1	*Exercise and Immunology Reviews*	2.0	*Applied Physiology, Nutrition, & Metabolism*
7.0	*International Journal of Epidemiology*		
5.3	*Exercise and Sport Sciences Reviews*	2.0	*Gait and Posture*
5.2	*Sports Medicine*	1.9	*Behavior Research Methods*
4.8	*Journal of Applied Psychology*	1.9	*Clinical Biomechanics*
4.5	*American Journal of Physiology—Endocrinology and Metabolism*	1.9	*International Journal of Sport Nutrition and Exercise Metabolism*
4.5	*Medicine & Science in Sports & Exercise*	1.9	*Journal of Aging and Physical Activity*
4.4	*American Journal of Sports Medicine*	1.9	*Journal of Occupational and Environmental Medicine*
4.4	*Acta Physiologica Scandinavica*	1.9	*Journal of Physical Activity and Health*
4.4	*Journal of Physiology*	1.8	*Journal of the International Society of Sports Nutrition*
3.7	*British Journal of Sports Medicine*		
3.6	*American Journal of Physiology—Heart and Circulatory Physiology*	1.8	*Journal of Strength and Conditioning Research*
3.5	*Journal of Applied Physiology*	1.7	*Applied Ergonomics*
3.4	*Journal of Epidemiology and Community Health*	1.7	*Psychology of Sport and Exercise*
		1.7	*Journal of Athletic Training*
3.2	*Scandinavian Journal of Medicine and Science in Sports*	1.7	*Ergonomics*
3.0	*Journal of Orthopaedic and Sports Physical Therapy*	1.6	*Journal of Electromyography and Kinesiology*
		1.6	*Clinical Journal of Sport Medicine*
2.9	*Journal of Science and Medicine in Sport*	1.6	*Pediatric Exercise Science*
2.7	*Journal of Biomechanics*	1.5	*Applied Psychology-International Review*
2.5	*Journal of Sport and Exercise Psychology*	1.5	*Current Sports Medicine Reports*
2.4	*Clinics in Sports Medicine*	1.4	*Motor Control*
		1.4	*Physical Therapy in Sport*
2.3	*International Journal of Sports Medicine*	1.3	*Physician and Sports Medicine*
2.3	*International Journal of Sports Physiology and Performance*	1.3	*Journal of Sport and Social Issues*
		1.3	*Journal of Applied Biomechanics*
2.1	*High Altitude Medicine and Biology*	1.2	*Sport, Education, and Society*
2.1	*Journal of Sports Sciences*	1.2	*Journal of Applied Sport Psychology*
2.1	*Human Movement Science*	1.2	*European Journal of Sport Science*

Table 22-1 Impact Factors for Exercise and Sports Medicine Journals with Impact Factors ≥1 (Continued)

Impact Factor	Journal	Impact Factor	Journal
1.1	*Research in Sports Medicine*	1.1	*Journal of Applied Behavioral Science*
1.1	*Adapted Physical Activity Quarterly*	1.0	*Journal of Motor Behaviour*
1.1	*Research Quarterly for Exercise and Sport*	1.0	*Leisure Sciences*
1.1	*Applied Psychological Measurement*	1.0	*(The) Sport Psychologist*

From Hopkins WG Impact factors and article influence scores for journals in sports medicine and science in 2013. *Sportscience* [Internet]. 2013;17:20–23. Available from: http://sportsci.org/2013/wghif.htm.

that the papers published in 2012 and 2011 each received an average of 4.5 citations in 2013. The 2013 impact factor for *MSSE* was calculated as follows:

A = total number of published manuscripts in *MSSE* in 2012 and 2011 cited by indexed publications in 2013

B = total number of citable published manuscripts in *MSSE* in 2012 and 2011

2013 Impact Factor = A/B

Table 22-1 lists the impact factors for sport medicine and science journals equal to or greater than 1 (8). Note that two of the top five journals (*i.e., Exercise and Sport Science Review* and *MSSE*) are official research journals for the ACSM. To publish in these respected journals, it is essential to report important new information that informs the reader of a complete story that is of interest to the journal's audience. It is not sufficient to submit a manuscript that reports only incremental advancements to publish in the top-tier journals.

Another important metric of an individual scientist's scholarly acumen is the **h-index**. The h-index is a metric that measures both impact and productivity of a scientist. The h-index is calculated by citation databases such as the Web of Knowledge. It is the number of publications that have been cited X or more times. For example, an h-index of 20 indicates that a scientist has 20 publications that have been published 20 or more times.

Table 22-2 Useful Website Information for Apprentice Scholars in Navigating the Demands of the Peer Review Process

Website	Content
www.acsm-msse.org	*MSSE* content page
www.editorialmanager.com/msse/	*MSSE* author and submission information
http://www.icmje.org/	Information on manuscript writing
http://abacus.bates.edu/~ganderso/biology/resources/writing/HTWsections.html	How to write biologic papers
http://www.columbia.edu/cu/biology/ug/research/paper.html	How to write biologic papers
http://advan.physiology.org/cgi/content/full/29/2/59	Ethics and scientific publications

MSSE, *Medicine & Science in Sports & Exercise.*

Other less critical factors for selecting a journal should include the timeliness of the journal for providing the first review, the timeliness of the journal for providing the final decision, the timeliness of the journal for publishing accepted manuscripts, the acceptance rate, the readership of the journal, and abstracting and indexing services for the journal, among others.

Journal Handling of a Manuscript

Upon receipt of a manuscript, the managing editor and the editorial staff will ensure that the manuscript meets the submission guidelines and the style and format requirements as specified in the instructions to authors (4). The managing editor and editorial staff are typically full-time employees and will communicate electronically with the author if deficiencies are noted, and they will ask for corrections.

If all submission requirements are satisfied and the manuscript is considered a fit for the journal, the **editor-in-chief** will assign the manuscript to an associate editor based on subject matter expertise. The editor-in-chief is typically a preeminent scholar in the field and holds this position as a part-time duty. One of the most important responsibilities for an editor-in-chief is to appoint other scholars in the field to the journal's **editorial board**. An editorial board typically consists of associate editors and editorial board members. Other positions on the editorial board can include consulting editors and associate editors-in-chief. The associate editors are assigned manuscripts based on subject area and content and have the responsibility of subsequently inviting reviewers to peer review the manuscript. Associate editors of journals can invite anybody in the field who they feel can offer an authoritative and fair critique, but they tend to heavily rely on appointed members of the editorial board as these members have agreed to review a minimum number or manuscripts a year. They have also been designated by the editor-in-chief as eminently qualified authorities who may peer review for the journal.

The number of reviewers invited and actually agreeing and completing the peer review can vary by circumstance and situation, but authors typically receive two to three reviewers for their manuscript. Once the reviewers have completed their reviews, they then can make recommendations to the associate editors. These recommendations typically fall into one of four categories: accept, revise (major revisions), revise (minor revisions), or reject. Once the associate editor receives the reviews back from the reviewers along with their recommendations, the associate editor is charged with making a determination and decision and informing the submitting author of the decision. The associate editor makes this decision based on the collective information provided by the reviewers as well an assessment by the associate editor himself or herself. It is important to note that reviewers are typically asked to provide two sets of written comments: (a) to the author and (b) confidential comments to the associate editor. The reviewer comments to the author are provided to the author in his or her entirety whether the manuscript is accepted, rejected, or in need of revisions. The author does not see the confidential comments to the associate editor, and these typically convey the degree or lack thereof for the reviewer's enthusiasm for the manuscript.

If an author is invited to make revisions, it is important to keep in mind that this is not a guarantee that the manuscript will be accepted, only that further revision is required before a final decision is to be made. The revising author should consider each reviewer comment and suggestion carefully. Efforts should be made for revision before attempting rebuttal.

If an author absolutely disagrees with a reviewer's suggestions, tact and deference should be exercised when explaining the counterargument thoroughly and respectfully. A detailed cover letter with a point-by-point explanation of how each review comment was addressed in the revision should be included.

If the associate editor finally makes a decision that the manuscript is suitable for acceptance, the author is notified and the journal will start processing the manuscript for publication. The publisher will generate a **galley proof** and provide the authors an opportunity for a final check before the manuscript goes to print. Figure 22-1 illustrates the current peer review process that *MSSE* employs.

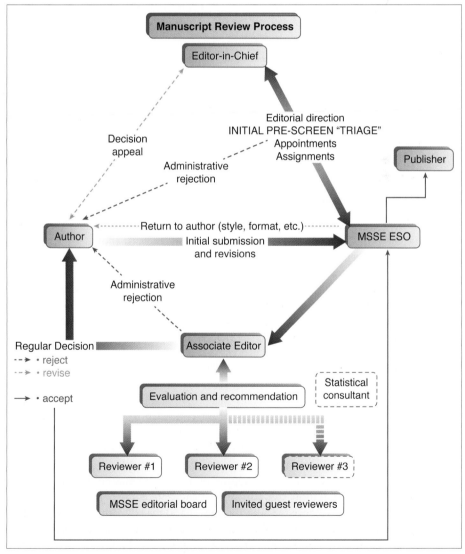

FIGURE 22-1: The manuscript peer review process for *MSSE*.

Successfully Navigating the Peer Review Process

The major determinant in successfully navigating the peer review process is to conduct a quality study resulting in a well-written and organized manuscript. Keys to writing a quality manuscript involve a firm grasp of the scientific literature; a passion for knowledge, reading, and writing; and discipline in time management. Keys for having a manuscript accepted for publication include having a novel and important scientific question, using cutting edge and innovative methodologies, having compelling and provocative arguments, and, finally, having polished writing. High-impact journals are highly selective, and it is not uncommon for journals to have acceptance rates below 30%. For example, the 2012 acceptance rate in *MSSE* was 29%.

As you learned in Chapter 20, the organizational structure of a peer reviewed manuscript consists of a title page, an abstract, an introduction, a methods section, a discussion section, references, tables, and figures. The title page will list the title of the manuscript, the authors, the authors' affiliations, the contact information for the corresponding author, and a running head. The abstract should provide enough information to stand alone on retrieval by an electronic search. The purpose and rationale for research should be clearly written. The methods section can be limited but should describe the research design and major procedures. Only data addressing the primary purpose and most significant finding should be provided. The conclusion should highlight the scientific importance of the findings.

Recommending Editors and Reviewers

There are several strategies authors can employ to increase their likelihood of receiving a fair and thorough review. For example, most journals allow submitting authors to suggest reviewers. Submitting authors are strongly encouraged to seize this opportunity. Authors should identify other scientists active in research similar to their own, and this can be achieved by having a solid understanding of the field via the published work in the references section or the authors of the works found during the initial literature search. Additionally, submitting authors should identify other scientists who are members of the journal's editorial board as well as experts in the author's line of research. Providing three names during the submission process is generally a good rule of thumb. These suggestions should also be of qualified scientists who are likely to accept the review invitation. Although you will want to invite scientists who will be inclined to provide a fair and balanced review, you should avoid scientists such as collaborators, supervisors, mentors, students, or family members who may have a conflict of interest when reviewing your work. Additionally, a submitting author can also identify scientists who they do not wish to review the manuscript. A compelling reason is usually required for justification. When presenting study results at a professional conference, a researcher can at times get a sense for fellow researchers who would fairly critique the work and of others who may not.

Submitting authors can also suggest associate editors. This is an underused strategy that can be of assistance for both the author and the editor-in-chief. The masthead page of journals provides the names of associate editors and submitting authors are encouraged to suggest associate editors whose line of research closely aligns with their own scientific work.

How Does a Reviewer Evaluate a Manuscript?

Upon acceptance of an invitation to serve as a reviewer, the journal will send instructions to the reviewer describing the manner in which they are to critique the manuscript (1,2,8,9,12). Typical of most modern scientific journals, *MSSE* uses an online system. For *MSSE*, reviewers are asked to rate the manuscript on four major focus areas: (a) research impact, (b) results originality, (c) data quality and methodology, and (d) overall rank. For each of the areas, the reviewer is asked to select one of six ratings: (a) top 10% (best), (b) top 25%, (c) top 50%, (d) bottom 50%, (e) bottom 25%, and (f) bottom 10% (worst).

Additionally, the reviewer must respond to the following questions:

1. Do you have major concerns regarding the data analysis and interpretation that warrant a focused statistical review for this manuscript (yes or no)?
2. Evaluate the use and quality of figures and tables (options include not applicable; figures/tables and text are complementary; figure/table quality is unsatisfactory; figures/tables are insufficient to illustrate concepts/results; some figures/tables are redundant; figures/tables are not needed for the subject matter; figures/tables are irrelevant to subject matter; figures/tables repeat data; some figures/tables may be removed from paper and published online as supplemental content)
3. If the associate editor invites the authors to revise the manuscript, do you want to review the revised work (yes or no)?
4. Is there a financial or other conflict of interest between your work and that of the author (yes or no)?

The reviewer is further asked to provide written comments to the author and confidential comments to the associate editor. Finally, the reviewer is asked to provide an overall recommendation: acceptance, minor revisions, major revisions, or rejection.

Revising a Manuscript

If the associate editor asks an author to make revisions, the author has an opportunity to significantly improve the manuscript and should view this as an opportunity to excel. The author should work to revise the manuscript in a timely manner and within the time period stated in the decision letter. *MSSE* allows two months to make revisions and resubmit. In your rebuttal letter, it is important to address all points raised by the reviewers. The rebuttal letter to the reviewers should specify exactly what revisions were made in the manuscript and exactly where these changes were made. It is recommended that you use track changes within the manuscript so that the reviewers can easily identify where revisions were made.

Handling Rejection

All scientists experience having a manuscript rejected. As stated previously, many top-tier journals have rejection rates exceeding 70% to 80%. Authors should thoroughly read the decision and all review comments to understand the primary flaws, concerns, and criticisms of the study. Critical review of one's science should be taken seriously but never personally. Authors should feel free to ask an associate editor for clarification if needed, but it is important to take the decision gracefully and use the reviews to rewrite the manuscript and submit elsewhere. If the author feels that there was an egregious factual misunderstanding by the reviewers, a request can be made to the associate editor to reconsider the decision. An appeal could also be made to the editor-in-chief if there is a flawed review. At times, reviewer comments might suggest alternate journals for the author to consider in resubmission; these suggestions are usually good ones.

Serving as a Peer Reviewer

Being asked to review a scholarly manuscript should be considered an honor and a privilege. You should normally only accept review invitations within your particular area of expertise, as this will be most beneficial to you as the reviewer and fairest to the author(s). Serving as a reviewer will sharpen your critical thinking skills and broaden your understanding of a given scientific topic area. There is usually little formal training on how to serve as a reviewer and most is by experience (1,8,12). More important, you must work to meet the deadlines for the journal. Many journals maintain internal ratings of their reviewers, and future opportunities to review are based on these ratings.

For *MSSE*, reviewers are asked to recommend acceptance only if the paper ranks in the top 25% of all papers or can be with appropriate revisions. If the paper's issues are unlikely to be resolved by revisions, the reviewer should recommend rejection. For apprentice scholars who are starting their professional careers, it is permissible to approach journals and volunteer services as a reviewer.

CONCLUSION

In summary, peer review is an integral step of the scientific method. A scientist's career success and professional reputation are largely influenced by how well a scientist can successfully navigate the demands of the peer review process. By completely understanding the peer review process, carefully considering a peer's critique of one's scientific work, and actively participating as a peer reviewer, a scientist can maximize the likelihood of publication success.

GLOSSARY

Editorial board: the editorial board is a group of selected and distinguished scientists that are affiliated with a peer reviewed journal and are unpaid volunteers that assist in setting journal policy and reviewing manuscripts to select for publication

Editor-in-chief: the editor-in-chief is a publication's editorial leader having responsibility for all operations and policies. Responsibilities of an editor-in-chief include selecting the editorial board, assigning manuscripts to associate editors and/or reviewers, developing policies and the direction for a journal, editing content, and handling author and reader's complaints and concerns

Galley proof: in printing and publishing, galley proofs are the preliminary versions of publications meant for review by authors, editors, and proofreaders

H-index: h-index is a measure that attempts to quantify both the productivity and citation impact of the published body of work of a scientist or scholar

Impact factor: the impact factor of an academic journal is a measure reflecting the average number of citations to recent articles published in that journal

REFERENCES

1. Benos DJ, Kirk KL, Hall JE. How to review a paper. *Adv Physiol Educ.* 2003;27(1-4):47–52.
2. Gura T. Peer review, unmasked. *Nature.* 2002;416(6878):258–260.
3. Henneberg M. Peer-review: the Holy Office of modern science. *Natural Science.*1997;1(2).
4. Hopkins WG Impact factors and article influence scores for journals in sports medicine and science in 2013. *Sportscience* [Internet]. 2013;17:20–23. Available from: http://sportsci.org/2013/wghif.htm.
5. International Committee of Medical Journal Editors Web site [Internet]. Recommendations for the conducting, reporting, editing and publication of scholarly work in medical journals. Vancouver (Canada): International Committee of Medical Journal Editors; [cited December 2014]. Available from: http://www.icmje.org/icmje-recommendations.pdf
6. Kassirer JP, Campion EW. Peer review. Crude and understudied, but indispensable. *JAMA.* 1994;272(2):96–97.
7. Kronick DA. Peer review in the 18th-century scientific journalism. *JAMA.* 1990;263(10):1321–1322.
8. Lovejoy TI, Revenson TA, France CR. Reviewing manuscripts for peer-review journals: a primer for novice and seasoned reviewers. *Ann Behav Med.* 2011;42(1):1–13.
9. Raff H, Brown D. Civil, sensible, and constructive peer review in APS journals. *J Appl Physiol.* 2013;115(3):295–296.
10. Sense About Science Web site [Internet]. Peer review: the nuts and bolts. London, United Kingdom: Sense About Science; [cited July 2012]. Available from: http://www.senseaboutscience.org/data/files/resources/99/Peer-review_The-nuts-and-bolts.pdf
11. Medicine & Science in Sport & Exercise Web site [Internet]. Indianapolis (IN): American College of Sports Medicine; [cited 2015 Jun 6]. Available from: http://www.acsm-msse.org
12. Vintzileos AM, Ananth CV. The art of peer-reviewing an original research paper: important tips and guidelines. *J Ultrasound Med.* 2010;29(4):513–518.

Building the Science Buzz: Working with Media to Create a Lay Translation of Your Discovery

Daniel J. Henkel, BA, APR

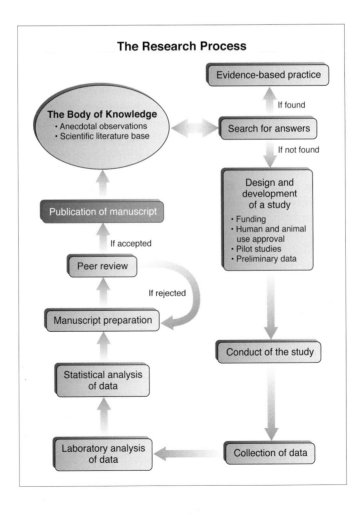

The Research Process

INTRODUCTION

Why share your research with the public? If you are a junior scientist on a research team, your efforts are part of a larger collaboration—perhaps a study to be submitted for publication in a journal (see Chapters 20–22) or presented at a conference. Your work contributes to the collective project. You're doing your job, and somebody else (senior scientist, project manager, lead author) will worry about reporting the results. You're all about the science, right?

Maybe it's not that simple. Think back to why you decided to become a scientist. Were you fascinated by bugs in your backyard? Did you wonder why you were told (correctly or incorrectly) not to swim right after eating, or whether some people were just born to run fast? What speculation and questions led you to a life of study and inquiry? The impulse to discover, to understand, and to *explain* courses through the veins of every scientist and simmers below the surface of every published study. It lies—latent, at times—just under the skin of every scientific project. We may talk in terms of objective measurement, of data, and rational observation, but the real force behind scientific discovery is that same impulse that leads the kid craning to watch a meteor shower cry, "Wow!"

Many a scientist began as a child showing her mother an unusual insect or asking about colors or foods or her sibling's behavior. That curiosity is the essence of critical investigation. It's the spark that fuels scientific enterprise. Sponsoring institutions may crave data and measure success by counting published articles and gauging influence factors, but the most basic, human, and compelling motivation behind science is "Wow!" and "Why?"

That may be enough to lead you to share your discoveries with the world. But even if adding new knowledge is enough for you, you have many reasons to explain your work and have it understood. Unless you're independently wealthy or an heir gifted with the resources to pursue your whims and interests, you are probably beholden to those who sponsor your research. Funding (discussed in Chapter 13) comes with expectations.

Many see dissemination of learning as a sacred obligation of the academy; it is the cycle of learning from masters and mentors, adding to the body of knowledge, and passing one's expertise along to the next generation of scientists and to society at large. Then there is the pressure to "publish or perish," with its ramifications on tenure, reputation, and career trajectory. Those whose work is seen as widely influential are generally in better professional stead. This means one should strive to reach an audience outside the circles of one's professional colleagues, adding to the ocean of information in the public media. Being accepted and published by an established journal is gratifying, validating, and professionally important, but compare the readership of even a top journal with that of a major newspaper or magazine and the numbers suggest a two-pronged approach to sharing your work. Thus, in addition to allowing one's colleagues to read of your discovery, it is important to gain some attention by the lay public when appropriate. Many universities and professional organizations such as the American College of Sports Medicine have public relations departments who can help authors share their work with a wider audience.

The realm of feature writers and TV newsrooms may be well outside the comfort zone of one who is at home behind a laboratory bench or proctoring an undergraduate exam. Given the importance of sharing one's discoveries through the media, however, the emerging scientist would do well to gain some level of competence in this arena.

This is the focus of this chapter: sharing your discovery not through scientific journals and presentations but with the general public through the way they get their information—from newspapers and broadcasts to podcasts and social media. Marie Curie would be intrigued.

AUDIENCES, CHANNELS, AND MESSAGES

Let's begin by exploring in turn:

1. **Audiences**—to whom you're talking
2. **Channels**—the medium or means by which the conversation takes place
3. **Journalists**—the reporters, editors, and producers who work in the media
4. **Messages**—how to tailor what you're saying to suit the audience and channel

Audiences

Did you ever try explaining the thesis of a scientific paper to an elderly relative? You probably used a somewhat different set of words than when explaining it to a classmate or the kid next door. Unless that great uncle was a scientist himself, he likely didn't have the background to understand all the terms and concepts you covered. He might have known what a hypothesis was, whereas your explanation to your young neighbor was that you had an idea you were testing. Each of them had a different set of understandings, a different frame of reference, and probably a different level of interest in your work. If you were to successfully get across to them some knowledge of your topic and findings, you had to put it to them in terms they knew, starting with the level of knowledge of each.

Think of your great uncle and your young neighbor as two different audiences; each is an audience of one with unique characteristics. Broadening out from there, you can identify one audience after another, grouping them by factors such as:

- Their interest in your topic: Why is it relevant to them? Why should they care about it? How does it relate to their occupations or daily lives? Are they passionate about the subject, or do you first have to get their attention and explain why this should matter to them?
- Their level of understanding: Are they in middle school, or do they have master's degrees? Are they likely to know the terms and concepts you use, or will they need explanation? Are they familiar with research methods and the literature in the field?
- Their attitudes and opinions about your subject matter: Is this a topic of current debate? Do you know where they're coming from on the subject? What else are they hearing or reading about it?
- How they get their information and form opinions: Do they read the daily paper? Do they listen to talk radio? Do they watch nature documentaries or sitcoms? What's trending on their social media feeds?

You can parse these audiences many ways, filtering them according to any number of factors. Everyone is a distinct individual, of course, but you're generally not writing or speaking to an audience of one. Look for the characteristics that members of a group have in common, and use that information to help you form your message.

The list of possible audiences is open-ended, but here's a starting point to get you thinking about them:

- The scientific community, including many subgroups such as those in your field, conference attendees, journal editors and publishers, research funders, faculty colleagues, etc. (You get the idea; examine your relationship with each and what you would like them to understand about you and your work.)
- The general public: an immense and inappropriately comprehensive bucket, but think of the readers of a typical daily newspaper. Don't assume much scientific literacy; reading levels may be from about middle school to high school level.
- Educated professionals, somewhat learned and accomplished, although maybe not in your field
- Science enthusiasts: curious people who may watch science-related documentaries and read science-focused consumer magazines
- Elected and appointed officials who make public policy that can affect you as a citizen and a scientist
- The business community: entrepreneurs, executives, and business owners in industries that are affected by scientific and technical developments

Taking a page from Web developers, you might invent avatars for each important audience. This is an exercise whereby a series of descriptive terms becomes a specific, fictional individual with particular characteristics, needs, preferences, predilections, and experiences. For example, the reference earlier to "elected and appointed officials" becomes "a middle-aged, religiously conservative school board member in a Midwestern city serving on a panel that selects science textbooks." This reveals ways in which an understanding of your work could inform those decisions. The stakes could be significant.

In considering how best to reach this specific audience, you might construct an avatar such as:

Name: Darrell Phillips, Jr.

Age: 43

Residence: Ames, Iowa

Marital status: married 19 years; two children in public high school

Occupation: franchisee and business manager, office supply store in suburban Ames

Community service: member, local chamber of commerce and several youth-serving organizations; member, township school board; serves on textbook selection committee

Religion: Evangelical Christian, serves as elder and religious education teacher

Education: BS in Business Management, Iowa State University; continuing education in Accounting, Human Resources, and Marketing

Interests: historical fiction, American history, economic development, collegiate sports, physical fitness

Although these descriptors relate only to one, hypothetical individual, they may help put a human face on what can seem like an impersonal, mass audience. Furthermore, they may prompt insights that help you tailor your message so that your audience can focus attention, hear it in context, and relate it to what they already know and value.

This technique is akin to your speech teacher's suggestion to address your remarks to an individual rather than to the masses gathered in the auditorium. Rather than speaking to an indistinct, generalized "someone," you're in a conversation with someone you know. Being aware of his or her background and mindset can help you explain yourself in a way that helps him or her better understand what you're telling him or her—and isn't that the point of communication?

Channels

Similarly, think of the array of media or channels by which we get information (Fig. 23-1). You can group them in large buckets (print, broadcast, social media) or slice and dice them as closely as suits your purpose. To name a few:

- Newspapers ranging from big-city dailies such as *The New York Times* to small-distribution community weeklies and everything in between. Think of newspaper beats and sections: breaking news, international, lifestyle, health, local politics, opinion, etc.
- Television: Once dominated by NBC, ABC, and CBS, TV now has numerous networks that may focus on particular topics such as home improvement, shopping or travel, or particular political leanings. Local stations add their own programming, such as news, public affairs, or lifestyle shows.
- Radio: A big, fragmented genre. Large cities may have dozens of stations, each serving up a specific style of music or information. In smaller media markets, one station may

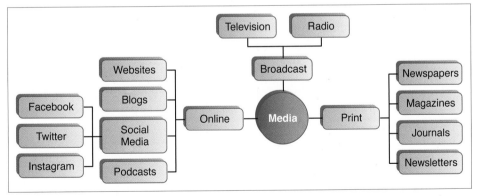

FIGURE 23-1:   The ability to preserve any publication, broadcast, image, or performance and to make it available on demand has transformed the way we share and access information. In the past, only those who listened or watched a radio or television show when it was broadcast could experience it. Podcasts, downloads, time-shifting, and on-demand availability now put consumers of media in control of a burgeoning array of choices. Traditional media, such as newspapers, magazines, and television news, are still important, but they compete with blogs and podcasts for mindshare and access.

offer news during the day, classical music in the evening, and classic rock overnight. Few stations have the fully staffed news departments that were common in years past. Online radio stations present a wealth of options, including live streaming of programs and download of podcasts to be heard at the listener's convenience.

- Magazines: Another diverse group, comprising everything from national newsweeklies to trade publications and periodicals on almost any conceivable interest or hobby. Even more than radio stations, periodicals are often targeted to niche audiences (*e.g.*, golfers, poodle breeders, yacht owners, paint retailers, astronomy buffs, etc.).

- Wire services provide content for stations and publications that subscribe to their services. You may be familiar with the Associated Press, United Press International, or Thomson Reuters, among others. Wire service staff may originate a news story or feature, or they may pick it up from a local paper, making it available to run in news outlets nationally or internationally.

- Websites may be managed by a company, government agency, or non-profit organization (university, professional society hospital, foundation, etc.). Many have online press rooms with news releases and stories relating to the issues that pertain to them. Websites with health information are among the most popular on the internet, offering opportunities for researchers, clinicians, and other professionals to share their knowledge.

- Mobile platforms are specially designed or adapted for smartphones, tablets, and other similar devices. Savvy publishers, broadcasters, and website sponsors make sure their products work well with the different screen sizes and functionalities of mobile devices, as increasing numbers of users get their information this way.

- Social media proliferate, with a handful dominating in a survival-of-the-fittest competition for eyeballs and engaged users. Facebook and Twitter are among the most popular, claiming a billion users between them. Among the scores of others are LinkedIn, YouTube, and Pinterest. Each offers unique appeal to users and opportunities for content providers.

Social media are an important, and growing, source of news for many users. According to a report from the Pew Research Center, Facebook is by far the largest social networking site among U.S. adults, and with half of its users getting news there, is also the largest among U.S. adults when it comes to getting news. As discussed in an earlier report, roughly two-thirds (64%) of U.S. adults use the site, and half of those users get news there—amounting to 30% of the general population. YouTube has the next greatest reach in terms of general usage, at 51% of U.S. adults (4).

YouTube, claiming more than 1 billion users worldwide, is inherently a visual medium. This underscores a shift toward visual rather than verbal literacy, the ability to take meaning from images rather than words.

- Infographics present data and images in a compelling, easily digested format. Successful infographics can make complex ideas and relationships more understandable, especially to visual learners. Often, a strong infographic will be shared by those who find it helpful or interesting. This may be done without express permission or attribution, so make sure to include appropriate source of information within the graphic itself.

- Blogs (web logs) abound, allowing anyone online to be a publisher. They may attract millions of visitors or just a handful, depending on the quality of their content (typically, of the opinion/essay/commentary variety) and their promotion.
- Podcasts make audio content downloadable at will. Radio programs are available on the listener's schedule; subscribers can automatically access every episode. Podcasts epitomize the evolution from content provider control to consumer control.
- Other channels include almost anywhere ideas can be expressed. Ever notice health information on food or product packaging? How about billboards or automated phone messages? Wherever words are used, there may be an opportunity to share relevant, evidence-based information.

Changing Channels: The Media, Technology, and Competition

The media universe is very different than it was even a few years ago. Ongoing restructuring driven by technology, audience preference, and economics has led to upheaval. Many daily newspapers have closed, as subscribers and advertisers migrated to online platforms. Cable television and more recently internet radio have fragmented broadcasting. Some commentators lament the lack of singularly important shared stories that in the past may have bonded large segments of the population together. In the last century, iconic events such as the first manned moon landing—even the final episode of the popular TV series "M*A*S*H"—drew huge television audiences and provided a nearly universal touch point for conversation. In this age of cable TV and viewing on demand, even the most popular televised events seldom attract such cross-cutting audiences.

At the same time, some celebrate the democratizing effects of technology, allowing anyone to be a publisher, producer, or journalist. Back in the day, magnates such as Hearst and Pulitzer were said to have bought ink by the barrel, giving them outsized influence in public discourse. Now, with information expressed as digits and pixels and with the price of devices dropping as they improve, anyone can be a publisher (and seemingly everybody is). Although publicly expressing one's opinion in years past may have meant submitting letters to the editor in hopes of getting published occasionally, blogging and social media today offer platforms by which all but the digitally disenfranchised can opine at length.

Journalists

Journalists are the professionals who research and write news, features, and other stories for publication or broadcast. We'll broaden the term a bit to include the editors or producers with whom you may work. (Producers coordinate the planning for a segment on radio, TV, or the web.)

The last decade or so has not been kind to print publishing. Although the hemorrhaging of American newsrooms is a real phenomenon (and much lamented), there are still thousands of journalists reporting the news. They may be fewer in numbers, reinventing themselves on the internet, and stretched across several beats, but they are there, covering local government, crime and economic development, reporting on health and environmental issues, developing lifestyle features, and trying to freshly cover evergreen topics such as holiday weight gain and back-to-school shopping. Professional journalists are a breed apart from the typical citizen blogger or the activist with a cause-related Facebook page. A journalism degree signifies a curious but skeptical nature and training in reporting techniques as well as adherence to a strict code of ethics that stresses transparency, impartiality, and responsibility to the truth. Few journalists would claim to be candidates for sainthood, and examples of lapses and bad apples abound. However, the professionalism of a trained, conscientious reporter can be especially notable in its absence—for example, when a glowing profile of a company turns out to be placed for payment by that company's PR department. (There's no harm in touting your company's virtues, but failing to disclose the connection is an ethical lapse.)

The shrinking of news staffs means they are more dependent than ever on content that comes to them ready to go or that can quickly be rendered into suitable form for a news story or feature. The closer your message is to meeting a news staff's needs, the more likely it is to get air time, print, or web space. Although reporters may need your content (be it a meeting announcement, research finding, or policy recommendation, if it helps to meet a deadline, it's content), they probably are not sitting around the newsroom, waiting for the phone to ring so that a brilliant young scientist can educate them. They are doing their jobs—checking out leads, verifying quotes, and drafting and editing stories as the next deadline nears. Help them do that difficult job and you become an essential part of the enterprise. The more you understand the needs and constraints of the medium and the process by which its journalists develop their stories, the more likely you are to become a valued contributor—perhaps an oft-consulted source or even a regular contributor.

Scientist Versus Journalist: A Tug of Words?

Journalists and their sources sometimes circle one another warily, each bent on doing the job right, aware of the need to work together, but unsure of the other's motives and methods. Such tension makes for good movie plots (think Katharine Hepburn and Humphrey Bogart in "The African Queen" or Michael Douglas and Kathleen Turner in "Romancing the Stone") but can be disconcerting for both parties and can interfere with optimal outcomes.

The perennial rub between journalist and expert typically stems from the expert's desire to explain fully and accurately and the journalist's need to do so concisely and in a way the audience will understand. The scientist, for example, may seek to offer new knowledge in a carefully defined context with references to established convention and a precise explanation of what the new findings mean. The journalist, by contrast, may attempt to convey the most relevant points to a scientifically naïve audience in a comfortable, approachable style and with a very limited word count. Add to that an increasing need for visual appeal, and the cultural clash between researcher and writer is enhanced.

Although there are many instances of happy collaborations between writers and the experts who serve as their sources, a more cynical look listing of worst-case grievances might look like the following:

The Journalist to the Scientist	The Scientist to the Journalist
• Ill-prepared to cover this topic	• Incapable of straightforward communication
• Superficial, satisfied with partial explanations	• Boring, verbose
• Overlooks important points; distracted by side issues	• Unable to summarize
• Throwing together a story to make deadline	• Insistent on qualifying and explaining, endlessly drawing minor distinctions
• Unwilling to commit to the rigor of getting it right	• Blind to metaphor and larger meaning

NOTE: These generalizations are meant to illustrate conflicts that sometimes arise between scientists and journalists. They are provided to foster understanding in hopes that appreciating one another's perspective can enhance communication.

Messages

In order to best help a journalist convey your information through the medium and to the audience, you need to understand the request/need/opportunity and determine how to fill that need—how to effectively tell the story. Say the phone rings, and it's a reporter who has been referred to you for a story she's just beginning to develop. Maybe she has seen a news release about a study on which you collaborated. Or perhaps her main source is another scientist doing related research, and she hopes you can comment from an independent perspective. How can you work with this journalist to share the results of your study? In short:

1. *Understand her focus, approach, and deadline* as well as the givens of her medium. Is she doing a 200-word news brief that will post this afternoon, or is she developing an in-depth feature story to run several months from now? What has she learned so far about the topic? What has she read, and with whom else has she talked? You need to know the "angle" of her story or help her determine it. The angle—also called the "hook" or "peg"—is the reporter's perspective on the topic. It identifies which facet she will emphasize or the approach from which she'll cover it. Although the notion of story angles may seem to indicate a lack of objectivity, it is essential given the impossibility of covering any complex subject in its entirety and the need to be selective in presenting it to her audience.

2. *Tell the story.* Help her understand why your research matters to her audience and how she can convey it to them. Relate your study to other topics of current discussion. If you study the health benefits of exercise, and healthcare costs are front-page news, that issue underscores the relevance of your research. If your topic is exercise motivation, the perennial stories about holiday recipes and resolutions, for instance, offer a perfect tie-in.

Scientist or Storyteller?

Most scientists would likely say they deal with facts; theirs is a world of observation and deduction in which objectivity and evidence-based statements are the rule. This is the foundation of peer-reviewed publishing. Asked to explain his research, a scientist might want to say, "It's all there in my published study. The data and conclusions speak for themselves."

Do they? Perhaps the data and conclusions speak to other scientists, but that dialect is probably unintelligible to the vast majority of people—even those for whom the information could be especially relevant or interesting. To convey your findings and understandings, you need to talk to people in a language they understand using terms and concepts with which they are familiar. Jargon—the use of specialized terms with precise meanings within a particular shared context—serves a purpose, but it can be off-putting to anyone who isn't in on it. Your goal is to communicate, not to impress, confuse, or frustrate. As Randy Olson, the marine biologist-turned-filmmaker, puts it, "The 'Why waste time? Just tell 'em what it is' philosophy may work for science students, but it doesn't for the broader audience. This is where so much of the art of communication resides"(6).

The hyperspecialization of all fields of knowledge has led to a situation in which only those working in your particular discipline can be assumed to understand it. Even fellow scientists may have to explain assumptions or summarize the tenets that underlie your work. Picture a neurobiologist talking to a psychometrist. Surely they have common ground, but they likely would need to avoid jargon and could not assume that each was familiar with the literature in each other's discipline. For some purposes, it's best to treat even a fellow scientist as a curious layman: respect, explain, and listen.

Stories, Not Fact Lists

It's important to understand how most people get their information, develop understandings, form opinions, and make decisions. Although we may like to think we are rational, objective, and impartial, the reality is that humans are emotional and impulsive by nature. Intuition and instinct can easily trump reasoned argument. How many automobiles have been purchased impulsively after a shopper fell in love with one model's svelte lines or throbbing audio system? How often has a voter selected a candidate based not on a careful review of his positions on all the issues but because of a gut feeling about his trustworthiness?

We crave stories and respond powerfully to them. A mountain of unassailable data may be formidable and impressive, and it lacks the motivating power of a simple story well told. Every habitual smoker knows that research has strongly linked the habit to deadly diseases, but that knowledge is no match for the addictive power of nicotine. Yet, hearing of a patient with emphysema struggle to take her last breath may be what compels a smoker to quit.

What's the lesson here for scientists? Reams of data, along with your careful explanation of methodology, results, and conclusions, may be just the ticket for explaining your work to a roomful of peers. That approach will cause most lay audience's eyes to glaze over, though, and they will fail to grasp your point. If you can succinctly get to the gist of your message and relate it to your audience's interests and experience, they are more likely to come away with a kernel of understanding. For example, people need to know that your study of physical activity levels and student achievement involved solid methodology on an appropriate sample, but the takeaway they'll remember is that "the kids who walked to school and had regular physical education classes scored higher on standard achievement tests and had fewer sick days and discipline problems than the less active students." This sort of summary statement doesn't tell the whole story, of course—you'd like to go into more detail, provide specific numbers, and provide context—but people tend to retain one or two basic points, and by stating things in a vivid, straightforward manner, you can help them get it right. The tables and citations that strengthen your journal article won't get the job done in a brief interview.

Nanci Hellmich of *USA Today* has spent decades writing for a lay audience about diet, nutrition, and fitness. She is a veteran at working with experts to distill what her readers want to know. "Most audiences don't want to be buried in the details of the study," she writes, "but they want the take-home message from the findings. Readers need to know how the research might help them live a better, healthier life" (3). Dorene Internicola of Reuters advises scientists to "Keep it simple. Boil down the methods and findings to the bare bones, and explain as simply as possible why it's important and how it changes the argument" (5).

Those working for a large corporation, hospital, university, or other institution may have a communications or media department to help as a go-between with the media. These colleagues can be invaluable in helping share your research with the larger world. They have one foot in the realm of science and evidence and one in the roiling maelstrom of the media and public affairs. It's their job to tell your story, endeavoring to have the main points come across accurately while dealing with the limitations of each medium and fighting for attention in a fragmented, competitive environment. Make sure your communications department is aware of your work and your willingness to help them share your institution's expertise. These professionals, whose core skills typically are in journalism or public relations and who may or may not have a strong science background, can help you identify what's newsworthy in your findings and determine how to express it effectively.

Calling university press departments "a great resource," Edward Archer, PhD, of the University of South Carolina's Arnold School of Public Health, recommends that scientists "use simple but powerful terms" (1). A news release on his research carried the headline, "Four Decades of Federally Funded Nutrition Research Fatally Flawed" (8). Propelled by this provocative headline, Archer's research trended at the very top of social media site Reddit for two days; the open-access paper drew more than 3,000 hits in 24 hours.

Your institutional media department can work with you to craft your message into a news release, which then can be distributed to any number of audiences. Depending on the subject matter, this may include general media such as newspapers and broadcast newsrooms as well as technical and scientific/medical writers. The headline is all-important, as illustrated by the example earlier. The release will likely include quotes from you as lead researcher, a brief description of the research, and a summary of relevant findings. This is where publicists can be tempted to go overboard, leading to sensationalized claims and a distortion of the facts. In an attempt to draw attention and stoke interest, health and science communication can lapse into hyperbole. You may need to rein them in a bit to keep things in perspective. The public is done a disservice when correlation is presented as causation, when preliminary results of a small sample are projected across an entire population, or when research discussed at a professional meeting is given equal weight to a study published in a respected, peer-reviewed journal. Reuters' Dorene Internicola observes that due to changes in technology and the media as a business, "Stories have gotten shorter; journalistic overstatement has become, in my humble opinion, sadly more acceptable, so it's more important than ever that researchers are clear and precise, lest their findings be distorted" (5).

Keeping the Story Accurate

As important as it is to tell a story effectively, it is supremely important not to let a good story get in the way of the truth. News releases from the American College of Sports Medicine (ACSM) carry a notice that ACSM "supports the 10 criteria for responsible health reporting as articulated by www.healthnewsreview.org" (7). The criteria, although most directly relevant to discussions of health interventions, are helpful for anyone seeking to communicate accurately and ethically about scientific, technical, or medical matters:

1. Does the story adequately discuss the costs of the intervention?
2. Does the story adequately quantify the benefits of the treatment/test/product/procedure?
3. Does the story adequately explain/quantify the harms of the intervention?
4. Does the story seem to grasp the quality of the evidence?
5. Does the story commit disease-mongering?
6. Does the story use independent sources and identify conflicts of interest?
7. Does the story compare the new approach with existing alternatives?
8. Does the story establish the availability of the treatment/test/product/procedure?
9. Does the story establish the true novelty of the approach?
10. Does the story appear to rely solely or largely on a news release?

Gary Schwitzer, publisher of *Health News Review*, told an ACSM audience that "even in 300 words, you can explain that in healthcare more isn't always better, newer isn't always better, and screening doesn't always make sense. . . . We don't expect the story to talk about a drug that's in phase 1 clinical trials as if it's available at the corner drugstore" (7). Numerous professional societies have codes of ethics to foster accurate communication in the public interest.

Although they take a fair number of hits from experts who feel they've been misquoted or their findings distorted, most journalists want to get it right. "Most good journalists want the same thing as you, that is, to be accurate," says veteran journalist John Hanc. He advises scientists to avoid acronyms and explain clearly. "When talking to journalists," he says, "scientists should not assume they are talking to colleagues . . . but also not to imbeciles either" (2). Even an experienced reporter with a graduate degree in science may be covering a beat ranging from healthcare economics to the space program, starting with a clean slate each time and needing to quickly research and write a story on a new topic each time. Without being insulting, you can ask a reporter what she understands about a topic and offer to provide an explanation when needed or to refer to reference sources.

Those new to working with the media (or those who are cynical about a reporter's competence or intent) may ask to review a story before publication. This is rarely allowed due to the need to preserve an independent press. Sometimes, a writer will allow or even ask a source to verify his or her direct quotations to ensure accuracy. Occasionally, a journalist who has been relying heavily on one particular source will ask that expert to review the article before it's published. Feel free during an interview (but not, obviously, during a live broadcast) to ask the journalist to read a quote back to you or whether your explanation was satisfactory. If you can explain something several different ways, you're more likely to convey it accurately to a reporter. Like most of us, they have a range of learning styles and frames of reference. Responsible journalists want to get it right. Suggest before the interview that someone fact-check each of your quotes or statements to ensure accuracy. If the reporter is reluctant to agree to this mutually protective practice, consider that a warning sign and be prepared to be misquoted. Don't take the reporter to task for not getting everything 100% right. If a news story on your work contains a significant error of fact, although, you can respectfully point it out and request that the archived and online versions be corrected. Don't ask for a retraction; those are reserved for rare cases such as flagrant or egregious journalistic misconduct. But the story may live forever online, and it's important to set the record straight so that those who find it in a future search will have accurate information.

Conveying Your Message on Television

Although many of us spend most of our time in the world of words and printed information, television is a primary source of information for millions of Americans. Whether it's a quick item on a news show, an extended in-studio interview, or a segment for a feature or documentary, TV offers an opportunity to share your expertise with a large audience. In order to do this effectively, you should understand the medium and prepare.

For example, say a news release on your research prompts a local TV science reporter to call you and ask for an interview—perhaps that same day. Unless the request came through your institution's press office, notify them immediately so they can help you prepare. Most often, the reporter will arrive with a videographer who will handle the camera and audio equipment and then work with the reporter to edit the footage into a brief news story.

The most salient fact to remember is that television is an overwhelmingly visual medium. Studies show that up to 80% of what people remember about a news story is visual. This means your carefully worded explanation of methodology may be upstaged by a shot of you nervously tapping your fingers as you speak. Take advantage of this intensely visual medium (and take the focus off yourself) by offering graphics that will enhance the story, such as a simple chart or graph, or data that the station's crew can use to develop an accompanying table.

The interview may take place in your lab or perhaps outside with your building in the background. The crew may shoot footage of you working on the computer or with lab equipment or perhaps talking with colleagues or walking down the hall. These shots are known as "B-roll" footage, providing visual interest as you talk with the reporter.

If you're answering questions from an off-camera news reporter, your responses may be edited down into one or two eight-second sound bites. Be pithy and complete, leaving pauses after sentences to make for easy editing. Give them tight phrases that tell the story in a few words. The reporter's questions may not be included, so start your response with helpful cues. For example, if she asks, "What are the relevant conclusions from your research?" you might respond with "What this study tells us is that . . ."

Most often, a producer or reporter will discuss the topic with you before the interview. This could be over the phone, in the studio before your segment, or at the site of the news interview before the camera is turned on. This discussion can help the reporter tease out the important threads in a subject of which he may have only a cursory understanding. Feel free to suggest what you think are the main points or takeaways; after all, you're the expert! For a studio interview (not necessarily a quick news story), the journalist may appreciate a list of suggested questions or topics for her to ask you. Make sure to mention limitations to your study and point out areas where further research is needed.

Preparing for the TV Interview

What you say will be supported or undermined by how you look and how you say it. Practice so that you are comfortable and credible. Dress appropriately and wear clothes in which you're comfortable. Have notes to refer to and to give you something to hold. Sit up straight and don't fidget, as this can be distracting to the viewer. Focus on sitting or standing comfortably and confidently. If you're wearing menswear, sit on the tail of your suit coat so that it doesn't balloon over your shoulders. If you're more comfortable sitting with your legs crossed, cross them at the ankles (never ankle-over-thigh, which looks ungainly on camera).

Be aware of how to dress for television; avoid distracting jewelry and very light or very dark garments. Small patterns such as herringbone can be problematic to the eye on screen. Medium brown or blue is usually safe. (Exception: On some occasions, a medical gown or lab coat may be more appropriate.) Observe how skilled TV personalities dress, sit, move, and speak.

For an on-camera interview, look at the host, not at the camera. The host/interviewer may address the audience. ("Welcome back. We're here with Dr. Terwilliger, discussing her research on the connection between exercise and mood.") Your job is to answer the host's questions and explain things to him or her. You might ask ahead of time "what the shot is," which will tell you, for example, that you'll be seen from the waist up. Any gestures, then, need to be above your waist to be seen. Speaking of gestures, keep them under control. Many people tend to talk with their hands, which can be distracting or downright irritating to the viewer. Ignore distractions such as crew members moving around off the set. Know how long the segment will be and make sure to get your key information in early and repeat it as appropriate. Assume you're on camera all the time, even when another guest is talking. Help focus attention by looking at whomever is talking at that time. Be aware that they may superimpose graphics as you're talking—perhaps based on the information you supplied.

If it is a recorded interview, ask in advance when it will air. You may record a segment midafternoon to air the following morning or possibly several times. If you say "this Friday" or "this morning," make sure that will be accurate for those who are watching or listening.

Still, even experienced professionals can feel a wave of panic when the recording begins or the TV interview goes live. Even a more relaxed discussion with a print reporter can go off track, leading you to forget key points. Plan your message points and write them down. Bullet points may make for more natural-sounding responses than fully scripted paragraphs. Practice in front of the mirror, into a recorder, or before friends. You may feel silly doing it, but it may help you feel more at ease during the interview itself. Most people are more comfortable doing radio interviews, which give you the opportunity to look at the notes on hand and not worry about your appearance.

It's OK to not always know the answer. We all have limits on what we know, and viewers will empathize with you if you're asked a question outside your knowledge or expertise. Feel free to say, "That's a good question, and I want to make sure to get you the correct figure. Let me check on that and get back to you." Then, of course, make sure you follow up as promised.

As mentioned previously, your institution's media relations staff can be staunch allies in all of this. Make sure to notify them when you're asked for an interview. Take any opportunities for media training to help you relax, prepare, and come across effectively.

CONCLUSION

The opportunity to share widely your research and expertise is part of your role as a scientist in the modern world. To do so effectively requires you to know your audiences and the channels by which they get their information and to prepare and deliver the appropriate message—to "tell the story." Working with journalists and other professionals, you can convey to the wider world the learning prompted by your early fascination with science and the natural world, giving your research a broad and enduring reach and impact.

GLOSSARY

Audiences: to whom you're talking

Channel: the medium or means by which the conversation takes place

Journalists: the reporters, editors, and producers who work in the media

Message: an expression of an idea, crafted to suit the audience and channel

Stakeholder: someone with an identifiable interest in the matter at hand

REFERENCES

1. Archer E. Personal communication. October 12, 2013.
2. Hanc J. Personal communication. October 8, 2013.
3. Hellmich N. Personal communication. October 10, 2013.
4. Holcomb J, Gottfried J, Mitchell A. News use across social media platforms; [cited 14 November 2013]. Available from: http://www.journalism.org/2013/11/14/news-use-across-social-media-platforms/
5. Internicola D. Personal communication. October 7, 2013.
6. Olson R. *Don't Be Such A Scientist: Talking Substance in an Age of Style.* Washington (DC): Island Press; 2009. 206 p.
7. Schwitzer G. American College of Sports Medicine takes public stand supporting HealthNewsReview.org criteria; [cited 22 Jul 2011]. Available from: http://www.healthnewsreview.org/2011/07/american-cvollege-of-sports-medicine-takes-public-stand-supporting-healthnewsrevieworg-criteria/
8. University of South Carolina. 40 years of federal nutrition research fatally flawed; [cited 9 Oct 2013]. Available from: http://www.eurekalert.org/pub_releases/2013-10/uosc-4yo100913.php

Index

Page numbers followed by *f*, *t*, or *b* indicate material in figures, tables, or boxes respectively.